Musculoskeletal Disorders

Musculoskeletal Disorders

Editor: Daphne Horton

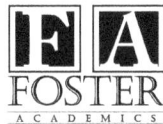

FOSTER
ACADEMICS

www.fosteracademics.com

www.fosteracademics.com

F A
FOSTER
A C A D E M I C S

Cataloging-in-Publication Data

Musculoskeletal disorders / edited by Daphne Horton.
     p. cm.
Includes bibliographical references and index.
ISBN 978-1-63242-762-5
1. Musculoskeletal system--Diseases. 2. Musculoskeletal system--Abnormalities.
3. Musculoskeletal system--Wounds and injuries. I. Horton, Daphne.
RC925 .M87 2019
616.7--dc23

Foster Academics,
118-35 Queens Blvd., Suite 400,
Forest Hills, NY 11375, USA

ISBN 978-1-63242-762-5 (Hardback)

Contents

Preface

The muscles, joints, nerves, tendons, ligaments and the structures supporting the back, neck and limbs together comprise the human musculoskeletal system. The pain, injuries and disorders of the musculoskeletal system are called musculoskeletal disorders. Such disorders usually arise from sudden exertion, repetitive strain or repeated exposure to force. Carpal tunnel syndrome, hand-arm vibration syndrome, tendinitis, epicondylitis and tension neck syndrome are some of the common examples of musculoskeletal disorders. X-ray and magnetic resonance imaging (MRI) are used to diagnose musculoskeletal disorders. This book brings forth some of the most innovative concepts and elucidates the unexplored aspects of musculoskeletal disorders. It consists of contributions made by international experts. For all those who are interested in musculoskeletal disorders, this book can prove to be an essential guide.

After months of intensive research and writing, this book is the end result of all who devoted their time and efforts in the initiation and progress of this book. It will surely be a source of reference in enhancing the required knowledge of the new developments in the area. During the course of developing this book, certain measures such as accuracy, authenticity and research focused analytical studies were given preference in order to produce a comprehensive book in the area of study.

This book would not have been possible without the efforts of the authors and the publisher. I extend my sincere thanks to them. Secondly, I express my gratitude to my family and well-wishers. And most importantly, I thank my students for constantly expressing their willingness and curiosity in enhancing their knowledge in the field, which encourages me to take up further research projects for the advancement of the area.

Editor

Functions, disabilities and perceived health in the first year after total knee arthroplasty; a prospective cohort study

Danielle D. P. Berghmans[1,4]* (iD), Antoine F. Lenssen[1,4], Pieter J. Emans[2,4] and Rob A. de Bie[3,4]

Abstract

Background: In end-stage knee osteoarthritis total knee arthroplasty (TKA) is an effective intervention to reduce pain and improve functioning in the majority of patients. However, after TKA some patients still experience pain, loss of function, deficient muscle strength or reduced walking speed. This study systematically assesses patients' functions, disabilities and health before TKA and at short- (3 months) and long-term (12 months) on all International Classification of Functioning, Disability and Health domains.

Methods: In this prospective cohort study 150 patients underwent the following tests before and at 3 and 12 months after surgery: Western Ontario and McMaster Universities Arthritis Index, Short Form 12, Knee Society Score, Patient Specific Functioning Scale, knee range of motion, quadriceps and hamstring strength, gait parameters, global perceived effect (only after surgery). All data was analyzed with repeated measures ANOVA for all measurement time points.

Results: Despite increased gait speed, quadriceps strength and scores on questionnaires being above pre surgical levels, patients do not reach levels of healthy persons. Walking speeds approach normal values and are higher in our study compared with the literature. Quadriceps strength stays at around 70 till 80% of norm values. However, dissatisfaction rates are below 10%, which is low compared to the literature.

Conclusions: Quality of life, activities, muscle strength and gait parameters improve significantly after TKA. However, some complaints regarding activities and walking speed remain. Most striking outcome is the remaining deficit in quadriceps strength.

Keywords: Osteoarthritis, TKA, Total knee arthroplasty

Background

Osteoarthritis (OA) is one of the ten most disabling diseases in developed countries: 9.6% of all men and 18.0% of all women over 60 years of age have symptomatic osteoarthritis [1]. While pain is the most prominent symptom, 80% of these patients have limitations in movement, and 25% cannot perform daily activities [1]. An increase in prevalence is expected due to ageing and obesity [1–5].

In end-stage osteoarthritis, joint replacement is an effective intervention to reduce pain and improve functioning in the majority of patients [3, 6–9]. However, it has been reported that 15–30% of patients still experience pain and loss of function after total knee arthroplasty (TKA) [7, 9–12].

Several studies have investigated recovery after TKA. Although most describe a 10–20% improvement in quadriceps strength and gait parameters in comparison to the pre-operative status, values remained lower than in healthy peers or the uninvolved leg [11–19]. A correlation between quadriceps strength and functional performance after TKA [18, 19] seems logical, for functional performance can be assumed to improve with quadriceps strength. Several studies found improvements in patient-reported

* Correspondence: danielle.berghmans@mumc.nl
[1]Department of Physical therapy, Maastricht University Medical Center +, PO 5800, 6202, AZ, Maastricht, The Netherlands
[4]Maastricht University/CAPHRI School for Public Health and Primary Care, P.O. Box 616, 6200, MD, Maastricht, The Netherlands
Full list of author information is available at the end of the article

outcome measures (PROMs), functional status and quality of life. [12–14, 20, 21]. However, patients often did not regain optimal health [22]. No relation with strength is investigated in these studies.

Although several studies investigated aspects of recovery after TKA, no study yet has incorporated all domains of the International Classification of Functioning, Disability and Health (ICF) in their assessment. Interesting findings in the ICF domains may be missed by the limited follow-up, population size and incompleteness of ICF domains of other studies. We therefore performed a prospective cohort study in which 150 patients scheduled for TKA were followed till 1 year after surgery, and in which we systematically assessed all domains of the ICF. Our first objective was to provide a more complete overview of current physical recovery rates of patients with TKA in the first year after surgery in the Netherlands. We hypothesize that the patients in our study will improve on all parameters in the first year after surgery. Our second objective is to generate normative quadriceps and hamstrings strength values for patients receiving a TKA in the Netherlands.

Methods

Study design

This prospective cohort study assessed all patients with the same set of measurement instruments during personal follow-up consultations at three time points before and after surgery. We chose as an endpoint a follow-up time of 1 year, as no further major improvement can be expected after this time period [7, 23].

Patients

Between March 1, 2011 and March 1, 2013, all consecutive patients with knee osteoarthritis scheduled for a TKA at the osteoarthritis clinic of Maastricht University Medical Centre (MUMC+) were informed about the study in writing and verbally at least 1 week before the planned surgery. On the day before surgery, when patients arrived at the hospital, they were contacted by the researcher, and written informed consent was obtained.

At the start of the study, we performed a sample size calculation. Based on the number of determinants and the pragmatic rule of thumb to include ten cases for each determinant we would need at least 120 cases to obtain adequate power (10×12 determinants = 120). Since we expected a lost of follow up of 15% we would need 140 subjects. To be on the safe side we included 10 patients more ($N = 150$).

Inclusion criteria were: Dutch speaking patients between 18 and 80 years at the time of surgery, diagnosed with knee osteoarthritis for which primary TKA was indicated. Patients were excluded if they underwent a unicondylar knee arthroplasty (UKA), had a neurological problem influencing ambulation or had an immobile hip or ankle arthrodesis. Severe comorbidities were excluded since all patients had to be eligible for surgery.

The local medical ethics committee of the MUMC+ reviewed and approved the study (NL33015.068.10 / METC 10–2-083). The rights of the subjects were protected under the Helsinki Declaration.

Surgery

All patients received a cemented Scorpio or Scorpio NRG TKA (Stryker, Kalamazoo, Michigan, USA). After performing a medial parapatellar approach a bony referenced, tibia first technique was used. A tourniquet was only used during the cementation period of the prosthesis. A previous study reported no differences in Range of Motion (ROM), function or Quality of Life between these to prosthesis [24].

Procedure

After signing informed consent, patients were enrolled in the cohort study. All assessments were performed by the research team the day before surgery and 3 and 12 months after surgery. We chose these time points because of scheduled appointments, enabling us to have personal contact with the patients without involving extra travel time. The patients were not shown the answers or the values obtained in previous sessions.

Measurements

In addition to the demographic patient characteristics (age, sex, height and weight), the following questionnaires and measurements were performed by a research team using a standardized protocol.

Health status questionnaires

The *Western Ontario and McMaster Universities Osteoarthritis Index (WOMAC)* is a self-administered disease-specific health questionnaire designed to measure the functional ability of the osteoarthritic hip and knee [25]. The WOMAC provides aggregate scores for each of three subscales: joint pain, joint stiffness and function. The WOMAC is a responsive instrument that yields reliable and valid measurements in patients with hip and knee osteoarthritis and has been extensively used to evaluate this patient population [9, 25–27]. The 5-point Likert version of this measure was used in our study. The scale was transformed to a range from 0 to 100 points (100 being the best score).

The *Patient Specific Functional Scale (PSFS)* records patients' perceptions of their disabilities [28]. Patients define their main complaints (i.e. difficulties performing certain activities) and rate the difficulty of performance on an 11-point numerical rating scale (NRS) (10 = no problems; 0 = impossible) [28] The three main complaints had to be defined as specifically as possible, and had to cause difficulties related to the osteoarthritis of the knee. The PSFS is a reliable and responsive measure in this population, [29, 30] and its validity has been confirmed in a population of patients with knee problems [29].

The *Knee Society Score (KSS)* is a knee-joint specific questionnaire and consists of two parts: a knee score (0–100, 100 being the best score) and a function score (0–100, 100 being the best score) [31]. The KSS is a valid and responsive measure in a population of patients after TKA [32].

The *Short Form 12 (SF12)* is a generic multidimensional questionnaire measuring quality of life from a patient's perspective. It is a short version of the SF36 and includes two components (physical and mental health), representing these respective domains (scale 0–100,100 being the best score). It is a valid, reliable and responsive measure in a general population and easy to administer [33].

The *global perceived effect (GPE)* is a 2-item scale on which patients can rate their overall recovery since a predefined point (in this study pre-surgical function) in time and their satisfaction with the treatment, on 7-point Likert scales (ranging from 2 [satisfied] to 14 [dissatisfied]). Its reliability and validity are good in patients with musculoskeletal disorders [34].

Physical performance tests

Muscle strength was assessed with a Biodex® System 3 Pro dynamometer (Biodex System 3 Pro Dynamometer, Biodex Medical Systems, Inc., Biodex Medical Systems, USA). Isokinetic strength (60^0/s and 180^0/s, in Nm) of the quadriceps and the hamstrings was measured using respectively five and ten repetitions. The peak volitional values were used in the analysis. The Biodex® is a reliable and valid isokinetic dynamometer [35].

ROM was measured with a long-arm goniometer, (Goniometer, Long Arm, Gymna, Belgium), according to Lenssen et al. [36] Extension and flexion were measured in supine position, with hyperextension noted as a positive value. Measuring ROM with a long-arm goniometer has been reported to be valid and reliable at group level [36].

The *gait parameters* of step length and walking speed were measured with the GAITRite® system (CIR systems, PA, USA), a highly valid and reliable tool to assess temporospatial gait parameters in patients undergoing a TKA [37].

Statistical analyses

Analyses were performed with SPSS for Windows version 23. [38] Means and standard deviations were

calculated to describe characteristics. Repeated Measures ANOVA were performed to test for significant differences between baseline till 3 months after surgery and between 3 and 12 months after. A significance level of *p* < .05 was used. A Bonferroni correction was used to correct for multiple testing.

Patients who dropped out during the test period were not replaced. All available data was analyzed; in case data was missing, the mean value of the parameter at that time point was imputed.

We also compared the strength of the quadriceps and hamstrings measured in our population with that of controls. We built a norm data set, consisting of 245 patients, 166 women (mean age 58.4 years [10.1], weight 69.6 kg [10.9]) and 129 men (56.2 years [10.7], weight 83.9 kg [10.6]). We tested their isokinetic quadriceps and hamstrings strength at an angular speeds of 60°/s and 180°/s. We calculated formulas (Table 1) for both sexes in both angular speeds for the quadriceps and hamstrings. These formulas were used to calculate the mean norm values for our population. These values and the percentage of the norm values are presented.

Results

Between March 1, 2011 and March 1, 2013, we included 150 patients, 71 men and 79 women, with a mean age of 64.7 ± 8.0 years. The majority of patients had surgery of the right knee (right 89, left 61) and mean BMI was 31.2 kg/m^2 for men and 30.7 kg/m^2 for women (Table 2). We lost 4 patients at 3-months follow-up and an additional 3 at the 12-month measurement. Not all patients were able to come to the hospital for the follow-up measurements, so data on physical tests (strength, temporospatial gait parameters and ROM) were unavailable for 7 patients at 3-months and for 9 patients at the 12-month measurement (4 of whom were the same as those at the three-month measurement).

With the exception of the SF12, patients improved significantly on all questionnaires over 3 and 12 months. The largest improvement occurred within the first 3 months. The largest and significant improvement of the SF12 Physical component was only between baseline and 3 months (Table 3).

Table 1 Isokinetic strenght formula

		Men	Women
Quadriceps	*60°/s*	305–2,67×age	172–1,42×age
	180°/s	207–1,96×age	108–0,94×age
Hamstrings	*60°/s*	193–1,66×age	116–1,01×age
	180°/s	149–1,36×age	89–0,81×age

Table 1 shows the fomula for calculating the isokinetic strength for a healthy population. Age in years

Table 2 Patient Characteristics

	Men	Women
Age (y) (sd)	64.2 (8.8)	65.1 (7.4)
Height (m) (sd)	1.75 (0.06)	1.66 (0.06)
Weight (Kg) (sd)	95.7 (13.6)	84.6 (15.5)
Body Mass Index (Kg/m^2) (sd)	31.2 (4.2)	30.7 (5.5)

Age, height, weight and body mass index for men and women. *sd* standard deviation

The GPE is shown in Fig. 1. After 3 months, 5.3% of all patients reported to have fully recovered from surgery, and after 1 year 25.3% did so. After 3 months, 2.7% of all patients were totally dissatisfied with the result and the treatment, against 1.3% after 1 year. Overall, the majority of patients were satisfied with the result, but had some residual complaints.

Figure 2 and 3 show respectively the 60°/s isokinetic quadriceps and hamstrings muscle strength in the peri-operative phase of men and women. After 3 months the quadriceps isokinetic strength measured at 60°/s speed is back on pre-surgical level for women (baseline 43.4 Nm [27.8]; 3 months 46.1 Nm [17.1]; *significance 1.000*) and for men (baseline 67.9 Nm [35.5]; 3 months 73.3 Nm [26.2]; *significance 0.521*). The quadriceps 180°/s only improved significantly in men in 3 3 months (baseline 43.3 Nm [23.0]; 3 months 50.5 Nm [17.4]; *significance 0.005*), women were back on pre-surgical level (baseline 29.2 Nm [16.4]; 3 months 30.0 Nm [11.7]; *significance 1.000*). Over 12 months a significant improvement was demonstrated, at both angular speeds and for both sexes (women 60°/s: 64.5 Nm [18.9] 180°/s: 38.2 [11.8]; men 60°/s: 95.2 Nm [30.5] 180°/s: 61.8 [19.1]). 60°/s Isokinetic Hamstrings strength in men and women

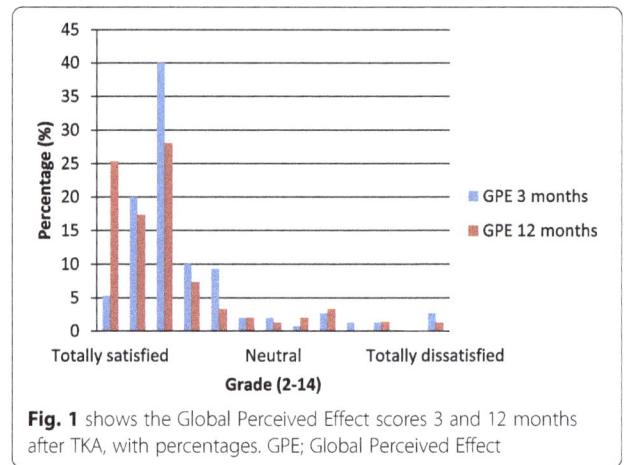

Fig. 1 shows the Global Perceived Effect scores 3 and 12 months after TKA, with percentages. GPE; Global Perceived Effect

improved significantly in the first year after surgery, compared to pre-surgical values (women; baseline 33.3 Nm [18.9]; 3 months 39.8 Nm [16.7]; *significance 0.009*; 12 months 50.7 Nm [16.2]; *significance 0.000*; men; baseline 48.0 Nm [23.4]; 3 months 65.6 Nm [22.8]; *significance 0.000*; 12 months 77.2 Nm [26.1]; *significance 0.000*). 180°/s Isokinetic Hamstrings strength only improved significant in in men in both time periods (baseline 37.8 Nm [18.6]; 3 months 47.1 Nm [17.8]; *significance 0.000*; 12 months 54.4 Nm [20.9]; *significance 0.002*. and in women only between 3 and 12 months (baseline 24.4 Nm [12.6]; 3 months 27.1 Nm [11.3]; *significance 0.263*; 12 months 33.3 Nm [11.6]; *significance 0.000*.)

We also compared muscle strength of our patients with that of healthy individuals. At baseline, our patients had 51.6 to 63.3% of the quadriceps strength of healthy persons, and 56.8–69.5% of the hamstrings strength. At

Table 3 Questionnaires

	Baseline	3 months	sig.	12 months	sig.
Short Form - 12; Physical (sd)	33.5 (7.9)	38.8 (7.7)	*0.000*	39.3 (9.2)	*1.000*
Short Form - 12; Mental (sd)	44.7 (10.6)	45.0 (9.6)	*1.000*	46.4 (9.2)	*0.164*
WOMAC Pain (sd)	10.6 (4.1)	16.0 (4.1)	*0.000*	17.6 (4.4)	*0.000*
WOMAC Stifness (sd)	4.1 (1.9)	4.9 (1.9)	*0.000*	5.8 (1.9)	*0.000*
WOMAC Function (sd)	39.0 (12.3)	54.4 (13.0)	*0.000*	58.2 (12.9)	*0.000*
WOMAC Total (sd)	54.1 (16.2)	75.4 (17.6)	*0.000*	81.7 (18.0)	*0.000*
PSFS 1 (sd)	1.9 (2.0)	2.8 (3.4)	*0.000*	6.6 (3.7)	*0.000*
PSFS 2 (sd)	2.2 (2.1)	4.8 (3.6)	*0.000*	6.8 (3.4)	*0.000*
PSFS 3 (sd)	2.4 (2.4)	4.9 (3.6)	*0.000*	6.9 (3.4)	*0.000*
Knee Society Score; Knee (sd)	52.5 (16.4)	76.1 (17.3)	*0.000*	84.1 (17.5)	*0.000*
Knee Society Score; Function (sd)	57.2 (13.1)	69.4 (15.4)	*0.000*	74.8 (18.5)	*0.000*

N number, *sd* standard deviation, *WOMAC* Western Ontario and McMaster Universities Osteoarthritis Index, *PSFS* Patient Specific Functional Complaint, *Sig* p-value
The scores on the questionnaires are given at baseline and 3 and 12 months after surgery. Significance of progression from baseline to 3 months and from 3 till 12 months

Quadriceps and Hamstrings strenght Men

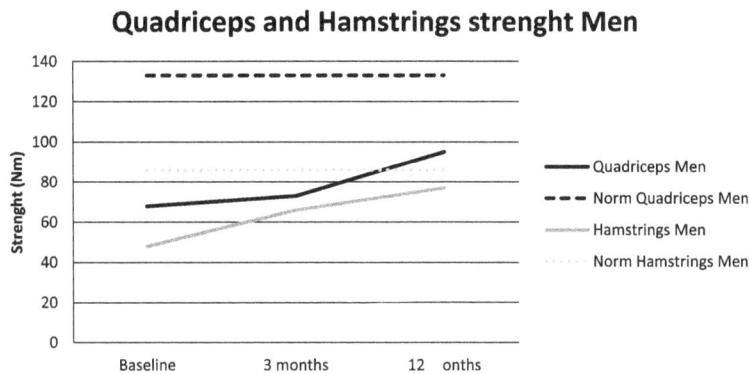

Fig. 2 Strength men.
Present the development of the Isokinetic Quadriceps and Hamstrings strength in the first year after a TKA in men and the reference values for this population

3 months, values were 55.7 to 64.4% of the quadriceps and 76.1–79.5% of the hamstrings, respectively, and at 12 months 72.0 to 81.7% and 88.4 to 100.7%, respectively.

Table 4 lists the ROM values. The mean baseline flexion was 120°. Flexion was limited immediately after surgery, but increased again during the first weeks. After three months, flexion had returned almost to baseline value, although there was still a significant difference. At 12 months, the flexion had returned to baseline level. Overall, extension ROM did not change significantly after a TKA.

Table 5 shows walking speed and step length. The step length of the healthy and surgical leg increased significantly over time. With increasing step length, walking speed also increased significantly over time after TKA (98.9 cm/s at baseline, 108.4 cm/s at 3 months and 117.0 cm/s at 12 months). Improvement of walking speed between baseline and the 3-month measurement was comparable to that between the 3- and 12-month measurements. The largest improvement in step length was between baseline and 3-month measurements.

Discussion

This study reports on the first year of physical recovery of patients undergoing a TKA in the Netherlands and could therefore be useful in informing patients about prognostic consequences of a TKA.

The most remarkable finding in this study is the persistent limited muscle strength. Whilst other outcome measures improved to nearly normal values compared to the healthy population, quadriceps strength lagged behind. Before surgery, strength was half of that of matched healthy persons, a higher deficit than reported in the literature [12, 15]. Three months after surgery, mean strength was comparable to pre-surgical values. Although strength increased from 3 till 12 months after TKA, it never reached 'healthy' values. We do not expect that pain has a role in the muscle strength deficit since a large amount of patient did not experienced pain during strength measurement after the surgery, in contrast with the measurement pre-surgically. One reason could be the changed kinematics of the knee (altered patellofemoral kinematics) and/or muscle loss due to surgery. A change in strength was seen in an in vitro study by

Quadriceps and Hamstrings strenght Women

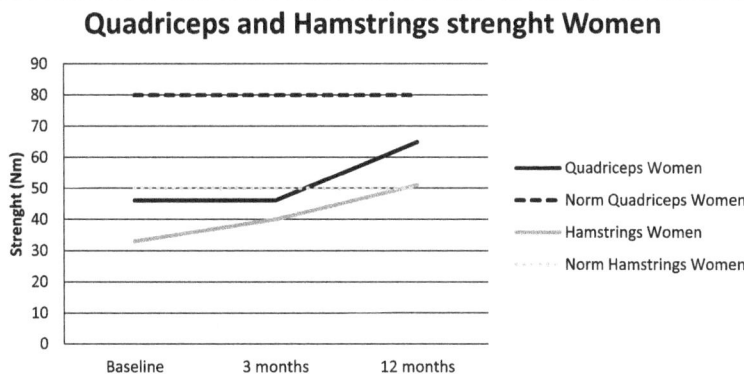

Fig. 3 Strength women.
Present the development of the Isokinetic Quadriceps and Hamstrings strength in the first year after a TKA in women and the reference values for this population

Table 4 ROM

	Baseline	3 months	sig.	12 months	sig.
Flexion (°) (sd)	120.1 (12.6)	114.9 (13.7)	0.001	120.6 (14.7)	0.000
Extension (°) (sd)	−2.3 (5.7)	−2.5 (5.3)	1.000	−1.3 (5.7)	0.085

n number, Sig. p -value
Flexion and extension values prior to surgery and 3 and 12 months after surgery, in degrees. Significance of progression from baseline to 3 months and from 3 till 12 months

Ostermeier et al., who compared hinged and non-hinged TKAs [39]. Further, during therapy focus is on functional training and isokinetic strength measurement is not performed standardly. Our large study population underlined the muscle deficit already reported in other studies with a smaller sample size [12, 15–19]. In these studies even a higher deficit was described 3 months after surgery [12, 18]. Further, the total gain in muscle strength in the first year was higher in our study compared to the literature [15]. This could be due to the larger improvement in the first months compared with the literature. A reason could be the health care system in the Netherlands. The main part of all patients receive routinely a prescription for physical therapy after the TKA surgery for 1 year physical therapy. Generally, they have therapy twice a week. This could result in a faster and larger improvement of muscle strength which focuses on activity level, like walking with and without crutches and walking stairs. This is in contrast with the amount of physical therapy patients receive in other countries worldwide. Bade et al. described only that 26% of all patients receive outpatient physical therapy [12]. This could also possibly explain the smaller deficit of walking speed in our study. Walking speed in our pre-surgical [12, 13] and post-surgical patients is higher than reported in the literature in which patients with a TKA walked 20% more slowly than healthy individuals 1 year after surgery [8, 13, 17]. Before surgery, the walking speed of patients in our study (98,9 cm/s) was 20.0–26.1% lower than in a healthy population (healthy walking speed for women [60–69 years] 1.24 m/s and for men [60–69 years] 1.34 m/s) [40]. After surgery, walking speed (108.4 cm/s) increased but remained lower than in healthy persons (between 81.0–87.3% of the healthy walking speed) [40]. After 12 months, walking speed

(117.0 cm/s) still increased, but did not reach the healthy level (attaining between 87.3 and 94.2% of the walking speed of healthy individuals). However, in terms of managing pedestrian street crossings with lights (which are designed for 1.2 m/s), 81% of our population were unable to cross the street safely before their surgery. After 3 months, this percentage had decreased to 65%, but after 12 months it was still 49%.

Pua et al. [41] investigated the relationship between walking speed and physical parameters in the first 16 weeks after TKA. They found ipsilateral quadriceps strength as strongest predictor for walking speed. No linear relationship existed till 111 N, a steep rise in gait speed was observed with every gain in muscle strength. After 111 Newton the speed increased more gradually [41]. However, according to Alnahdi et al. [42], the influence of quadriceps strength on gait patterns is only moderate till 6 months and in the period till 1 year it even decreases.

All questionnaires regarding level of functioning, quality of life and patient-specific complaints yielded lower scores compared to healthy controls, both pre- and post-surgical. (For healthy peers, we assumed highest possible score on the WOMAC, KSS and PSFS [related to knee problems] may be expected. For the SF12 we used reference data from the United states of America in which the healthy population had a score on the mental part of 51.6 and 43.9 on the physical part [43]). However, a large and significant increase was reported on all questionnaires over the 12 months following surgery. This is in agreement with previous studies [4, 9, 12–15, 18, 20–22]. Only, our population seemed to recover faster; they performed on pre-surgical level at 3months, while in other studies this took about 6 months [12]. Again, this could be due to the amount of physical therapy in the Netherlands, focused on activities like walking, walking stairs and making transfers.

Possible due to the faster increase in strength, walking speed and questionnaires, our patients were more satisfied compared to those in other studies, as seen on the GPE (8.7% dissatisfied at 3 months, 7.9% dissatisfied at 12 months, whereas in other studies 15–30% of the patients were dissatisfied) [7, 9–12]. However, a relation between satisfaction and improvement in pain, function and handicap is difficult, and therefore, according to

Table 5 Walking speed and step length

		Baseline	3 months	sig.	12 months	sig.
Walking speed (cm/s) (sd)		98.9 (23.3)	108.4 (19.9)	0.000	117.0 (19.9)	0.000
Step lenght	Surgical leg (cm) (sd)	57.6 (11.2)	61.9 (8.3)	0.000	64.1 (8.5)	0.000
	Healthy leg (cm) (sd)	58.0 (9.9)	62.2 (8.6)	0.000	64.8 (8.7)	0.000

n number, Sig. p- value
Walking speed and step length pre-surgical and 3 and 12 months after TKA with the significance level

Genet et al. satisfaction should be investigated as an independent parameter [14].

Nonetheless, patients' physical capability can be satisfying, their spare capacity could be less, giving a higher risk for frailty in case of a trauma or hospitalization. Therefore, despite of the importance of their satisfaction as success indicator for surgery, measuring their functional activity level is an important indicator.

Limitations

We decided to use performance tests to assess functions and questionnaires to measure activities, so the results regarding activities are from the patients' view and could therefore be subjective.

Another limitation is that we do not have information about osteoarthritis in other joints of the patients. Which might have an influence on the functional performance.

Our findings confirm that a TKA improves quality of life for patients with knee osteoarthritis and can be used to inform patients about possible prognostic consequences of a TKA, which is imported in patient-centered care. However, patients do not reach the values attained by healthy persons, and complaints persist in the first year after surgery. Quadriceps strength in particular remains limited, which may be a reason for persistent complaints. In our opinion most muscle deficits are not noticed during daily activities. However, in case of illness of (surgical) stress patients have less spare capacity and will have a higher chance to become frail. Physical therapy focuses on ROM and daily activities, but testing and training quadriceps strength until normal values are attained (if possible) is an important part of the therapy. As mentioned earlier, further research should focus on the effect of more progressive resistance training on the remaining muscle strength deficits in the first year after TKA. Besides this, further investigation in pathophysiology of muscle weakness is necessary.

Conclusions

Quality of life, activities, muscle strength and gait parameters improve significantly after a TKA. However, complaints on activities and walking speed remain. Most striking was the limited quadriceps strength, which we believe may restrict patients in daily life. Therefore, future studies should address the impact of strength training after a TKA on the improvement in muscle strength and daily activities.

Abbreviations

GPE: Global Perceived Effect; ICF: International Classification of Functioning, Disability and Health; KSS: Knee Society Score; MUMC: Maastricht University Medical Centre; OA: Osteoarthritis; PROM: Patient-Reported Outcome Measures; PSFS: Patient Specific Functional Scale; ROM: Range of Motion; SF12: Short Form 12; TKA: Total Knee Arthroplasty; UKA: Unicondylar Knee Arthroplasty; WOMAC: Western Ontario and McMaster Universities Osteoarthritis Index

Acknowledgements

We would like to thank the following persons for their contributions to this study: Nick Coenen, Lotte van Delft, Simone Engels, Anja Großek, Aniek Heldens, Peter Hilgers, Elena Issigonis, Ramon Janssen, Patrick Lebeck, Michael Leroy, Dennis Linden, Maarten Neuhaus, Laura Niggebrugge, Hugo van Nuland, Hannah Pallubinski, Ineke Salemans, Pia Stadler, Sanne Vijgen, Marwin Weber and Mandy Welters.

Funding

This research did not receive any specific grant from funding agencies in the public, commercial, or not-for-profit sectors.

Authors' contributions

Study conception and design: DB, AL, RB. Acquisition of data: DB, AL. Analysis and interpretation of the data: DB, AL, RB, PE. Drafting of the manuscript: DB. Critical revision: AL, RB, PE. Read and approved the manuscript: DB, AL, RB, PE.

Competing interests

The authors declare that they have no competing interests.

Author details

[1]Department of Physical therapy, Maastricht University Medical Center +, PO 5800, 6202, AZ, Maastricht, The Netherlands. [2]Department of Orthopedics, Maastricht University Medical Center +, PO 5800, 6202, AZ, Maastricht, The Netherlands. [3]Department of Epidemiology, Maastricht University, P.O. Box 616, 6200, MD, Maastricht, The Netherlands. [4]Maastricht University/CAPHRI School for Public Health and Primary Care, P.O. Box 616, 6200, MD, Maastricht, The Netherlands.

References

1. Chronic rheumatic conditions [http://www.who.int/chp/topics/rheumatic/en/]. Accessed 26 Feb 2018.
2. Köke A, van den Ende C, Jansen M, Steultjens M, Veenhof C: KNGF-standaard Beweeginterventie Artrose. 2008.
3. Kennedy DM, Stratford PW, Riddle DL, Hanna SE, Gollish JD. Assessing recovery and establishing prognosis following total knee arthroplasty. Phys Ther. 2008;88(1):22–32.
4. Papakostidou I, Dailiana ZH, Papapolychroniou T, Liaropoulos L, Zintzaras E, Karachalios TS, Malizos KN. Factors affecting the quality of life after total knee arthroplasties: a prospective study. BMC Musculoskelet Disord. 2012;13(1):116.
5. Priority Medicines for Europe and the World 2013 Update [http://www.who.int/medicines/areas/priority_medicines/Ch6_12Osteo.pdf]. Accessed 26 Feb 2018.
6. Beers MH, Berkow R. The Merck manual, vol. 2: Bohn Stafleu Van Loghum; 2003.
7. Zeni JA Jr, Snyder-Mackler L. Early postoperative measures predict 1- and 2-year outcomes after unilateral total knee arthroplasty: importance of contralateral limb strength. Phys Ther. 2010;90(1):43–54.
8. Mizner RL, Petterson SC, Stevens JE, Axe MJ, Snyder-Mackler L. Preoperative quadriceps strength predicts functional ability one year after total knee arthroplasty. J Rheumatol. 2005;32(8):1533–9.
9. Jones CA, Voaklander DC, Suarez-Alma ME. Determinants of function after total knee arthroplasty. Phys Ther. 2003;83(8):696–706.
10. Bourne RB, Chesworth BM, Davis AM, Mahomed NN, Charron KD. Patient satisfaction after total knee arthroplasty: who is satisfied and who is not? Clin Orthop Relat Res. 2010;468(1):57–63.
11. Yoshida Y, Mizner RL, Ramsey DK, Snyder-Mackler L. Examining outcomes from total knee arthroplasty and the relationship between quadriceps strength and knee function over time. Clin Biomech. 2008;23(3):320–8.
12. Bade MJ, Kohrt WM, Stevens-Lapsley JE. Outcomes before and after total knee arthroplasty compared to healthy adults. J Orthop Sports Phys Ther. 2010;40(9):559–67.

13. Bolink S, Grimm B, Heyligers I. Patient-reported outcome measures versus inertial performance-based outcome measures: a prospective study in patients undergoing primary total knee arthroplasty. Knee. 2015;22(6):618–23.

14. Genet F, Schnitzler A, Lapeyre E, Roche N, Autret K, Fermanian C, Poiraudeau S. Change of impairment, disability and patient satisfaction after total knee arthroplasty in secondary care practice. Ann Readapt Med Phys. 2008;51(8):671–6. 676-682

15. Meier W, Mizner R, Marcus R, Dibble L, Peters C, Lastayo PC. Total knee arthroplasty: muscle impairments, functional limitations, and recommended rehabilitation approaches. J Orthop Sports Phys Ther. 2008;38(5):246–56.

16. Rossi MD, Hasson S. Lower-limb force production in individuals after unilateral total knee arthroplasty. Arch Phys Med Rehabil. 2004;85(8): 1279–84.

17. Walsh M, Woodhouse LJ, Thomas SG, Finch E. Physical impairments and functional limitations: a comparison of individuals 1 year after total knee arthroplasty with control subjects. Phys Ther. 1998;78(3):248–58.

18. Mizner RL, Petterson SC, Snyder-Mackler L. Quadriceps strength and the time course of functional recovery after total knee arthroplasty. J Orthop Sports Phys Ther. 2005;35(7):424–36.

19. Silva M, Shepherd EF, Jackson WO, Pratt JA, McClung CD, Schmalzried TP. Knee strength after total knee arthroplasty. J Arthroplast. 2003;18(5): 605–11.

20. Dailiana ZH, Papakostidou I, Varitimidis S, Liaropoulos L, Zintzaras E, Karachalios T, Michelinakis E, Malizos KN. Patient-reported quality of life after primary major joint arthroplasty: a prospective comparison of hip and knee arthroplasty. BMC Musculoskelet Disord. 2015;16(1):1.

21. Poortinga S, Van den Akker-Scheek I, Bulstra SK, Stewart RE, Stevens M. Preoperative physical activity level has no relationship to the degree of recovery one year after primary Total hip or knee arthroplasty: a cohort study. PLoS One. 2014;9(12):e115559.

22. Finch E, Walsh M, Thomas SG, Woodhouse LJ. Functional ability perceived by individuals following total knee arthroplasty compared to age-matched individuals without knee disability. J Orthop Sports Phys Ther. 1998;27(4):255–63.

23. Lingard EA, Katz JN, Wright EA, Sledge CB. Predicting the outcome of total knee arthroplasty. J Bone Joint Surg. 2004;86(10):2179–86.

24. Lützner J, Hartmann A, Lützner C, Kirschner S. Is range of motion after cruciate-retaining total knee arthroplasty influenced by prosthesis design? A prospective randomized trial. J Arthroplast. 2014;29(5):961–5.

25. Bellamy N, Buchanan WW, Goldsmith CH, Campbell J, Stitt LW. Validation study of WOMAC: a health status instrument for measuring clinically important patient relevant outcomes to antirheumatic drug therapy in patients with osteoarthritis of the hip or knee. J Rheumatol. 1988;15(12):1833–40.

26. Collins NJ, Misra D, Felson DT, Crossley KM, Roos EM. Measures of knee function: international knee documentation committee (IKDC) subjective knee evaluation form, knee injury and osteoarthritis outcome score (KOOS), knee injury and osteoarthritis outcome score physical function short form (KOOS-PS), knee outcome survey activities of daily living scale (KOS-ADL), Lysholm knee scoring scale, Oxford knee score (OKS), western Ontario and McMaster universities osteoarthritis index (WOMAC), activity rating scale (ARS), and Tegner activity score (TAS). Arthritis Care Res. 2011;63(S11):S208–28.

27. Gill SD, de Morton NA, Mc Burney H. An investigation of the validity of six measures of physical function in people awaiting joint replacement surgery of the hip or knee. Clin Rehabil. 2012;26(10):945–51.

28. Stratford P. Assessing disability and change on individual patients: a report of a patient specific measure. Physiother Can. 1995;47:258–63.

29. Chatman AB, Hyams SP, Neel JM, Binkley JM, Stratford PW, Schomberg A, Stabler M. The patient-specific functional scale: measurement properties in patients with knee dysfunction. Phys Ther. 1997;77(8):820–9.

30. Berghmans DD, Lenssen AF, van Rhijn LW, de Bie RA. The patient-specific functional scale: its reliability and responsiveness in patients undergoing a Total knee arthroplasty. J Orthop Sports Phys Ther. 2015;45(7):550–6.

31. Insall JN, Dorr LD, Scott RD, Scott WN. Rationale of the knee society clinical rating system. Clin Orthop Relat Res. 1989;(248):13–4.

32. Lingard EA, Katz JN, Wright RJ, Wright EA, Sledge CB. Validity and responsiveness of the knee society clinical rating system in comparison with the SF-36 and WOMAC. J Bone Joint Surg. 2001;83-A(12):1856–64.

33. Ware JE Jr, Kosinski M, Keller SD. A 12-item short-form health survey: construction of scales and preliminary tests of reliability and validity. Med Care. 1996;34(3):220–33.

34. Kamper SJ, Ostelo RW, Knol DL, Maher CG, de Vet HC, Hancock MJ. Global perceived effect scales provided reliable assessments of health transition in people with musculoskeletal disorders, but ratings are strongly influenced by current status. J Clin Epidemiol. 2010;63(7):760–766.e761.

35. Drouin JM, Valovich-mcLeod TC, Shultz SJ, Gansneder BM, Perrin DH. Reliability and validity of the Biodex system 3 pro isokinetic dynamometer velocity, torque and position measurements. Eur J Appl Physiol. 2004;91(1):22–9.

36. Lenssen AF, van Dam EM, Crijns YH, Verhey M, Geesink RJ, van den Brandt PA, de Bie RA. Reproducibility of goniometric measurement of the knee in the in-hospital phase following total knee arthroplasty. BMC Musculoskelet Disord. 2007;8:83.

37. Webster KE, Wittwer JE, Feller JA. Validity of the GAITRite walkway system for the measurement of averaged and individual step parameters of gait. Gait Posture. 2005;22(4):317–21.

38. Field AP. Discovering statistics using SPSS: SAGE Publications Ltd; 2009.

39. Ostermeier S, Friesecke C, Fricke S, Hurschler C, Stukenborg-Colsman C. Quadriceps force during knee extension after non-hinged and hinged TKA: an in vitro study. Acta Orthop. 2008;79(1):34–8.

40. Bohannon RW, Andrews AW. Normal walking speed: a descriptive meta-analysis. Physiotherapy. 2011;97(3):182–9.

41. Pua Y-H, Seah FJ-T, Clark RA, Poon CL-L, Tan JW-M, Chong H-C. Factors associated with gait speed recovery after total knee arthroplasty: a longitudinal study. In: Seminars in arthritis and rheumatism: 2017: Elsevier; 2017. p. 544–51.

42. Alnahdi AH, Zeni JA, Snyder-Mackler L. Gait after unilateral total knee arthroplasty: frontal plane analysis. J Orthop Res. 2011;29(5):647–52.

43. Health UDo. Interpreting the SF12. In. 2001:1–17. http://health.utah.gov/opha/publications/2001hss/sf12/SF12_Interpreting.pdf. Accessed 31 Aug 2017.

2

Lantern-shaped screw loaded with autologous bone for treating osteonecrosis of the femoral head

Dasheng Lin[1,2]* , Lei Wang[1], Zhaoliang Yu[3], Deqing Luo[1], Xigui Zhang[4] and Kejian Lian[1]

Abstract

Background: Treatment for osteonecrosis of the femoral head (ONFH) in young individuals remains controversial. We developed a lantern-shaped screw, which was designed to provide mechanical support for the femoral head to prevent its collapse, for the treatment of ONFH. The purpose of this study was to investigate the efficacy and safety of the lantern-shaped screw loaded with autologous bone for the treatment of pre-collapse stages of ONFH.

Methods: Thirty-two patients were randomly divided into two groups: the lantern-shaped screw group (core decompression and lantern-shaped screw loaded with autogenous bone) and the control group (core decompression and autogenous bone graft). During 36 months follow-up after surgery, treatment results in patients were assessed by X-ray and computed tomography (CT) scanning as well as functional recovery Harris hip score (HHS).

Results: Successful clinical results were achieved in 15 of 16 hips (94%) in the lantern-shaped screw group compared with 10 of 16 hips (63%) in the control group ($p = 0.0325$). Successful radiological results were achieved in 14 of 16 hips (88%) in the lantern-shaped screw group compared with 8 of 16 hips (50%) in the control group ($P = 0.0221$).

Conclusion: The lantern-shaped screw loaded with autologous bone for the treatment of pre-collapse stages of ONFH is effective and results in preventing progression of ONFH and reducing the risk of femoral head collapse.

Keywords: Lantern-shaped screw, Autogenous bone graft, Core decompression, Osteonecrosis of the femoral head

Background

Hip-preserving surgery has been variable in treating osteonecrosis of the femoral head (ONFH), but there is a lack of consensus on the effectiveness of joint preserving procedures for ONFH. It is undesirable that hip replacement has been undertaken for the young individuals in whom hip prostheses have a limited survival. It is better to preserve the femoral head than replace it [1]. The exact mechanisms of femoral head collapse remain unclear. One hypothesis is based on the effects of shear stress at the boundary of necrotic and normal zones [2], and the other is in accordance with the grade of bone resorption at the boundary [3]. Karasuyama et al. [4] indicated that

sclerotic differences at the boundary may play a crucial role in the pathomechanism of femoral head collapse. Core decompression with or without bone grafting are the most common technique for the early stages of ONFH [5–8]. Nevertheless, the current clinical results were not very satisfactory for patients in the early stages of ONFH performed with core decompression due to the lack of the sufficient structural support [9–11]. Various osteotomies including transtrochanteric rotational osteotomy and curved varus osteotomy have been presented well-known to treat ONFH [12]. Nevertheless, some studies have described various clinical results and risk factors for failure of the osteotomies, such as nonunion of the osteotomy and postoperative fracture of the femoral neck [13]. Porous tantalum implant procedure has been used for the management of the early stages of ONFH [14]. However, this procedure is neither entirely effective nor can it obtain predictable results [15–17]. It has been demonstrated that

---

* Correspondence: linds@xmu.edu.cn
[1]Orthopaedic Center of People's Liberation Army, The Affiliated Southeast Hospital of Xiamen University, Zhangzhou 363000, China
[2]Department of Surgery, Experimental Surgery and Regenerative Medicine, Ludwig-Maximilians-University (LMU), 80336 Munich, Germany
Full list of author information is available at the end of the article

the implantation of a non-vascularized or vascularized fibula graft is a valuable treatment option for femoral head collapse prevention and hip function improvement in patients with pre-collapse osteonecrosis [18–21]. However, this technique may have certain drawbacks in that the implanted bone flaps would result in potential postoperative displacement. Improper post-operative weight-bearing onto the operated hip can also lead to the loosening of the implanted bone flaps, as well as poor bone regeneration and fusion [19, 22, 23].

In the actual practice, an ideal implant should be guaranteed to contact with the bone around the tunnel of the core decompression, as well as buttressing the subchondral bone of the femoral head. Collapse of femoral head will be less likely to occur when the implant contacted with the subchondral bone maximally [24]. Therefore, based on this principle, researchers have designed numerous devices for mechanical support of the femoral head, such as the super elastic cage implantation [25], the biomaterial-loaded allograft threaded cage [26], the umbrella-shaped memory alloy femoral head support device [27], PLGA/TCP scaffold [28], and cementation [29]. In our study, we developed a lantern-shaped screw, which was designed to provide the achievement of surface at surface support for the femoral head to prevent its collapse, for the treatment of ONFH. The purpose of this study was to investigate the efficacy and safety of a lantern-shaped screw loaded with autologous bone for the treatment of pre-collapse stages of ONFH.

Methods
Designing of the lantern-shaped screw
In collaboration with Weigao Orthopaedic Device Co., Ltd. (Weihai, China) and Double Engine Medical Material Co., Ltd. (Xiamen, China), we have designed a lantern-shaped screw, for which we have obtained a patent (patent number: CN103445851B). This screw is made of titanium alloy and cannulated, which is able to be full of the autogenous bone. The titanium mesh installed outside the

lantern-shaped screw can be unfolded into the lantern shape to support the subchondral bone as much as possible. Furthermore, the tail cap of angle plate is a locking screw and can block the lantern-shaped screw back off (Fig. 1). Biomechanical tests of the lantern-shaped screws ($n = 10$) were done on the Dynacell, which is the truly dynamic load cell, designed from the outset for measuring dynamic loads (Instron, America). The results showed that the deformation behavior of the unfolded titanium mesh would not be varied until the strength of vertical compression was increased to 256.7 N (range 248–272 N). By acting the force of 500 N on the titanium mesh, the deformation was 1.9 mm (range 1.5–2.4 mm). These data demonstrated that the lantern-shaped screws have the sufficient mechanical strength to allow for the weight-bearing activities.

Inclusion and exclusion criteria for this study
Patients were eligible for inclusion that aged 16 years to 50 years, suffered from ARCO stage II to III ONFH [19], and necrotic lesions occupying more than the medial 2/3 of the weight-bearing area [30]. Bone marrow oedema on magnetic resonance imaging (MRI) in the ONFH represents a secondary sign of subchondral fracture and thus indicates ARCO stage III [31]. The extent of the necrotic lesion within the femoral head was graded as Type A, B or C using the classification on the mid-coronal T1-weighted MRI scans. Type A lesions occupy less than 1/3 of the medial weight-bearing area or show no lesion on the mid-coronal MRI scan, Type B lesions occupy between 1/3 and 2/3 of the weight-bearing area, and Type C lesions occupy greater than 2/3 of the weight-bearing area [30]. Patients were excluded that had previous pathological fracture, or infection, or severe metabolic diseases, or cognitive impairment.

From January 2011 to December 2013, thirty-two patients with ONFH were eligible and enrolled into this study. There were twenty-five males and seven females that between 16 and 47 years of age. The duration from

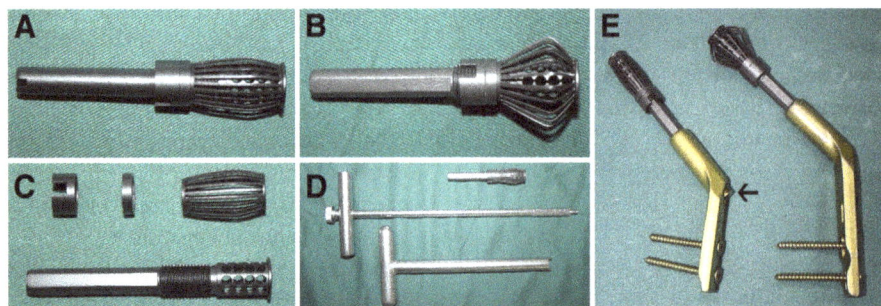

Fig. 1 The lantern-shaped screw. **a** Photo of the folding lantern-shaped screw. **b** Photo of the unfolding lantern-shaped screw. **c** Photo of the structure and composition of the lantern-shaped screw. **d** Photo of the supporting equipment for the lantern-shaped screw. **e** Photo of the lantern-shaped screw and the angle plate with a locking tail cap (black arrow)

symptom onset to surgery treatment was 9 months to 38 months (Table 1). Patients who met the inclusion criteria were randomly divided into two groups: the lantern-shaped screw group (core decompression and lantern-shaped screw loaded with autogenous bone) and the control group (core decompression and autogenous bone graft). The randomization of the patients was done based on randomized numbers generated by sealed-envelope method.

Detailed baseline patient characteristics are shown in Table 1. No significant differences were found in the baseline characteristics of the two groups, including patients' age, gender, side of treated hip, body mass index, etiology, duration of illness, ARCO stage, and preoperative Harris hip score (HHS) [32].

Surgical technique

All patients underwent surgery under spinal anesthesia or general anesthetic. After positioning of the patient in the supine position on an orthopedic traction table, the hip was exposed through a lateral approach, and a longitudinal incision was applied. With an incision of the subcutaneous tissue and the lateral fascia, the vastus lateralis muscle was separated by blunt dissection, and the proximal lateral femoral cortex was exposed. Core decompression was performed under C-arm fluoroscope using the standard technique [5, 6]. And then, the necrotic bone was removed locally.

In the control group, the autogenous iliac-crest grafts were implanted into the region of the necrotic core through the bone channel. In the lantern-shaped screw group, the autogenous iliac-crest grafts were filled into the cannulated screw, and the rest of the autogenous bones were implanted into the region of the necrotic core. The bearing position of the lantern-shaped screw was a depth of approximate 7 mm beneath the articular cartilage surface. Then, the lantern-shaped screw was unfolded into the lantern shape using our designed reamer. Intraoperative C-arm fluoroscope confirmed the adequacy of positioning of the implant in the whole process (Fig. 2). Finally, the angle plate was fixed prior to closing the wound.

Postoperative management and follow-up assessment

Antibiotic treatment was intravenously used within 24 h after surgery. The patients were rapidly mobilized and educated to be non-weight-bearing for 6 weeks. Partial weight-bearing with crutches or a walking aid was permitted for the following 6 weeks, and full-weight-bearing walking was allowed at 12 weeks postoperatively.

Clinically they were evaluated immediately after surgery and at 3, 6, 12, 24, and 36 months postoperatively. The HHS, which was acquired preoperatively and at 12, 24, and 36 months postoperatively, was used to evaluate the function of the hips. X-ray and computed tomography (CT) scans of the hips were experienced at the

Table 1 Baseline patient characteristics

Characteristic	Lantern-shaped screw group (n = 16)	Control group (n = 16)	p value
Mean age (range), yr.	31.5 ± 1.9 (16–47)	32.6 ± 1.7 (18–44)	0.6622
Female/ male, n	3/ 13	4/ 12	1.0000
Right/ left hip involved, n	9/ 7	10/ 6	0.7189
Body mass index (range), kg/cm^2	24.9 ± 0.5 (21–27)	24.3 ± 0.5 (21–26)	0.3978
Etiology			0.4652
Nontraumatic, n	9	11	
Traumatic, n	7	5	
Duration of illness (range), mo	18.8 ± 2.0 (9–36)	20.5 ± 1.8 (11–38)	0.5379
ARCO stage (II/ III)	7/ 9	8/ 8	0.7232
Bone marrow edema of hip (III)	5	6	0.7097
Mean operation time (range), min	80.13 ± 3.3 (56–105)	71.4 ± 3.1 (45–90)	0.0621
Mean blood loss (range), mL	180.6 ± 14.9 (110–350)	158.8 ± 13.7 (90–280)	0.2892
Harris hip score			
Pre-operation (range)	60.3 ± 1.8 (48–72)	61.1 ± 2.0 (48–76)	0.7457
12 months (range)	86.3 ± 0.98 (81–94)	80.8 ± 1.5 (67–90)	0.0054
24 months (range)	85.6 ± 1.3 (70–92)	79.4 ± 1.7 (64–91)	0.0078
36 months (range)	85.2 ± 1.7 (68–95)	78.2 ± 2.2 (64–93)	0.0173
Successful clinical results (%)	15 (94)	10 (63)	0.0325
Successful radiological results (%)	14 (88)	8 (50)	0.0221

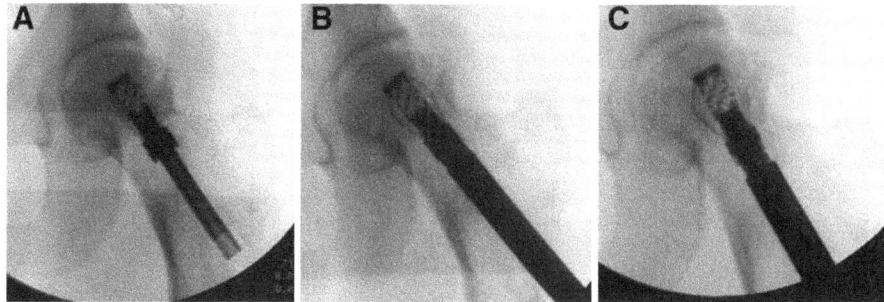

Fig. 2 Intraoperative radiography for evaluation of surgical procedure. **a** Insertion of the lantern-shaped screw. **b** The lantern-shaped screw was being unfolded. **c** The lantern-shaped screw was the achievement of surface at surface support for the subchondral bone of femoral head

same follow-up times. The primary results of this study were clinical and radiological failure. Clinical failure was defined as HHS < 75 points or a requirement for subsequent hip surgery. New occurrence of collapse or increased collapse of greater than 2 mm on X-ray during follow-up was defined as radiological failure [11, 33, 34].

Statistical analysis

SPSS 19.0 (SPSS Company, America) statistical software was used for statistical analysis. Baseline characteristics were assessed using descriptive statistics. The chi-square test was taken to compare nominal data. The t-test or Mann-Whitney U test was used to compare metric data. All statistical assessments were two-sided and evaluated at the 0.05 level of statistical significance.

Results

The control group required less operation time and blood loss, but was not statistically different from the lantern-shaped screw group (Table 1). At 36 months follow-up, there was a significant difference between the preoperative and the last follow-up HHS in the lantern-shaped screw group ($p < 0.0001$) and control group ($P < 0.0001$). HHS was significantly improved in the lantern-shaped screw group when compared to the control group ($P = 0.0173$). The proportion of successful clinical results was significantly higher in the lantern-shaped screw group compared with the control group. Successful clinical results were achieved in 15 of 16 hips (94%) in the lantern-shaped screw group (Fig. 3). One hip (HHS was 68 points) required total hip replacement because of secondary degenerative arthritis at 32 months postoperatively, and was considered clinical failure. In the control group, successful clinical results were achieved in 10 of 16 hips (63%). Of the 6 hips that were clinical failures, three hips (HHS were 64, 67, and 68 points) underwent total hip replacement because of secondary degenerative arthritis 13, 19, and 20 months after surgery. Two (HHS were 64 and 71 points) underwent vascularized fibular grafting at 16 and 21 months after

surgery and the remaining one (HHS was 73 points) had not undergone any further surgery at the last follow-up. The lantern-shaped screw group had a better radiological outcome than the control group ($P = 0.0221$). Successful radiological results were achieved in 14 of 16 hips (88%) in the lantern-shaped screw group compared with 8 of 16 hips (50%) in the control group (Table 1). The survival rates using requirement for further hip surgery as an endpoint were slight higher in the treatment group when compared with the control group ($P = 0.0628$; Fig. 4).

Discussion

Our primary study utilizing our designed lantern-shaped screw for the treatment of pre-collapse stages of ONFH has generated promising effectiveness, with salvage of femoral head and improvement of the hip joint function at 36 months follow-up. A certain advantage of this screw is the achievement of surface at surface support between the weight-bearing area and upper surface of the lantern-shaped screw. Meanwhile, autogenous bone grafting promotes the bone regeneration and reconstruction.

Preservation of the collapse of the femoral head is the great predominant principle to treat patients with pre-collapse stages of ONFH despite of the unestablished pathogenesis. The rareness of bone repair microcirculation will cause osteonecrosis, primarily occurring in weight-bearing region of the femoral head [35]. However, many studies have suggested that the occurrence of the collapse is associated with the period of repair of necrotic area instead of period of ischemic necrosis [36, 37]. The repair can make the femoral head necrotic area construct again but it can also make bone structure alter or the mechanical properties decline in the process. The decline of mechanical properties is correlated directly with the collapse of the femoral head. The process of resorption of necrotic bone and replacement with new bone happen simultaneously [38]. Motomura et al. [2] who studied 30 femoral head specimens, found that in all of the femoral heads, collapse consistently involved a fracture at the lateral boundary of the necrotic lesion and that collapse began at the lateral boundary of the necrotic lesion and the size of the necrotic lesion seemed to contribute to its distribution. Consequently, in the clinical practice, preventing the collapse of subchondral bone has to be given sufficient biomechanical support and suitable circumstances to fulfill bone repair.

For many decades, surgical interventions for the hip-preserving have been controversial. Besides those techniques mentioned above, Papanagiotou et al. [39] reported a safe and effective method that non-vascularised fibular grafting with recombinant bone morphogenetic protein-7 for the management of ONFH in five of seven hips. They noted early consolidation of the non-vascularised fibular grafting and preventing collapse in pre-collapse stages. Yamasaki et al. [40] thought that it appeared to confer benefit in the repair of osteonecrosis and in the prevention of collapse by the transplantation of bone-marrow-derived mononuclear cells with a porous hydroxyapatite scaffold on early bone repair. Malizos et al. [41] introduced a technique using two or three 4.2 mm (or later 4.7 mm) tantalum pegs

for the prevention of collapse of the necrotic lesion, finding that the estimated mean implant survival was 60 months. Chang et al. [42] reported that the poly (propylene fumarate) and calcium phosphate cement were combined to provide appropriate mechanical strength after core-decompressed femoral heads and offer the properties of osteoconductivity. Therefore, all the techniques are based on the mechanical support for the femoral head to prevent its collapse before the bone repair.

The goal of this procedure was to provide mechanical support of the articular surface while promoting bone healing and remodeling, and delay or avoid total hip replacement. The lantern-shaped screw is made of titanium with quite great intensity. Actually, the device is designed predominantly based on one of the characteristics of titanium, that is, it has great plasticity with a ductility property of up to 50–60%. The intensity allows the device to give sufficient support assistance and the plasticity is responsible for the transformation from the shape of cylinder into lantern. Furthermore, the tail cap of angle plate is locking screw and can block the lantern-shaped screw back off. The whole surgical

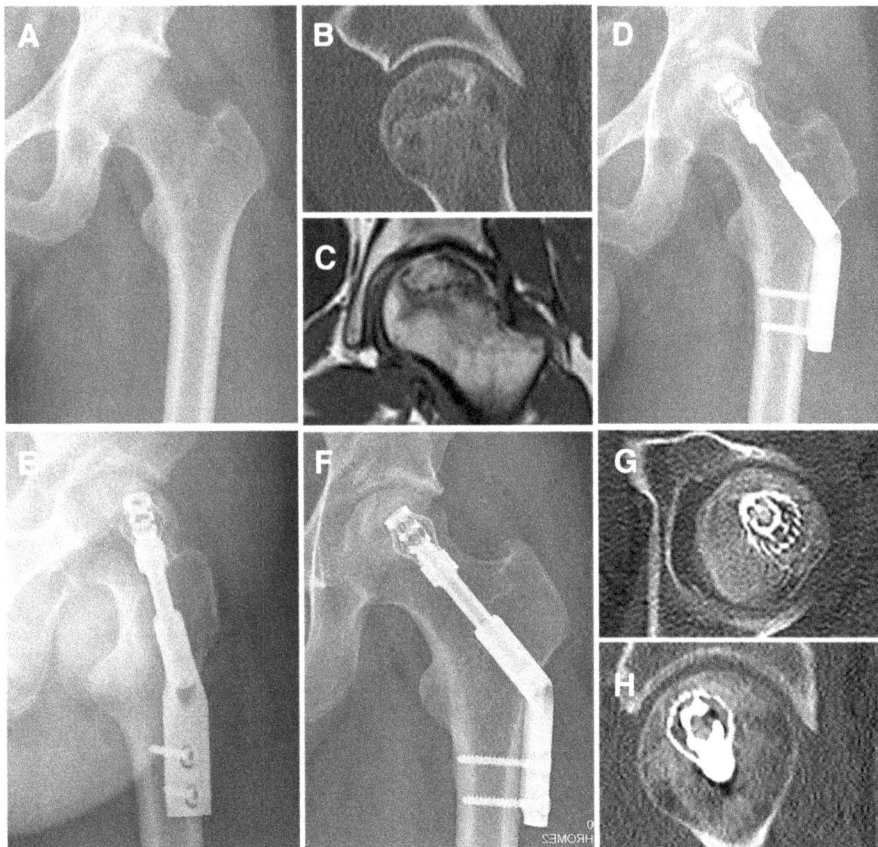

Fig. 3 Representative radiographic images from both preoperative and postoperative taken at immediately after the lantern-shaped screw implantation and 36 months. **a-c** Preoperative X-ray, CT and sagittal T2-weighted magnetic resonance image showing ARCO stage III ONFH in a man aged 29 years. **d** and **e** X-ray anteroposterior view on the day of surgery. **f-h** X-ray and CT scans at 36 months after surgery showing union

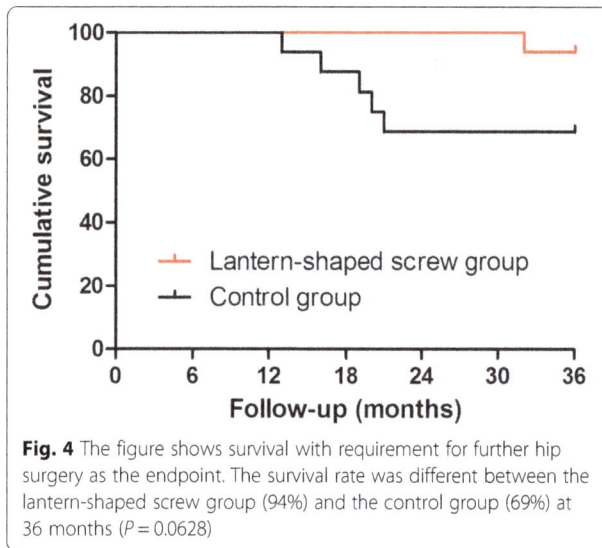

Fig. 4 The figure shows survival with requirement for further hip surgery as the endpoint. The survival was different between the lantern-shaped screw group (94%) and the control group (69%) at 36 months (P = 0.0628)

procedure via the support device involved core decompression by decreasing intraosseous pressure to prevent the ischaemia, reconstruction of necrotic bone beneath the weight-bearing region, mechanical support of the articular surface via the surface at surface contact achieved by the lantern-shaped screw. Therefore, the lantern-shaped screw can be used in pre-collapse stages of ONFH.

Limitations
This study has several limitations. Once the bone remodeling has occurred, the lantern-shaped screw has certain drawbacks in that it cannot be removed. Additionally, a small number of patients and short period of follow-up are the main limitations of this study. More studies with larger sample size and longer follow-up are required to accept the role of the lantern-shaped screw in ONFH.

Conclusion
In summary, the biomechanical property and the bone remodeling regarding the lantern-shaped screw was verified, and the features of this device were also assessed. It is shown that the lantern-shaped screw loaded with autogenous bone may delay or avoid the progression of the collapse of the cartilage for the pre-collapse stages. It can not only provide appropriate circumstance to facilitate new bone remodeling but also strengthen the biomechanical structure for the weight-bearing region. We believe that the lantern-shaped screw could be used not only for autogenous bone graft but also for injection drugs, growth factor, mesenchymal stem cells and so on to be effective in early stages of ONFH. Therefore, we predict that the lantern-shaped screw could provide mechanical support and have considerable potential for medical application.

Abbreviations
CT: Computed tomography; HHS: Harris hip score; MRI: Magnetic resonance imaging; ONFH: Osteonecrosis of the femoral head

Funding
This project was supported by the key projects from the Nanjing Military Region during the 12th Five-Year Plan Period (No. 10MA073 and No. 12MA067).

Authors' contributions
DSL: conceived the study, designed, and analyzed experiments and wrote the manuscript. LW and DQL: Data collection and analysis. ZLY and XGZ: manufactured the materials and tested the biomechanical strength of the materials. KJL: performed the surgery. All authors read and approved the final and submitted manuscript.

Competing interests
The authors declare that they have no competing interests.

Author details
[1]Orthopaedic Center of People's Liberation Army, The Affiliated Southeast Hospital of Xiamen University, Zhangzhou 363000, China. [2]Department of Surgery, Experimental Surgery and Regenerative Medicine, Ludwig-Maximilians-University (LMU), 80336 Munich, Germany. [3]Weigao Orthopaedic Device Co., Ltd, Weihai 264200, China. [4]Double Engine Medical Material Co., Ltd, Xiamen 361000, China.

References
1. Kose KC. Femoral head resurfacing for the treatment of osteonecrosis in the young patient. Clin Orthop Relat Res. 2004;425:290.
2. Motomura G, Yamamoto T, Yamaguchi R, Ikemura S, Nakashima Y, Mawatari T, et al. Morphological analysis of collapsed regions in osteonecrosis of the femoral head. J Bone Joint Surg Br. 2011;93(2):184–7.
3. Li W, Sakai T, Nishii T, Nakamura N, Takao M, Yoshikawa H, et al. Distribution of TRAP-positive cells and expression of HIF-1alpha, VEGF, and FGF-2 in the reparative reaction in patients with osteonecrosis of the femoral head. J Orthop Res. 2009;27(5):694–700.
4. Karasuyama K, Yamamoto T, Motomura G, Sonoda K, Kubo Y, Iwamoto Y. The role of sclerotic changes in the starting mechanisms of collapse: a histomorphometric and FEM study on the femoral head of osteonecrosis. Bone. 2015;81:644–8.
5. Hungerford DS. Core decompression of the femoral head for osteonecrosis. J Bone Joint Surg Am. 1988;70:474–5.
6. Warner JJ, Philip JH, Brodsky GL, Thornhill TS. Studies of nontraumatic osteonecrosis. The role of core decompression in the treatment of nontraumatic osteonecrosis of the femoral head. Clin Orthop Relat Res. 1987;(225):104–27.
7. Marker DR, Seyler TM, Ulrich SD, Srivastava S, Mont MA. Do modern techniques improve core decompression outcomes for hip osteonecrosis? Clin Orthop Relat Res. 2008;466(5):1093–103.
8. Kerimaa P, Väänänen M, Ojala R, Hyvönen P, Lehenkari P, Tervonen O, et al. MRI-guidance in percutaneous core decompression of osteonecrosis of the femoral head. Eur Radiol. 2016;26:1180–5.
9. Zalavras CG, Lieberman JR. Osteonecrosis of the femoral head: evaluation and treatment. J Am Acad Orthop Surg. 2014;22:455–64.
10. Tabatabaee RM, Saberi S, Parvizi J, Mortazavi SM, Farzan M. Combining concentrated autologous bone marrow stem cells injection with core decompression improves outcome for patients with early-stage osteonecrosis of the femoral head: a comparative study. J Arthroplast. 2015;30:11–5.
11. Yin H, Yuan Z, Wang D. Multiple drilling combined with simvastatin versus multiple drilling alone for the treatment of avascular osteonecrosis of the femoral head: 3-year follow-up study. BMC Musculoskelet Disord. 2016;17:344.
12. Lee YK, Park CH, Ha YC, Kim DY, Lyu SH, Koo KH. Comparison of surgical parameters and results between curved varus osteotomy and rotational osteotomy for osteonecrosis of the femoral head. Clin Orthop Surg. 2017; 9(2):160–8.

13. Ha YC, Kim HJ, Kim SY, Kim KC, Lee YK, Koo KH. Effects of age and body mass index on the results of transtrochanteric rotational osteotomy for femoral head osteonecrosis: surgical technique. J Bone Joint Surg Am. 2011; 93(Suppl 1):75–84.

14. Tsao AK, Roberson JR, Christie MJ, Dore DD, Heck DA, Robertson DD, et al. Biomechanical and clinical evaluations of a porous tantalum implant for the treatment of early-stage osteonecrosis. J Bone Joint Surg Am. 2005;87 (Suppl 2):22–7.

15. Tanzer M, Bobyn JD, Krygier JJ, Karabasz D. Histopathologic retrieval analysis of clinically failed porous tantalum osteonecrosis implants. J Bone Joint Surg Am. 2008;90:1282–9.

16. Varitimidis SE, Dimitroulias AP, Karachalios TS, Dailiana ZH, Malizos KN. Outcome after tantalum rod implantation for treatment of femoral head osteonecrosis: 26 hips followed for an average of 3 years. Acta Orthop. 2009;80:20–5.

17. Ma J, Sun W, Gao F, Guo W, Wang Y, Li Z. Porous tantalum implant in treating osteonecrosis of the femoral head: still a viable option? Sci Rep. 2016;6:28227.

18. Korompilias AV, Beris AE, Lykissas MG, Kostas-Agnantis IP, Soucacos PN. Femoral head osteonecrosis: why choose free vascularized fibula grafting. Microsurgery. 2011;31:223–8.

19. Zhao D, Huang S, Lu F, Wang B, Yang L, Qin L, et al. Vascularized bone grafting fixed by biodegradable magnesium screw for treating osteonecrosis of the femoral head. Biomaterials. 2016;81:84–92.

20. Korompilias AV, Lykissas MG, Beris AE, Urbaniak JR, Soucacos PN. Vascularised fibular graft in the management of femoral head osteonecrosis: twenty years later. J Bone Joint Surg Br. 2009;91:287–93.

21. Zhang CQ, Sun Y, Chen SB, Jin DX, Sheng JG, Cheng XG, et al. Free vascularised fibular graft for post-traumatic osteonecrosis of the femoral head in teenage patients. J Bone Joint Surg Br. 2011;93:1314–9.

22. Malizos KN, Quarles LD, Dailiana ZH, Rizk WS, Seaber AV, Urbaniak JR. Analysis of failures after vascularized fibular grafting in femoral head necrosis. Orthop Clin North Am. 2004;35:305–14.

23. Dailiana ZH, Toth AP, Gunneson E, Berend KR, Urbaniak JR. Free vascularized fibular grafting following failed core decompression for femoral head osteonecrosis. J Arthroplast. 2007;22:679–88.

24. Civinini R, De Biase P, Carulli C, Matassi F, Nistri L, Capanna R, et al. The use of an injectable calcium sulphate/calcium phosphate bioceramic in the treatment of osteonecrosis of the femoral head. Int Orthop. 2012;36:1583–8.

25. Wang Y, Chai W, Wang ZG, Zhou YG, Zhang GQ, Chen JY. Superelastic cage implantation: a new technique for treating osteonecrosis of the femoral head with mid-term follow-ups. J Arthroplasty. 2009;24:1006–14.

26. Yang S, Wu X, Xu W, Ye S, Liu X, Liu X. Structural augmentation with biomaterial-loaded allograft threaded cage for the treatment of femoral head osteonecrosis. J Arthroplast. 2010;25:1223–30.

27. Yu X, Jiang W, Pan Q, Wu T, Zhang Y, Zhou Z, et al. Umbrella-shaped, memory alloy femoral head support device for treatment of avascular osteonecrosis of the femoral head. Int Orthop. 2013;37:1225–32.

28. Qin L, Yao D, Zheng L, Liu WC, Liu Z, Lei M, et al. Phytomolecule icaritin incorporated PLGA/TCP scaffold for steroid-associated osteonecrosis: proof-of-concept for prevention of hip joint collapse in bipedal emus and mechanistic study in quadrupedal rabbits. Biomaterials. 2015;59:125–43.

29. Wood ML, McDowell CM, Kelley SS. Cementation for femoral head osteonecrosis: a preliminary clinic study. Clin Orthop Relat Res. 2003;412: 94–102.

30. Nishii T, Sugano N, Ohzono K, Sakai T, Haraguchi K, Yoshikawa H. Progression and cessation of collapse in osteonecrosis of the femoral head. Clin Orthop Relat Res. 2002;400:149–57.

31. Meier R, Kraus TM, Schaeffeler C, Torka S, Schlitter AM, Specht K, et al. Bone marrow oedema on MR imaging indicates ARCO stage 3 disease in patients with AVN of the femoral head. Eur Radiol. 2014;24:2271–8.

32. Harris WH. Traumatic arthritis of the hip after dislocation and acetabular fractures: treatment by mold arthroplasty. An end-result study using a new method of result evaluation. J Bone Joint Surg Am. 1969;51:737–55.

33. Lee MS, Hsieh PH, Chang YH, Chan YS, Agrawal S, Ueng SW. Elevated intraosseous pressure in the intertrochanteric region is associated with poorer results in osteonecrosis of the femoral head treated by multiple drilling. J Bone Joint Surg Br. 2008;90:852–7.

34. Kang P, Pei F, Shen B, Zhou Z, Yang J. Are the results of multiple drilling and alendronate for osteonecrosis of the femoral head better than those of multiple drilling? A pilot study. Joint Bone Spine. 2012;79:67–72.

35. Mont MA, Hungerford DS. Non-traumatic avascular necrosis of the femoral head. J Bone Joint Surg Am. 1995;77:459–74.

36. Brown TD, Way ME, Ferguson AB Jr. Mechanical characteristics of bone in femoral capital aseptic necrosis. Clin Orthop Relat Res. 1981;(156):240–7.

37. Ueo T, Tsutsumi S, Yamamuro T, Okumura H, Shimizu A, Nakamura T. Biomechanical aspects of the development of aseptic necrosis of the femoral head. Arch Orthop Trauma Surg. 1985;104:145–9.

38. Kim HJ. Hyperbaric oxygen therapy as a treatment for stage-I avascular necrosis of the femoral head. J Bone Joint Surg Br. 2004;86:150–1.

39. Papanagiotou M, Malizos KN, Vlychou M, Dailiana ZH. Autologous (non-vascularised) fibular grafting with recombinant bone morphogenetic protein-7 for the treatment of femoral head osteonecrosis: preliminary report. Bone Joint J. 2014;96-B:31–5.

40. Yamasaki T, Yasunaga Y, Ishikawa M, Hamaki T, Ochi M. Bone-marrow-derived mononuclear cells with a porous hydroxyapatite scaffold for the treatment of osteonecrosis of the femoral head: a preliminary study. J Bone Joint Surg Br. 2010;92:337–41.

41. Malizos KN, Papasoulis E, Dailiana ZH, Papatheodorou LK, Varitimidis SE. Early results of a novel technique using multiple small tantalum pegs for the treatment of osteonecrosis of the femoral head: a case series involving 26 hips. J Bone Joint Surg Br. 2012;94:173–8.

42. Chang CH, Liao TC, Hsu YM, Fang HW, Chen CC, Lin FH. A poly (propylene fumarate)--calcium phosphate based angiogenic injectable bone cement for femoral head osteonecrosis. Biomaterials. 2010;31:4048–55.

3

Use of The Global Alliance for Musculoskeletal Health survey module for estimating the population prevalence of musculoskeletal pain: findings from the Solomon Islands

D. G. Hoy[1,2,3*], T. Raikoti[3], E. Smith[1], A. Tuzakana[4], T. Gill[5], K. Matikarai[3], J. Tako[4], A. Jorari[3^], F. Blyth[1], A. Pitaboe[4], R. Buchbinder[6], I. Kalauma[4^], P. Brooks[7], C. Lepers[3], A. Woolf[2,8], A. Briggs[9] and L. March[1,2]

Abstract

Background: Musculoskeletal (MSK) conditions are common and the biggest global cause of physical disability. The objective of the current study was to estimate the population prevalence of MSK-related pain using a standardized global MSK survey module for the first time.

Methods: A MSK survey module was constructed by the Global Alliance for Musculoskeletal Health Surveillance Taskforce and the Global Burden of Disease MSK Expert Group. The MSK module was included in the 2015 Solomon Islands Demographic and Health Survey. The sampling design was a two-stage stratified, nationally representative sample of households.

Results: A total of 9214 participants aged 15–49 years were included in the analysis. The age-standardized four-week prevalence of activity-limiting low back pain, neck pain, and hip and/or knee pain was 16.8, 8.9, and 10.8%, respectively. Prevalence tended to increase with age, and be higher in those with lower levels of education.

Conclusions: Prevalence of activity-limited pain was high in all measured MSK sites. This indicates an important public health issue for the Solomon Islands that needs to be addressed. Efforts should be underpinned by integration with strategies for other non-communicable diseases, aging, disability, and rehabilitation, and with other sectors such as social services, education, industry, and agriculture. Primary prevention strategies and strategies aimed at self-management are likely to have the greatest and most cost-effective impact.

Keywords: Musculoskeletal, Pain, Survey, Global, Solomon Islands

Background

Musculoskeletal (MSK) conditions are common and the biggest global cause of physical disability [1]. A series of systematic reviews on the prevalence of MSK pain that were conducted as part of the Global Burden of Disease (GBD) 2010 Study [2–8] revealed a substantial shortage of data at the population level in most countries. Further, of the population-level studies available, there was substantial heterogeneity between the case definitions used, making it difficult to compare data across countries and over time.

Many other health conditions causing a large global burden of disease have standard surveys and/or survey modules for estimating population-wide prevalence. For example, for mental health, there is the World Mental Health Survey [9], and the WHO STEPs mental health module [10]. In the absence of a standard survey module for MSK health, characterized by the experience of MSK-related pain, the Global Alliance for MSK Health (GMUSC) embarked on a project to develop such a tool.

* Correspondence: damehoy@yahoo.com.au
^Deceased
[1]University of Sydney, Sydney, Australia
[2]Global Alliance for Musculoskeletal Health, Truro, UK
Full list of author information is available at the end of the article

The Solomon Islands is a nation that sits in the Pacific region. Like many areas of the world, there is very limited information on MSK pain in the Pacific [11]. The objective of the current study was to use the GMUSC MSK survey module to estimate the prevalence of pain at common MSK sites in the Solomon Islands.

Methods

Study setting

The Solomon Islands is a low-income country and is part of the Melanesian group of islands. It consists of nearly 1000 islands and has a tropical climate. English is the official language, but Pidgin is also widely used. Most of the country's labor force is engaged in subsistence crop and animal raising, hunting and fishing. In 2016, the population was estimated to be approximately 640,000 with approximately 80% living in rural areas. In 2009, life expectancy at birth was estimated to be 66 years for males and 73 years for females. While infectious diseases continue to be prominent in the Solomon Islands, non-communicable diseases (NCDs) are also rapidly increasing due largely to changing lifestyles [12].

Study design

The GMUSC MSK survey module was included in the 2015 Solomon Islands Demographic and Health Survey (SIDHS). The Global Demographic and Health Survey (DHS) Program has conducted the DHS more than 300 times in over 90 countries. It selects nationally-representative samples to study fertility, family planning, maternal and child health, gender, HIV/AIDS, malaria, and nutrition [13]. The SIDHS focused on these issues as well as pain of MSK aetiology (referred to as 'MSK pain').

The SIDHS was coordinated by the Solomon Islands National Statistics Office (SINSO) with assistance from the Pacific Community (SPC). Training for conducting the survey was conducted at three levels according to standard DHS training procedures: 1) Training of trainers; 2) Pilot training; and 3) Main training. Training of trainers included training of those who would lead subsequent trainings, as well as testing of the questionnaires for content, translation, skip procedures and filtering instructions. The pilot training of fieldworkers was provided to 70 field workers from five provinces and was also another opportunity to further test the questionnaires. The field workers consisted of SINSO staff, nurses, health technicians, and trained interviewers. All the field workers could read, speak and understand Pidgen, and most, but not all, were literate in English. The main training took 3 weeks and included 145 field workers. It included presentations, mock interviews, quizzes and role-playing. Data were collected by 14 teams, each of nine people. Data collection initially ran from April to September 2015, and a follow-up period ran from October to November 2015 to revisit those people who were not available

to respond to the survey at their initial visit. This was limited to the capital, Honiara, as this was the site where the majority of non-responders lived.

Participants

The sampling design was a two-stage stratified, nationally-representative sample of households. In the Solomon Islands, enumeration areas (EAs) are at the sub-village level and are considered by the SINSO to be the smallest geographical unit. The average size of an EA is 68 households. There are a total of 1342 EAs and 91,251 households in the Solomon Islands [12]. A target sample size of 5064 households was chosen by the SINSO for consistency with the previous SIDHS in 2006/7, and took into account an anticipated household response rate of 95%.

The sampling frame was a list of all EAs and their respective number of households. From this list, 211 EAs were selected using sampling with probability proportional to the estimated number of households in the EA. In each of the selected EAs, 24 households were selected using systematic random sampling. Consistent with standard DHS protocol, which has a focus on women's reproductive health, all women aged 15–49 in these households were eligible to be individually interviewed, while men aged 15 and over in every second household were eligible to be interviewed. For this reason, women aged 50 years and over were not sampled.

Variables, data sources and measurement

Three questionnaires (household, female, and male) were used [12]. All content except for the MSK module was based on previously developed modules by the Global DHS Program, which were adapted to the specific needs of the Solomon Islands.

The MSK survey module was constructed by the GMUSC Surveillance Taskforce and members of the GBD MSK Expert Group. The intention was to develop a one-page module that would not necessarily be used as a stand-alone tool, but rather as a component that could seamlessly integrate within other pre-existing and planned surveys such as national health surveys, or in this case, the DHS. Such purposive integration would likely increase its uptake, save resources, minimise survey burden from conducting multiple surveys on local communities, provide access to a larger range of covariates, and encourage responses that are integrated with other NCDs and other health issues such as healthy aging, and disability, rather than having 'siloed' MSK responses.

The MSK module was based on literature reviews and previous consensus exercises for establishing a standard approach to collecting population-based data on the epidemiology of various MSK conditions. The measures in the MSK module were prevalence of low back pain, neck pain, and hip and/or knee pain. For low back pain, we used the minimal definition of low back pain for face-to-face interviews from an international modified Delphi consensus study [14]. For neck pain, the results from a previous expert consensus exercise were used [15]. For hip and/or knee pain, the results from an expert consensus exercise for monitoring MSK problems in Europe were used [16]. Consistent with the methods of a previous systematic review of prevalence studies of low back pain [17], four key elements were specified in the module: the prevalence period (4 weeks), the anatomical location referred to; a minimum episode duration (1 day), and whether or not the question referred to activity-limiting pain. For hip and/or knee pain, it was felt a question on diagnosis for people with chronic symptoms was also important to include. It was felt this was less important for spinal pain given, for example, the importance of avoiding over-medicalization of back pain [18]. The module is shown in Additional file 1.

Using standard DHS protocols, the survey questionnaires were translated into Pidgin and back-translated into English in order to check the accuracy of the translation. Survey content, skip procedures and filtering instructions were pre-tested by staff from the SINSO.

Efforts to minimize study bias

To minimise risk of bias in the prevalence estimates of MSK pain we used a framework based upon a risk of bias tool for prevalence studies [19]. Specifically: 1) The MSK module items had been developed through extensive Delphi and other expert consensus exercises; 2) The case definitions used were in accordance with international recommendations; 3) Selection bias was minimized through selecting a nationally-representative sample using standard selection methods; 4) Non-response bias was minimized by conducting follow up visits to non-responders; 5) Data were collected directly from the subjects as opposed to from a proxy; 6) The same mode of data collection (face-to-face interviews) was used for all subjects; and 7) The recall period was 4 weeks – this length results in less recall bias than longer periods (e.g., 1 year).

Statistical methods

Data were entered into the CSPro computer package two times with 100% verification [20]. Analysis was performed in Microsoft Excel [21]. For the purpose of comparison between the genders, we only included males aged 15 to 49 years for most of the analysis. The outcome variables of interest were activity-limiting low back pain (AL-LBP), activity-limiting neck pain (AL-NP), activity-limiting hip or knee pain (AL-HKP), and hip or knee pain that had lasted for longer than 3 months (HKP > 3/12). There were relatively little missing data: 16 missing values (out of 9214) for AL-LBP, 14 for AL-NP, 4 for AL-HKP, and 39 for HKP > 3/12. These

were treated conservatively as a 'No' response in the analysis.

Proportions and confidence intervals (CIs) for each outcome variable of interest were calculated. An overall design effect (averaged over all variables) had been calculated for the SIDHS to account for the complex sampling design [12] – this value (1.393) was applied in the calculation of CIs. The age-standardized prevalence for the age-group 15–49 years for each outcome variable of interest was calculated using Solomon Islands national population data for 2015. Sub-group analyses were conducted for gender, age group, urbanicity (urban households were considered to be those in Honiara or provincial capital towns), maximum education level reached, and ethnicity. We performed further analysis on prevalence in males across all ages 15 years and above to assess whether prevalence estimates were likely to be under or over estimates for the population 15 years and above in the Solomon Islands.

Results

Study participants

Of the 5064 households selected in the sample, 5042 households (99.8%) (n = 9214 participants) were successfully interviewed. Among the households interviewed, 6657 eligible females 15–49 years were identified, of whom 6292 (95.0%) were successfully interviewed. For males, 3920 eligible males were identified, of whom 3628 (93.0%) were successfully interviewed. Of these, 2922 (80.6%) were aged 15–49 years (Fig. 1).

Of the interviewees, 5429 (59%) resided in rural areas, 3750 (41%) were educated to pre-school or primary level, 4032 (44%) to secondary level, and 721 (8%) to tertiary level. 8857 (96%) were Melanesian, 202 (2.2%) Polynesian, 131 (1.4%) Micronesian, and the remainder from some other ethnic group.

Activity-limiting low back pain

The four-week prevalence of low back pain was 50.5% (95% CI: 49.3 to 51.7). The four-week prevalence of activity-limiting low back pain was 16.8%; the four-week age-standardized prevalence of activity-limiting low back pain was 16.7% (95% CI: 16.4 to 16.9). Prevalence was significantly higher in females compared with males, and rural areas compared with urban areas. Across both sexes, prevalence generally tended to increase with age and decrease by education level. Prevalence was highest in Micronesians, followed by Melanesians, and then Polynesians (Table 1).

Activity-limiting neck pain

The four-week prevalence of neck pain was 29.6% (95% CI: 28.5 to 30.7). The four-week prevalence of activity-limiting neck pain was 8.92%; the four-week age-standardized

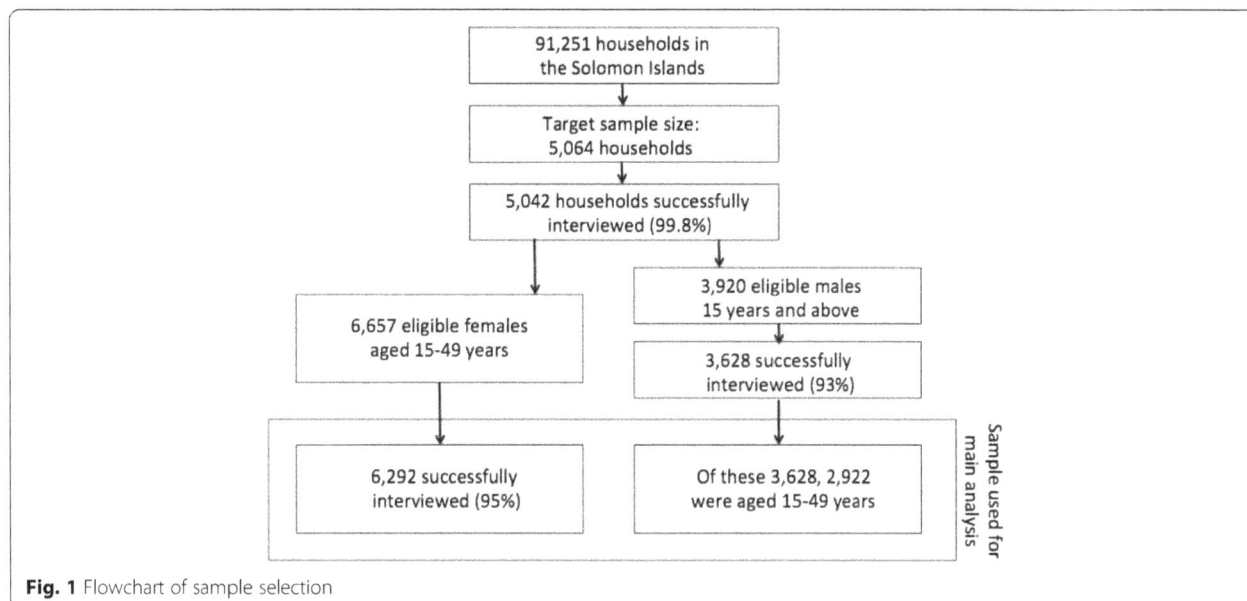

Fig. 1 Flowchart of sample selection

prevalence of activity-limiting neck pain was 8.9% (95% CI: 8.7 to 9.1). Prevalence was higher in females compared with males, although this was not significant at the 0.05 level. Prevalence was significantly higher in rural areas compared with urban areas. Again, prevalence generally tended to increase with age and decrease by education level across both sexes. Prevalence was highest in Melanesians, followed by Micronesians, and then Polynesians (Table 2).

Activity-limiting hip or knee pain
The four-week prevalence of hip or knee pain was 33.9% (95% CI: 32.8 to 35.1). The four-week prevalence of activity-limiting hip or knee pain was 10.8%; the four-week age-standardized prevalence of activity-limiting hip or knee pain was 10.8% (95% CI: 10.5 to 11.0). Prevalence was significantly higher in females compared with males, and rural areas compared with urban areas. Across both sexes, prevalence increased with age, and tended to decrease by education level. Prevalence was highest in Melanesians, followed by Micronesians, and then Polynesians (Table 3).

Hip or knee pain lasting longer than three months
The data collectors accidentally asked about *any* hip or knee pain that had lasted for 3 months or more, as opposed to *activity-limiting* hip or knee pain that had lasted for 3 months or more. The four-week prevalence of any hip or knee pain that had lasted for 3 months or more was 10.6% (95% CI: 9.9 to 11.4); the four-week age-standardized prevalence of any hip or knee pain that had lasted for 3 months or more was 9.9% (95% CI: 9.7 to 10.1). Prevalence was significantly higher in females (11.8%; 95% CI: 10.9 to 12.7) compared with males (8.0%; 95% CI: 6.9 to 9.2), and rural areas (12.5%; 95% CI: 11.5 to 13.6) compared with urban areas (7.9%; 95%

CI: 6.9 to 8.9). Prevalence increased with age in both sexes, and decreased by education level in males; there was no clear relationship between prevalence and education level in females. Prevalence was highest in Melanesians, followed by Micronesians, and then Polynesians.

Diagnosis given to those who had hip or knee pain over the past month
Similar to the previous question, the data collectors accidentally asked for the past-month diagnosis related to *any* hip or knee pain that had lasted for 3 months or more, as opposed to the diagnosis related to *activity-limiting* hip or knee pain that had lasted for 3 months or more. Of the 3125 people who had experienced hip or knee pain over the past 4 weeks, 18.2% (n = 570) reported they had received a diagnosis from a medical doctor. The most common diagnoses given were pneumonia (n = 228), common cold (n = 161), and bone dislocation (n = 14).

Activity-limiting MSK pain in multiple MSK sites
Of the 22.1% (n = 2035) of people who had activity-limiting MSK pain at one or more of the three sites examined, 11.7% (n = 1093) had activity-limiting MSK pain at one site only, 6.0% (n = 556) at two sites, and 4.2% (n = 386) at all three sites.

Age trends of activity-limiting pain
There was a substantial increase in the prevalence of pain at all MSK sites in the years beyond 49 years of age for males, suggesting that the estimates in the 15–49 year age group are likely to be an underestimate of prevalence for all people 15 years and above in the Solomon Islands (Fig. 2).

Table 1 Four-week prevalence of activity-limiting low back pain ("In the past 4 weeks, have you had pain in your low back? If yes, was this pain bad enough to limit your usual activities or change your daily routine for more than one day?"), both sexes, 15–49 year olds

Background characteristic	Numerator	Denominator	Prevalence (%)	LCL (95%)	UCL (95%)
Total	1543	9214	16.8	15.9	17.7
Sex					
Female	1166	6292	18.5	17.4	19.7
Male	377	2922	12.9	11.5	14.3
Age group					
15–19	182	1818	10.0	8.4	11.6
20–24	234	1582	14.8	12.7	16.9
25–29	240	1534	15.7	13.5	17.8
30–34	249	1341	18.6	16.1	21.0
35–39	240	1204	19.9	17.3	22.6
40–44	201	959	21.0	17.9	24.0
45–49	197	776	25.4	21.8	29.0
Urbanicity					
Urban	532	3785	14.1	12.8	15.4
Rural	1011	5429	18.6	17.4	19.8
Education					
Pre-school	2	9	22.2	0.0	54.3
Primary	723	3741	19.3	17.8	20.8
Secondary	597	4032	14.8	13.5	16.1
Tertiary	81	721	11.2	8.5	14.0
Vocational	25	148	16.9	9.8	24.0
Other	1	156	0.6	0.0	2.1
Missing	114	555	20.5	16.6	24.5
Ethnicity					
Melanesian	1488	8857	16.8	15.9	17.7
Polynesian	30	202	14.9	9.1	20.6
Micronesian	24	131	18.3	10.5	26.1
Other	1	21	4.8	0.0	15.5
Missing	0	3	0.0	0.0	0.0

LCL Lower 95% Confidence Limit, *UCL* Upper 95% Confidence Limit

Use of the MSK module

The SINSO and SPC staff reported that the GMUSC MSK module integrated well with the DHS survey, was easy to understand and use, and that it only added a few extra minutes to each interview. The use of the MSK module and analysis of MSK data for the Solomon Islands study cost a few thousand dollars compared to the tens or even hundreds of thousands of dollars a stand-alone survey of this size would have cost. Data analysis indicated only 1% of data were missing.

Discussion

The objectives of the current study were to derive standard and comparable estimates of the prevalence of common MSK pain in the Solomon Islands; and to use the GMUSC MSK module for the first time, and in particular, to determine whether it could feasibly be integrated within an existing population health survey.

Strengths and limitations

We surveyed a nationally representative sample of 15–49 year olds (and a wider age-range in males), and used a standardized tool, which integrated into an existing national survey instrument. A number of measures were taken to minimize study bias, and there was a very good response rate. The recall period of 4 weeks may have resulted in some recall bias. One minor error by data collectors occurred in that for question MSK 7 and MSK8, they used question MSK 5 as the entry point, rather than question MSK 6, thus including *any* hip or knee

Table 2 Four-week prevalence of activity-limiting neck pain ("In the past 4 weeks, have you had pain in your neck? If yes, was this pain bad enough to limit your usual activities or change your daily routine for more than one day?"), both sexes, 15–49 year olds

Background characteristic	Numerator	Denominator	Prevalence (%)	LCL (95%)	UCL (95%)
Total	822	9214	8.9	8.2	9.6
Sex					
Female	596	6292	9.5	8.6	10.3
Male	226	2922	7.7	6.6	8.9
Age group					
15–19	123	1818	6.8	5.4	8.1
20–24	134	1582	8.5	6.9	10.1
25–29	116	1534	7.6	6.0	9.1
30–34	118	1341	8.8	7.0	10.6
35–39	129	1204	10.7	8.7	12.8
40–44	101	959	10.5	8.2	12.8
45–49	101	776	13.0	10.2	15.8
Urbanicity					
Urban	287	3785	7.6	6.6	8.6
Rural	535	5429	9.9	8.9	10.8
Education					
Pre-school	2	9	22.2	0.0	54.3
Primary	391	3741	10.5	9.3	11.6
Secondary	320	4032	7.9	7.0	8.9
Tertiary	43	721	6.0	3.9	8.0
Vocational	15	148	10.1	4.4	15.9
Other	1	156	0.6	0.0	2.1
Missing	50	555	9.0	6.2	11.8
Ethnicity					
Melanesian	804	8857	9.1	8.4	9.8
Polynesian	10	202	5.0	1.4	8.5
Micronesian	7	131	5.3	0.8	9.9
Other	1	21	4.8	0.0	15.5
Missing	0	3	0.0	0.0	0.0

LCL Lower 95% Confidence Limit, *UCL* Upper 95% Confidence Limit

pain rather than *activity-limiting* hip or knee pain. This will be made clearer in future trainings.

MSKs in the Solomon Islands

The prevalence of pain was high at all the MSK sites that were evaluated. Low back pain had the highest prevalence, followed by hip or knee pain, and then neck pain. Our findings for the age-standardized prevalence of activity-limiting low back and neck pain in the Solomon Islands were substantially higher than those of GBD 2016 (low back pain: 5.1%; neck pain: 2.6%), which are based on models that extrapolate data from elsewhere [22]. This is partly, but not entirely, explained by the inclusion of all ages in GBD 2016 estimates. The ratio between the age-standardized

prevalence of activity-limiting low back and neck pain (1.87) was comparable to the same ratio for GBD 2016 (1.96) [22].

Consistent with previous research on MSK conditions, prevalence of MSK pain tended to increase with age in each of the sites that we evaluated [17, 23, 24]. The results were also consistent with previous findings that low back pain tends to be more prevalent in those with lower levels of education [25]. One of the most interesting findings was in regard to ethnicity. Generally, Polynesian countries have a higher prevalence of overweight and obesity compared to Melanesian and Micronesian countries [26]. Given this, and the fact that obesity is a risk factor for low back pain [25], and osteoarthritis of the knee [27], one may have expected higher rates of low back and knee pain in the Polynesian group in this

Table 3 Four-week prevalence of activity-limiting hip or knee pain ("In the past 4 weeks, have you had pain in your hips or knees? If yes, was this pain bad enough to limit your usual activities or change your daily routine for more than one day?"), both sexes, 15–49 year olds

Background characteristic	Numerator	Denominator	Prevalence (%)	LCL (95%)	UCL (95%)
Total	998	9214	10.8	10.1	11.6
Sex					
Female	779	6292	12.4	11.4	13.3
Male	219	2922	7.5	6.4	8.6
Age group					
15–19	116	1818	6.4	5.1	7.7
20–24	142	1582	9.0	7.3	10.6
25–29	142	1534	9.3	7.6	11.0
30–34	150	1341	11.2	9.2	13.2
35–39	164	1204	13.6	11.3	15.9
40–44	129	959	13.5	10.9	16.0
45–49	155	776	20.0	16.7	23.3
Urbanicity					
Urban	328	3785	8.7	7.6	9.7
Rural	670	5429	12.3	11.3	13.4
Education					
Pre-school	1	9	11.1	0.0	35.3
Primary	486	3741	13.0	11.7	14.3
Secondary	365	4032	9.1	8.0	10.1
Tertiary	48	721	6.7	4.5	8.8
Vocational	15	148	10.1	4.4	15.9
Other	1	156	0.6	0.0	2.1
Missing	82	555	14.8	11.3	18.3
Ethnicity					
Melanesian	971	8857	11.0	10.2	11.7
Polynesian	13	202	6.4	2.4	10.4
Micronesian	14	131	10.7	4.4	16.9
Other	0	21	0.0	0.0	0.0
Missing	0	3	0.0	0.0	0.0

LCL Lower 95% Confidence Limit, *UCL* Upper 95% Confidence Limit

study. However, this group had the lowest prevalence, although this was not significant at the 0.05 level. Further research is needed to better understand this.

The diagnoses reported for hip and/or knee pain were most commonly pneumonia and the common cold. There are high rates of communicable diseases in the Solomon Islands and it is possible that these symptoms reflect manifestations of infection [28]. While SPC report there was not an unusually high amount of influenza-like illnesses being reported in the Solomons at the time of the survey there was a dengue fever outbreak and reported cases of Zika virus [29], and both of these can result in arthralgia. [30, 31]. These self-reported diagnoses may also reflect a lack of knowledge about causes of MSK pain among the general population and/or communication gaps with health professionals.

This study has established that MSK pain is common, and given existing data on the burden of disease associated with MSK conditions, a significant burden of disease is likely to be present in the Solomon Islands. This likely current and future burden needs to be better addressed in order to maximise function, productivity and livelihoods, and ensure that health systems in the Solomons are not overwhelmed as the country's population ages. However, in upscaling efforts to address the burden of MSK in the Solomons, it is important that a vertical or 'siloed' approach to addressing MSKs is avoided.

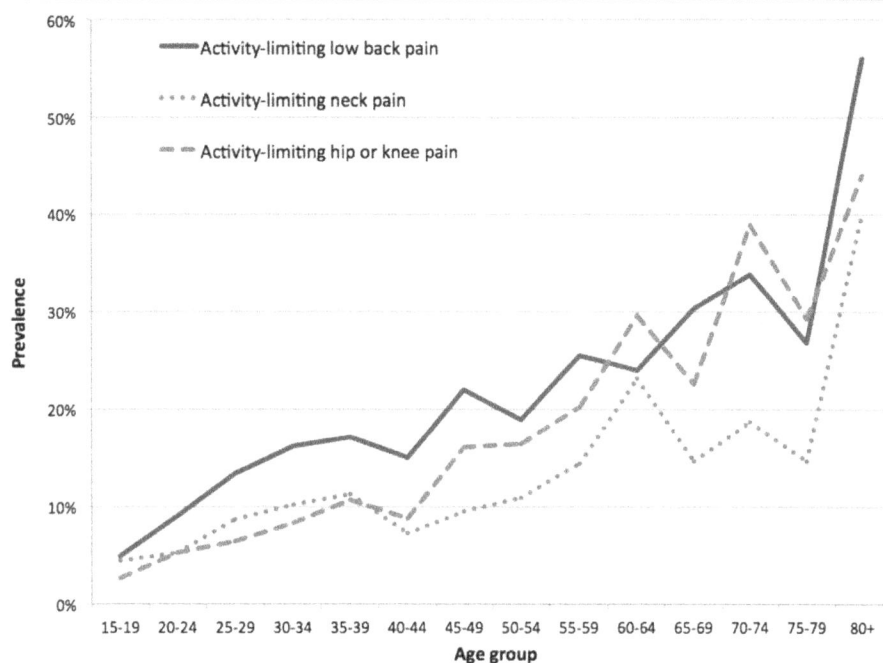

Fig. 2 Four-week prevalence of activity-limiting pain, males, 15 years and above

It is key that any approach addressing the burden of MSKs is underpinned by 'integration' [32, 33]. MSK pain shares risk factors that are common to other conditions such as diabetes and cardiovascular disease. Further, as people age, they are faced with multi-morbidities and require an integrated approach to health care to ensure the care is person-centred, holistic and efficient [34]. Consequently, an approach that is integrated with other non-communicable diseases, issues such as aging, disability, and rehabilitation, and other sectors such as social services, education, industry, and agriculture is likely to promote a more streamlined, cost-effective approach, avoid doubling of efforts and wasting of resources, and avoid ultimate damage to fragile health systems [32]. Integration should take place at macro- (policy) levels, meso- (health service) levels, and micro- (clinician/patient) levels [33].

Primary prevention strategies and strategies aimed at self-management are likely to have the greatest and most cost-effective impact in reducing the burden of MSK pain in the Solomon Islands. For example, Buchbinder et al. promote the concept of living well with low back pain through focusing on self-management and healthy lifestyles [18]. Where feasible, approaches should be integrated with those of other non-communicable diseases, and issues such as healthy aging, consistent with recommendations from the World Health Organization [34]. Locally relevant mass media campaigns encouraging healthy lifestyles, including obesity-reduction and physical activity, and improving population beliefs about

prevention and management of MSK health and persistent pain, are likely to have a positive impact [32, 33]. Models of Care need to be tailored to the specific capacities and needs of the specific setting. For example, it may be possible to have dedicated staff for treating MSK pain at the national level; however, at sub-national levels, this may become less realistic given the limited funding and number of staff in health services. Alternative approaches, such as having NCD generalists, inclusive of MSK health, who provide treatment and advice should be further explored.

MSK module
Staff reported the tool MSK module integrated well, was easy to use, and it was very affordable compared with the alternative of a stand-alone survey. Utilization of the module as part of existing surveys is therefore likely to be a relatively affordable way of improving data coverage across the globe, and thus improving the understanding of MSK pain, and informing ways of mitigating the growing global burden of MSK pain. While in-depth cognitive interviews and examination of inter-rater reliability of the tool was not possible in the current study due to resource constraints and heavy workloads of the data collection team, this is planned for the future.

The other benefit of including the module within other more general surveys, and consistent with the Principles of Development Effectiveness [35–37], is that it can help to facilitate integration of the MSK response across the broader health system. Translation of survey results into national policy and practice aimed at reducing MSK burden is paramount. A two-page summary of findings and key recommendations was prepared for the Solomon Islands government to assist with this process (Additional file 2).

The Global Alliance for Musculoskeletal Health have already used the results of the pilot to further refine the module for use in other countries throughout the world. Questions on upper limb pain have been added, and the tool has recently been piloted in a South Australian health survey. The latest version of the tool can be found at http://bjdonline.org/msk-survey-module/.

Conclusion

The prevalence of activity-limited pain was high in all measured MSK sites in the Solomon Islands. This indicates an important public health issue for the Solomon Islands that needs to be addressed. Efforts should be underpinned by integration with strategies for other non-communicable diseases, aging, disability, and rehabilitation, and with other sectors such as social services, education, industry, and agriculture. Primary prevention strategies and strategies aimed at self-management are likely to have the greatest and most cost-effective impact.

Abbreviations

AL-HKP: Activity-limiting hip or knee pain; AL-LBP: Activity-limiting low back pain; AL-NP: Activity-limiting neck pain; CI: Confidence interval; DHS: Demographic and Health Survey; EA: Enumeration Area; GBD: Global Burden of Disease; GMUSC: Global Alliance for Musculoskeletal Health; HIV/AIDs: Human immunodeficiency virus infection and acquired immune deficiency syndrome; HKP > 3/12: Hip or knee pain that had lasted for longer than 3 months; MSK: Musculoskeletal; NCDs: Non-communicable diseases; NHMRC: National Health and Medical Research Council; SIDHS: Solomon Islands Demographic and Health Survey; SINSO: Solomon Islands National Statistics Office; SPC: Pacific Community; UNICEF: United Nations Childrens' Fund; WHO STEPs: The World Health Organization stepwise approach to surveillance of non-communicable disease risk

Funding

The Solomon Islands Demographic and Health Survey was funded by the Australian Government, the Government of the Solomon Islands, and UNICEF Pacific. Analysis of musculoskeletal data was funded by the University of Sydney Institute and Bone and Joint Research. RB is funded by an NHMRC Senior Principal Research Fellowship. AMB is supported by a fellowship awarded by the Australian National Health and Medical Research Council (#1132548). The funders had no role in the study design. The authors declare that they have no competing interests.

Authors' contributions

DH, ES, TG, FB, RB, PB, AW, LM designed the module. TR, AT, KM, JT, AJ, AP, IK were involved in the data collection. DH analyzed and interpreted the data. DH drafted the manuscript. DH, TR, ES, AT, TG, KM, JT, AJ, FB, AP, RB, PB, CL, AW, AM, LM provided comment on the draft manuscript. DH, TR, ES, AT, TG, KM, JT, AJ, FB, AP, RB, PB, CL, AW, AM, LM read and approved the final manuscript.

Competing interests

The authors declare that they have no competing interests.

Author details

[1]University of Sydney, Sydney, Australia. [2]Global Alliance for Musculoskeletal Health, Truro, UK. [3]Pacific Community (SPC), Noumea, New Caledonia. [4]Solomon Islands National Statistics Office, Honiara, Solomon Islands. [5]University of Adelaide, Adelaide, Australia. [6]Monash University, Melbourne, Australia. [7]University of Melbourne, Melbourne, Australia. [8]Royal Cornwall Hospital, Truro, UK. [9]Curtin University, Perth, Australia.

References

1.   GBD 2016 Disease and Injury Incidence and Prevalence Collaborators. Global, regional, and national incidence, prevalence, and years lived with disability for 328 diseases and injuries for 195 countries, 1990–2016: a systematic analysis for the global burden of disease study 2016. Lancet. 2017;390(10100):1211–59.
2.   Smith E, Hoy D, Cross M, Merriman TR, Vos T, Buchbinder R, et al. The global burden of gout: estimates from the global burden of disease 2010 study. Ann Rheum Dis. 2014;73(8):1470–6.
3.   Cross M, Smith E, Hoy D, Nolte S, Ackerman I, Fransen M, et al. The global burden of hip and knee osteoarthritis: estimates from the global burden of disease 2010 study. Ann Rheum Dis. 2014;73(7):1323–30.
4.   Hoy D, March L, Brooks P, Blyth F, Woolf A, Bain C, et al. The global burden of low back pain: estimates from the global burden of disease 2010 study. Ann Rheum Dis. 2014;73(6):968–74.
5.   Hoy D, Smith E, Cross M, Sanchez-Riera L, Buchbinder R, Blyth F, et al. The global burden of musculoskeletal conditions for 2010: an overview of methods. Ann Rheum Dis. 2014; In press
6.   Hoy D, March L, Woolf A, Blyth F, Brooks P, Smith E, et al. The global burden of neck pain: estimates from the global burden of disease 2010 study. Ann Rheum Dis. 2014;73(7):1309–15.
7.   Smith E, Hoy DG, Cross M, Vos T, Naghavi M, Buchbinder R, et al. The global burden of other musculoskeletal disorders: estimates from the global burden of disease 2010 study. Ann Rheum Dis. 2014;73(8):1462–9.
8.   Cross M, Smith E, Hoy D, Carmona L, Wolfe F, Vos T, et al. The global burden of rheumatoid arthritis: estimates from the global burden of disease 2010 study. Ann Rheum Dis. 2014;73(7):1316–22.
9.   Harvard Medical School. World Mental Health Survey Inititative. 2005; Available from: https://www.hcp.med.harvard.edu/wmh/index.php. Cited 28 Oct 2017
10. World Health Organization. NCD STEPs Mental Health/Suicide Module. 2017; Available from: http://www.who.int/ncds/surveillance/steps/en/. Cited 28 Oct 2017
11. Hoy D, Roth A, Viney K, Souares Y, Lopez AD. Findings and implications of the global burden of disease 2010 study for the Pacific Islands. Prev Chronic Dis. 2014;11:E75.
12. Solomon Islands Statistics Office. Solomon Islands Demographic Health Survey 2015. 2017; Available from: https://sdd.spc.int/en/. Cited 28 Oct 2017
13. USAID. Demographic and Health Survey. 2017; Available from: https://dhsprogram.com/Who-We-Are/About-Us.cfm. Cited 28 Oct 2017
14. Dionne CE, Dunn KM, Croft PR, Nachemson AL, Buchbinder R, Walker BF, et al. A consensus approach toward the standardization of back pain definitions for use in prevalence studies. Spine. 2008;33(1):95–103.
15. Guzman J, Hurwitz EL, Carroll LJ, Haldeman S, Côté P, Carragee EJ, et al. A new conceptual model of neck pain: linking onset, course, and care: the bone and joint decade 2000-2010 task force on neck pain and its associated disorders. Spine (Phila Pa 1976). 2008;33(4 Suppl):S14–23.
16. eumusc.net. Musculoskeletal Health in Europe - Core Indicators: eumusc.net; 2013.
17. Hoy D, Bain C, Williams G, March L, Brooks P, Blyth F, et al. A systematic review of the global prevalence of low back pain. Arthritis Rheum. 2012;64(6):2028–37.
18. Buchbinder R, van Tulder M, Öberg B, Costa L, Woolf A, Schoene M, et al. Low pain pain: a call for action. Lancet. 2018;
19. Hoy D, Brooks P, Woolf A, Blyth F, March L, Bain C, et al. Assessing risk of bias in prevalence studies: modification of an existing tool and evidence of interrater agreement. J Clin Epidemiol. 2012;65(9):934 9.
20. United States Census Bureau. Census and survey processing system 2017; Available from: https://www.census.gov/. Cited 28 Oct 2017

21. Microsoft Corporation. Microsoft Excel 2010. 2010; Available from: https://products.office.com/en-au/excel. Cited 17 Sept 2015

22. Institute for Health Metrics and Evaluation (IHME). GBD Data Tool. 2016. Seattle, USA: IHME, University of Washington; 2016.

23. Hoy D, Protani M, De R, Buchbinder R. The epidemiology of neck pain. Best Pract Res Clin Rheumatol. 2010;24(6):783–92.

24. Hoy DG, Fransen M, March L, Brooks P, Durham J, Toole MJ. In rural Tibet, the prevalence of lower limb pain, especially knee pain, is high: an observational study. J Phys. 2010;56(1):49–54.

25. Hoy DG, Brooks P, Blyth F, Buchbinder R. The epidemiology of low back pain. Best Pract Res Clin Rheumatol. 2010;24(6):769–81.

26. Kessaram T, McKenzie J, Girin N, Roth A, Vivili P, Williams G, et al. Noncommunicable diseases and risk factors in adult populations of several Pacific Islands: results from the WHO STEPwise approach to surveillance. Aust N Z J Public Health. 2015;39(4):336–43.

27. Zheng H, Chen C. Body mass index and risk of knee osteoarthritis: systematic review and meta-analysis of prospective studies. BMJ Open. 2015 Dec 11;5(12):e007568.

28. Dai XQ, Liu M, Zhang TH, Yang XS, Li SL, Li XG, et al. Clinical predictors for diagnosing pandemic (H1N1) 2009 and seasonal influenza (H3N2) in fever clinics in Beijing, China. Biomed Environ Sci. 2012;25(1):61–8.

29. Christelle Lepers (personal communication). Secretariat of the Pacific Community. Noumea, New Caledonia. 2017.

30. Lozier MJ, Burke RM, Lopez J, Acevedo V, Amador M, Read JS, et al. Differences in prevalence of symptomatic Zika virus infection by age and sex-Puerto Rico, 2016. J Infect Dis. 2017;217(11):1678–89.

31. Hasan S, Jamdar SF, Alalowi M, Al Ageel Al Beaiji SM. Dengue virus: A global human threat: review of literature. J Int Soc Prev Community Dent. 2016;6(1):1–6.

32. Hoy D, Geere J-A, Davatchi F, Meggitt B, Barrero LH. A time for action: opportunities for preventing the growing burden and disability from musculoskeletal conditions in low-and middle-income countries. Best Pract Res Clin Rheumatol. 2014;28:377–93.

33. Briggs AM, Cross MJ, Hoy DG, Sanchez-Riera L, Blyth FM, Woolf AD, et al. Musculoskeletal health conditions represent a global threat to healthy aging: a report for the 2015 World Health Organization world report on ageing and health. The Gerontologist. 2016;56(Suppl 2):S243–55.

34. World Health Organization. Global Strategy and Action Plan for Ageing and Health. 2017; Available from: http://who.int/ageing/global-strategy/en/. Cited 28 Oct 2017

35. High Level Forum on Aid Effectiveness. Busan partnership for effective development co-operation. Busan, Republic of Korea; 2011.

36. High Level Forum on Aid Effectiveness. Accra agenda for action. Accra, Ghana; 2008.

37. High Level Forum on Aid Effectiveness. Paris declaration on aid effectiveness: ownership, harmonisation, alignment, results and mutual accountability. Joint Progress Towards Enhanced Aid Effectiveness. Paris; 2005.

4

Individuals with mild-to-moderate hip osteoarthritis have lower limb muscle strength and volume deficits

Aderson Loureiro[1,2,3], Maria Constantinou[1,4], Laura E. Diamond[1,5]* ⓘ, Belinda Beck[1] and Rod Barrett[1]

Abstract

Background: Individuals with advanced hip osteoarthritis (OA) exhibit generalized muscle weakness of the affected limb and so clinical practice guidelines recommend strength training for the management of hip OA. However, the extent and pattern of muscle weakness, including any between-limb asymmetries, in early stages of the disease are unclear. This study compared hip and knee muscle strength and volumes between individuals with mild-to-moderate symptomatic and radiographic hip OA and a healthy control group.

Methods: Nineteen individuals with mild-to-moderate symptomatic and radiographic hip OA ($n = 12$ unilateral; $n = 7$ bilateral) and 23 age-matched, healthy controls without radiographic hip OA or hip pain participated. Isometric strength of the hip and knee flexors and extensors, and hip abductors and adductors were measured. Hip and thigh muscle volumes were measured from lower limb magnetic resonance images. A full-factorial, two-way General Linear Model was used to assess differences between groups and between limbs.

Results: Participants in the hip OA group demonstrated significantly lower knee flexor, knee extensor, hip flexor, hip extensor and hip abductor strength compared to controls and had significantly lower volume of the adductor, hamstring and quadriceps groups, and gluteus maximus and gluteus minimus muscles, but not tensor fasciae latae or gluteus medius muscles. There were no between-limb strength differences or volume differences within either group.

Conclusions: Atrophic, bilateral hip and knee muscle weakness is a feature of individuals with mild-to-moderate hip OA. Early interventions to target muscle weakness and prevent the development of strength asymmetries that are characteristic of advanced hip OA appear warranted.

Keywords: Atrophy, Weakness, OA, MRI, Isometric

Background

People with hip osteoarthritis (OA) often experience joint pain, stiffness, reduced joint range of motion, and muscle weakness [1–4]. These deficits can limit performance of activities of daily living and diminish quality of life [5]. Hip OA has no cure, and progression to more advanced disease occurs in many patients. Conservative non-pharmacological interventions focus primarily on alleviating pain and improving function [6–11]. Individuals

with advanced hip OA exhibit generalized muscle weakness of the affected limb [12–19], which is underpinned by a combination of muscle atrophy [16, 18, 20–22], reduced muscle density [14, 21, 22], and muscle inhibition [22]. Clinical practice guidelines recommend land-based therapeutic exercise for the management of hip OA [23], most notably resistance training, which can reduce pain, stiffness and self-reported disability, and improve strength, physical function and joint range of motion [24, 25]. At present however, there is limited understanding of the extent and pattern of muscle weakness in earlier stages of the disease. If muscle weakness were also found to be a feature of mild-moderate hip OA, then interventions such as resistance training that target muscle weakness and prevent the development of strength asymmetries

* Correspondence: l.diamond@griffith.edu.au
[1]Menzies Health Institute Queensland, School of Allied Health Sciences, Griffith University, Gold Coast, QLD 4222, Australia
[5]Centre of Clinical Research Excellence in Spinal Pain, Injury & Health, School of Health & Rehabilitation Sciences, The University of Queensland, Brisbane, QLD, Australia
Full list of author information is available at the end of the article

characteristic of advanced hip OA [26] may be warranted in earlier stages of the disease.

Most investigations of muscle properties in hip OA have included individuals in advanced stages of the disease [14, 16, 18, 20–22]. Studies that included patients across the early spectrum of disease severity [12, 27] reported lower gluteal muscle volumes in individuals with unilateral hip OA compared to their contralateral side and a group of healthy controls. Deficits in hip abduction and internal rotation strength of the affected leg compared to healthy controls were also noted and suggest that muscle weakness could also be a feature of earlier stages of the disease than previously reported. It therefore remains unclear whether muscle weakness and atrophy that precede advanced stages of the disease extend beyond the abductor muscle group of the affected leg to other prime movers (i.e. quadriceps, hamstrings, adductors) within the most affected leg or the contralateral leg. Evidence of between-limb differences in hip and knee muscle strength and/or muscle volume have been reported in advanced hip OA [12, 22] and following total hip replacement [21]. While Grimaldi et al. [20, 28] reported an absence of asymmetry in the volume of the gluteal, piriformis, and tensor fascia latae muscles in mild hip OA, symmetry of other important hip and knee muscles is yet to be assessed. An improved understanding of whether muscle weakness and atrophy in mild-to-moderate hip OA is generalized or specific to certain muscles or muscle groups in the lower extremity is required to appropriately inform and optimise management programs.

The purpose of this study was to compare hip and knee muscle strength and volumes between individuals with mild-to-moderate symptomatic and radiographic hip OA and a healthy control group. Based on evidence from studies which report muscle weakness and atrophy in knee OA [29], it was hypothesized that individuals with mild-moderate hip OA would similarly exhibit muscle weakness and lower limb muscle atrophy, particularly in their (more) affected limb, compared to healthy age-matched controls.

Methods

Participants

Individuals aged 45 to 80 years with symptomatic unilateral or bilateral hip osteoarthritis were recruited from local hospital orthopaedic waiting lists to participate in this case-control study. Healthy controls were recruited through advertising and word-of-mouth. All participants were screened through radiographic examination (anterior-posterior radiographs of the pelvis and hips) and self-reported measures of pain and function (modified Harris Hip Score (HHS) [30]). Unilateral and bilateral hip OA participants were required to have hip pain and/or functional limitations during activities of daily living (HHS ≤ 95; 0 = extreme hip

problems, 100 = no hip problems) and had a Kellgren-Lawrence (KL) grade [31] for their affected hip(s) of 2 or 3 and/or joint space width (JSW) ≤ 3 mm). Unilateral hip OA participants had KL scores of 0 or 1 for their contralateral hip. Healthy controls were required to have no hip pain or functional limitations during activities of daily living (HHS > 95) and had KL grades ≤1 and JSW > 3 mm for both hips. KL scores were determined by a single radiologist in a blinded manner from bilateral weight-bearing radiographs performed in 15 degrees of femoral internal rotation [32]. The same radiologist electronically measured supero-medial, apical and supero-lateral hip JSW [33]. Exclusion criteria for both groups included: (i) previous lower limb or back fracture or surgery; (ii) history of trauma to the hip joint or pelvis region; (iii) other forms of arthritis, diabetes, cardiac or circulatory conditions; and (iv) use of corticosteroid medication. All individuals were able to walk without physical assistance or devices.

An a priori power analysis using hip abduction strength data from Zacharias et al. [27] (hip OA = 0.15(0.09); controls = 0.25(0.10)) estimated a minimum of 12 participants were required in each group (significance level was set at α= 0.05 and power at 0.80 (one tail)). Participants were enrolled concurrently in another study [34]. This study was approved by the institutional Human Research Ethics Committee and written informed consent was obtained from the participants prior to participating in the study.

Procedures

Participants initially attended a laboratory session to assess bilateral isometric strength of the lower extremity muscles. Anthropometric measures including height (m) and body mass (kg) were also taken. Body mass index (BMI) was determined as weight divided by the square of height (kg/m^2). Within 48 h of attending the strength testing session, participants underwent bilateral magnetic resonance imaging (MRI) of their lower extremity in a private radiologic clinic. This study conformed to the STROBE statement for reporting case-control studies [35].

Maximal voluntary isometric hip and knee muscle strength was measured using an isokinetic dynamometer (Biodex System 4, Biodex Medical Systems, USA) using a protocol adapted from Carty et al. [36]. Hip flexor, extensor, adductor and abductor strength were assessed while standing in 0° of hip flexion and adduction (neutral position), with the knee constrained in 60° of flexion using a post-surgical orthopaedic knee brace, and the ankle in 5° of plantar flexion. Participants were allowed to apply a light force against the dynamometer head for the purpose of maintaining balance. Knee flexor and extensor strength tests were performed while seated. Knee flexor strength was assessed at 30° of knee flexion with the hip in 90° of flexion and the ankle in 5° of plantar flexion. Knee extensor strength was assessed at 60° of knee flexion with the hip in 70° of flexion and the ankle in 5° of plantar flexion. The order of strength measurements was from hip to knee randomized by limb. Participants performed a 5-s practice trial at 75% of maximal effort for each exercise, followed by a 60-s rest and a 5-s maximal contraction. Prior to each maximal effort trial, participants were instructed to contract as hard as they could for 5-s, with verbal encouragement provided to help maximize effort. The instantaneous peak isometric torque for each exercise was adjusted to account for the torque due to the dynamometer attachment and lower limb segments distal to the joint being tested in accordance with the recommendations of Kellis and Baltzopoulos [37], using body segment parameters estimated from Dempster [38]. Isometric strength at each joint, in each direction, was defined as the peak torque measured normalized to body mass (Nm/kg).

A 3.0 T MRI whole body scanner (Phillips Ingenia, Phillips Medical, Netherlands), was used to image bilateral lower limbs of all participants. Axial plane scans were performed with participants positioned supine in the scanner using body coil arrays placed superiorly on the limbs with contiguous slices taken from approximately 2-cm superior to the iliac crest to approximately 2-cm inferior to the proximal tibio-fibula joint. Both lower limbs were scanned simultaneously with T1 weighted 2-dimensional gradient-recall acquisition in the steady state; slice thickness 10-mm, inter-slice gap 1-mm, flip angle 90^0; repetition time 677 msec, echo time 6.5 msec; field of view $280 \times 500 \times 219$ mm; 352×499-pixel matrix; acquisition time 1 min 29 s. Volumes of individual muscles (tensor fasciae latae (TFL), gluteus maximus (GMax), gluteus medius (GMed), gluteus minimus (GMin)) and muscle groups (adductors (i.e. magnus, gracilis, brevis, and longus) (Add), quadriceps (i.e. vastus medialis, vastus intermedius, vastus lateralis, rectus femoris) (Quad), hamstrings (i.e. semimembranosus, semitendinosus, biceps femoris) (Hams)) were then calculated using Mimics software (Materialise N.V., Belgium). The ilopsoas muscle was not assessed as it was only partially visible in the MRI scans obtained. Muscles were segmented on a slice-by-slice basis by a single reader (AL) using the semi-automated lasso tool (Fig. 1a). These data were then combined to create the final 3-dimensional (3D) rendering. The 3D-volume object was wrapped using finest detail of 0.50 mm and a gap closing distance of 1.00 mm, followed by a smoothing process with a factor of 1.0 and 4 iterations. Finally, the muscle volumes were determined by summing all pertinent pixels within the resultant binary volume (Fig. 1b-c). Individual and group muscle volumes were normalized to body mass (cm^3/kg). Reliability of muscle segmentation was assessed following the approach described by Grimaldi et al. [20]. In brief this involved the same investigator (AL) segmenting the same image slices from all muscles for a single randomly selected participant on 2 occasions, approximately 2 weeks apart. Intra-rater reliability, as assessed using the intra-class correlation coefficient (ICC) was high, with ICCs for all muscles in excess of 0.985.

Statistical analysis

Shapiro-Wilk tests were used to examine data normality. Demographic and clinical variables were compared between groups using independent t-tests or Pearson's chi-square. A full-factorial, two-way General Linear Model was used to assess the effect of a between subject factor (Group) and a within subject factor (Leg) on muscle strength and volume. A priori contrasts were used to assess differences between limbs within each group. Leg was defined as affected/contralateral for participants with unilateral OA and most affected (on the basis of symptoms)/less affected for participants with bilateral OA. The test limb was randomly selected (left/right) for control participants. Effect sizes for main group effects were computed using Cohen's d. Statistical analyses were performed using SPSS version 17.0 for Windows (SPSS Inc., Chicago, USA) with significance level set at $p < 0.05$.

Results

There were no differences in age, height, or body mass between the hip OA and control groups. On average, participants in the hip OA group had a higher BMI than participants in the control group ($p < 0.01$) (Table 1).

Lower limb strength

No group by leg interaction effects were detected for any measure of lower-limb strength. A significant main effect of group was detected for knee flexor, knee extensor, hip flexor, hip extensor, hip abductor strength (Table 2 and Fig. 2a), but not hip adductor strength. No significant strength differences were detected between legs within each group.

Hip and knee muscle volume

No group by leg interaction effects were detected for any measure of hip or knee muscle volume. A significant main effect of group was detected for GMax, GMin, Add, Hams, and Quad volume (Table 2 and Fig. 2b), but not TFL and GMed. No significant volume differences were detected between legs within each group.

Discussion

This study compared bilateral isometric hip and knee muscle strength and hip and knee muscle volume between individuals with symptomatic and radiographic mild-to-moderate hip OA and healthy controls. Consistent with our hypothesis, individuals with hip OA tended to be weaker and have less muscle volume than those in

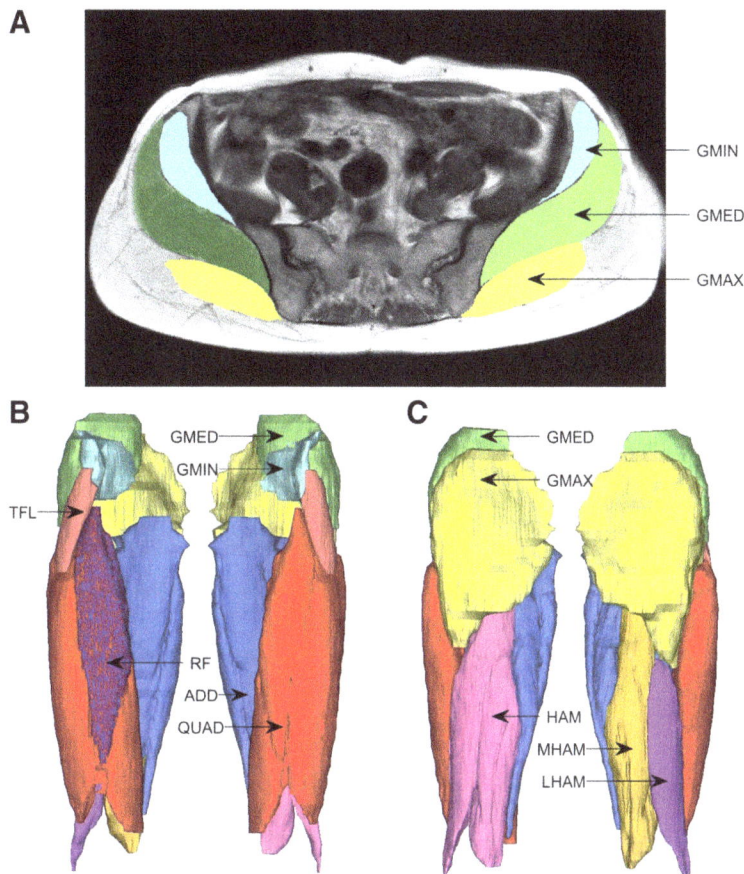

Fig. 1 Muscle and muscle group segmentation from magnetic resonance images of a representative healthy control participant; **a** superior view of muscle masks segmented from an individual transverse plane slice; **b-c** anterior and posterior views, respectively, of 3D rendering of thigh and hip muscles (GMIN-gluteus minimus; GMED-gluteus medius; GMAX-gluteus maximus; TFL-tensor fasciae latae; ADD-adductors; QUAD-quadriceps; HAM-hamstrings)

Table 1 Participant characteristics of hip osteoarthritis and control groups

Characteristic	Unilateral hip OA $n = 12$		Bilateral hip OA $n = 7$		Hip OA $n = 19$		Control $n = 23$	
Age (years)	62.9 ± 10.0		63.0 ± 6.4		62.8 ± 8.6		58.2 ± 8.6	
Males, n (%)	3 (25%)		3 (42%)		6 (32%)		8 (35%)	
Height (m)	1.65 ± 0.09		1.69 ± 0.14		1.66 ± 0.10		1.69 ± 0.08	
Body mass (kg)	77.3 ± 14.0		77.2 ± 15.0		77.2 ± 14.0		69.9 ± 10.0	
Body mass index (kg/m^2)	28.2 ± 3.5		27.1 ± 3.5		27.8 ± 3.5[*]		24.4 ± 3.0	
Harris Hip Score (HHS)[ab]	69.9 ± 12.9		66.2 ± 13.5		68.6 ± 12.9		99.9 ± 0.7	
	Affected	*Contralateral*	*Most affected*	*Less affected*	*(Most) affected*	*Contralateral/Less affected*	*Left*	*Right*
Joint space width (mm)	2.3 ± 1.1	3.5 ± 0.7	2.9 ± 0.5	3.0 ± 0.5	2.5 ± 1.0[*]	3.3 ± 0.7[*]	4.0 ± 0.5	3.9 ± 0.6
Kellgren-Lawrence grade	2, $n = 4$ 3, $n = 8$	0, $n = 4$ 1, $n = 8$	2, $n = 4$ 3, $n = 3$	2, $n = 5$ 3, $n = 2$	2, $n = 8$ 3, $n = 11$	0, $n = 4$ 1, $n = 8$ 2, $n = 5$ 3, $n = 2$	0, $n = 12$ 1, $n = 11$	0, $n = 18$ 1, $n = 5$

Values are mean (standard deviation) unless otherwise stated

OA osteoarthritis

[*]$p < 0.05$ hip OA compared to control group

[a]HHS scale – 0 = extreme hip problems and 100 = no hip problems; [b]Most symptomatic hip for participants with bilateral hip osteoarthritis and randomly assigned hip for control participants; Kellgren-Lawrence grading scale – 0 = no radiographic features of hip osteoarthritis and 4 = large osteophytes

Table 2 Summary statistics for the effect of group (hip osteoarthritis versus control) on muscle strength and volume measures

	Hip OA (mean ± SD)	Control (mean ± SD)	F, p	Mean difference (mean ± SD)	95% CI of mean difference	Effect size
Strength (Nm/kg)						
Knee flexors	0.977 ± 0.292	1.255 ± 0.281	9.579, 0.004*	0.278 ± 0.392	0.096, 0.460	0.71
Knee extensors	1.286 ± 0.344	1.664 ± 0.328	12.450, 0.001*	0.378 ± 0.462	0.164, 0.593	0.82
Hip flexors	0.898 ± 0.331	1.216 ± 0.314	9.866, 0.003*	0.319 ± 0.440	0.113, 0.524	0.73
Hip extensors	0.908 ± 0.292	1.216 ± 0.281	11.652, 0.02*	0.307 ± 0.392	0.125, 0.490	0.78
Hip abductors	0.662 ± 0.209	0.905 ± 202	14.34, 0.001*	0.244 ± 0.279	0.113, 0.374	0.87
Hip adductors	0.639 ± 0.323	0.834 ± 0.314	3.794, 0.06	0.194 ± 0.436	−0.008, 0.397	0.44
Volume (cm³/kg)						
TFL	0.909 ± 0.324	0.816 ± 0.300	0.986, 0.327	0.094 ± 0.410	−0.285, 0.098	0.23
GMax	9.560 ± 2.336	11.119 ± 2.153	5.268, 0.028*	1.558 ± 2.995	0.182, 2.934	0.52
GMed	4.031 ± 0.722	4.241 ± 0.666	1.001, 0.324	0.209 ± 0.911	−0.216, 0.634	0.23
GMin	1.006 ± 0.380	1.525 ± 0.352	22.048, < 0.001*	0.520 ± 0.484	0.295, 0.744	1.07
Add	10.827 ± 2.111	12.489 ± 1.947	7.380, 0.01*	1.662 ± 2.668	0.420, 2.940	0.62
Hams	7.444 ± 1.548	9.117 ± 1.426	13.899, 0.001*	1.673 ± 1.957	0.762, 2.583	0.85
Quad	16.114 ± 4.512	20.769 ± 4.160	12.666, 0.001*	4.655 ± 5.701	2.001, 7.311	0.82

Add adductors, *CI* confidence interval, *Hams* hamstrings, *GMax* gluteus maximus, *GMed* gluteus medius, *GMin* gluteus minimus, *OA* osteoarthritis, *Quad* quadriceps, *TFL* tensor fasciae latae
*Significant difference between groups ($p < 0.05$)

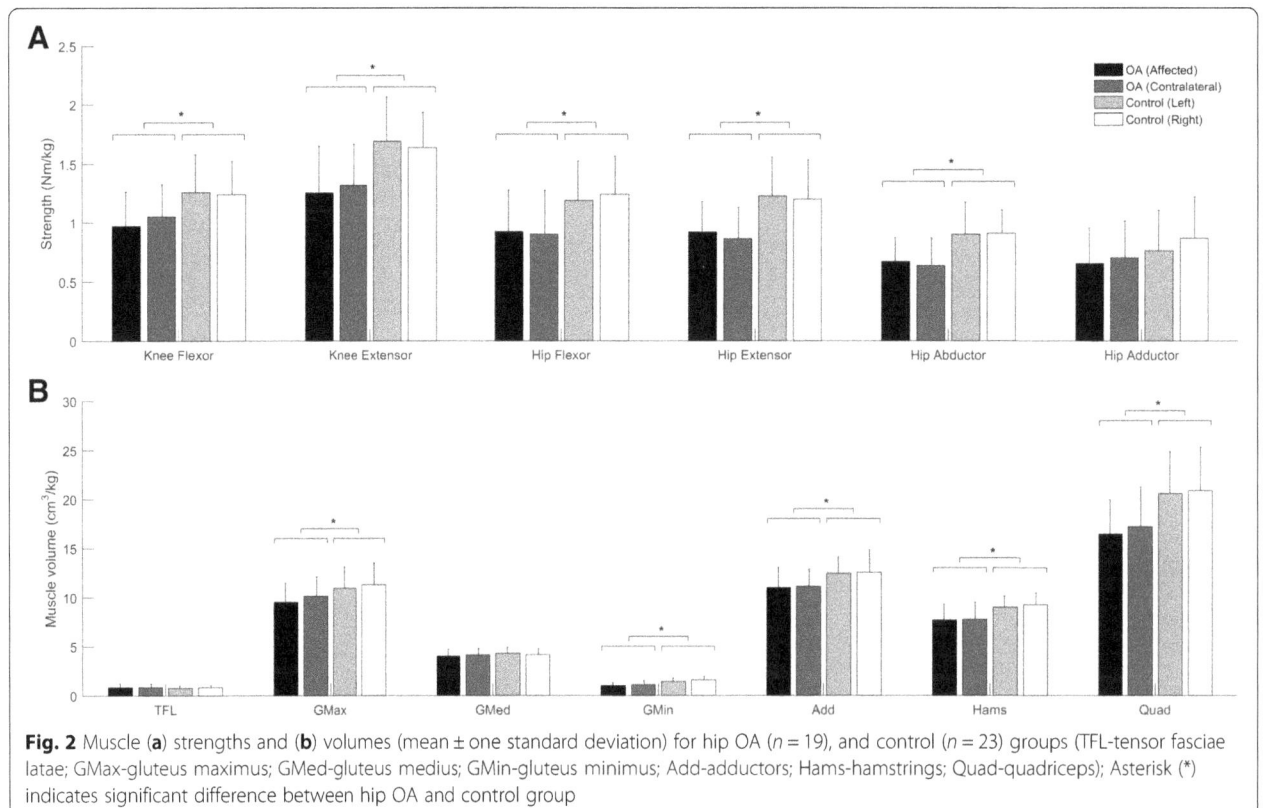

Fig. 2 Muscle (**a**) strengths and (**b**) volumes (mean ± one standard deviation) for hip OA ($n = 19$), and control ($n = 23$) groups (TFL-tensor fasciae latae; GMax-gluteus maximus; GMed-gluteus medius; GMin-gluteus minimus; Add-adductors; Hams-hamstrings; Quad-quadriceps); Asterisk (*) indicates significant difference between hip OA and control group

the healthy control group. Defics in strength were detected for the hip flexors, extensors and abductors, and the knee flexors and extensors, but not the hip adductors. Smaller muscle volumes were detected for gluteus maximus, gluteus minimus, and the adductor, hamstring and quadricep muscle groups, but not for tensor fascia latae or gluteus medius. Previous research has demonstrated generalized lower limb muscle weakness and atrophy in advanced stages of hip OA [26], and in the hip abductors in earlier stages of the disease [27]. The main and novel finding of the present study was that pervasive deficits in lower limb muscle strength and size are also present in mild-to-moderate stages of the disease process. In contrast to our hypothesis, no between-limb differences in muscle strength or volume were found in our mild-to-moderate hip OA group. Between-limb asymmetries in muscle strength and volume instead appear to primarily be a feature of advanced stage hip OA [26].

Muscle strength and volume in individuals with mild-to-moderate hip OA

Individuals with hip OA exhibited strength deficits in the hip and knee flexors and extensors and hip abductors relative to control participants. Hip and knee muscle strength in the directions assessed was on average 22–26% lower than the control group. In general, the strength deficits in the hip OA group fall within the range reported (13–37%) in previous investigations of hip muscle strength in hip OA [12, 39]. Only hip adduction strength was not significantly lower in the hip OA group, but approached significance ($p = 0.06$) with an effect size of 0.44, which may be clinically meaningful. We therefore interpret these findings to indicate that muscle weakness in the most affected limb in mild-to-moderate hip OA tends to be generalized rather than specific to individual muscles or muscle groups and that the magnitude of weakness is similar between mild-to-moderate and advanced hip OA. The underlying cause of muscle weakness in hip OA remains unclear but could arise from decreased physical activity and/or unloading of the lower extremity during physical activity [34], perhaps driven by some combination of pain and motor dysfunction. Unresolved questions that will require further investigation concern whether muscle weakness precedes or follows the onset of hip OA, and whether weakness is a contributing cause or consequence of hip OA.

Hip and knee muscle volumes were on average 5–30% lower in individuals with hip OA across all muscle groups and individual muscles assessed, with the exception of tensor fascia latae and gluteus medius. The smaller muscle volumes in individuals with mild-to-moderate hip OA likely underpin their generalized deficits in hip and knee muscle strength, and coincide with reports of advanced

hip OA [26]. In general, there was a correspondence in the amount of weakness detected at the joint level, and the atrophy of muscles that contributed to the measured strength. For example, the 22–26% lower strength of the knee flexors and extensors in the hip OA group, corresponded with 18–22% reductions in muscle volume of the hamstrings and quadriceps respectively, and suggest that muscle atrophy in hip OA is a major mechanism of underlying muscle weakness in these muscles. Our findings of lower gluteal (maximus and minimus) muscle volumes in individuals with hip OA compared to healthy controls are consistent with Zacharias et al. [27]. Further, our observations are broadly consistent with findings from a systematic review of muscle strength and size in hip OA relative to controls [26], which suggest that advanced unilateral hip OA is characterized by generalized muscle weakness and atrophy of muscles in the affected limb. Although gluteus medius had a 5% lower volume in the hip OA group, this mean group difference was not statistically significant. The tensor fascia latae muscle volume was similarly not significantly different between groups. The absence of group differences in muscle volume for these muscles could be explained by possible group differences in hip abductor muscle activation capacity, force sharing between synergistic abductor muscles and muscle quality. A further possibility is that some muscles may compensate for reduction in strength of synergistic muscles as has been observed in individuals with knee muscle pathology following anterior cruciate ligament reconstruction [40]. Indeed Grimaldi et al. [20] reported larger volumes for gluteus medius compared to healthy controls in early stages of hip pathology compared to atrophy in later stages.

Muscle strength and volume in the affected and less-affected/contralateral limbs of individuals with mild-to-moderate hip OA

Lower muscle strength and volume did not differ significantly between-limbs in individuals with hip OA. Although 12 of 19 (63%) of our cohort had unilateral hip OA (between-limb KL grade difference ≥1), it is possible that the inclusion of 7 bilateral participants prevented asymmetries from being detected. However, a post hoc analysis of the unilateral hip OA sub-group did not reveal any clear trends to support strength or volume asymmetry (data not presented). Grimaldi et al. [20], who evaluated gluteal muscle size in individuals with mild and advanced unilateral hip OA, similarly observed no difference in muscle size between the affected and contralateral limb in the mild hip OA group. However, our observations contradict those of Zacharias et al. [27], who reported lower gluteal muscle volumes in individuals with moderate unilateral hip OA (KL grade 2: $n = 7$; KL grade 3: $n = 13$) compared to their contralateral side. When participants from Zacharias et al.

[27] were dichotomized based on OA severity, only those with KL grade = 3 demonstrated atrophy in the gluteal muscles. Our cohort was comprised of 42% of individuals with KL grade = 2, which in light of the findings of Zacharias et al. [27], may suggest that muscle related asymmetry becomes more prominent with disease progression. A possible explanation for the lack of difference is muscle strength between limbs in hip OA is that rather than favouring the contralateral limb during the performance of functional tasks, individuals with mild-to-moderate hip OA unload both limbs through a reduction in overall physical activity.

Reduced muscle strength and volumes in the affected compared to contralateral limb are well documented in individuals with end-stage hip OA [14, 16, 18, 20–22]. In general, it is difficult to compare the findings from the present study to those from the literature due to differences in participant characteristics (single versus mixed sex, pre- versus post-total hip replacement), strength measurements (e.g. isometric versus isokinetic), and muscles assessed. However, findings from Zacharias et al. [27] and Grimaldi et al. [20], where a subset of lower limb muscle strength and/or muscle volumes were measured in participants with hip OA from across the disease spectrum using a consistent approach, suggest that asymmetries in strength and volume become more pronounced with disease progression. Interventions to retain bilateral muscle strength during early-middle stages of the disease therefore appear warranted in the management of hip OA. This recommendation is consistent with the evidence-based clinical practice guidelines for therapeutic exercise in the management of hip OA which recommend land-based therapeutic exercise, most notably strength training, to reduce pain, stiffness and self-reported disability, and improve physical function and range of motion [41].

Strengths and limitations
A strength of this study was that eligibility was based on radiographic and symptomatic criteria, which minimized the well-known risk of participant misclassification [42]. There were also several limitations to the study. First, the study was not sufficiently powered to perform a sub-group analysis of unilateral and bilateral participants. A future study with a larger sample size is required to more definitively determine whether strength and muscle volume asymmetry is evident within these hip OA sub-groups. More females were recruited to the hip OA and control groups than males (hip OA: 13 female, 6 male; control: 15 female, 8 male), which may be a source of experimental bias. While the hip OA group in our study had a significantly higher BMI than controls, strength and volume measures were normalised to body mass. We chose this method as it is common and therefore

facilitates comparison of findings with other studies that have used the same approach and it also has physical meaning. Strength was assessed in the present study under isometric conditions, which may not reflect muscle function during dynamic conditions including activities of daily living. It was not possible to segment boundaries for some smaller muscles (e.g. internal/external hip rotators) or muscles with insertions outside the imaged segments (e.g. iliopsoas), and thus only large hip/knee spanning muscles and muscle groups were evaluated. Further, reliability of muscle segmentation from MRI scans was established using data from a single participant. It is important for future studies to more fully elucidate the implications of reduced muscle strength and volume in mild-to-moderate hip OA for motor function and disease progression. Multiple statistical comparisons were made in the present study, which has the potential to increase the risk of type 1 error. A statistical correction was not performed due of the exploratory nature of this study [43, 44]. It is noteworthy that the hip OA cohort from the present study also exhibited reduced self-selected walking speed and altered hip joint mechanics, including lower net hip joint loading over a reduced range of hip motion for a longer proportion of the gait cycle, when walking at their preferred gait speed relative to healthy control participants [34]. These findings are consistent with an underloading hypothesis for hip OA progression, perhaps due in part to muscle weakness, which could have implications for disease progression through altered mechano-biological processes within the joint [45].

Conclusions
The main conclusion from this study is that atrophic hip and knee muscle weakness is a distinct feature of mild-to-moderate hip OA. These strength and muscle size deficits tended to be generalized rather than localised to individual muscles and/or muscle groups in the lower limb, and have possible implications for daily function, quality of life and OA disease progression. While no evidence of between-limb asymmetry in muscle strength or volume was found in the present study, intervention early in the disease process to prevent the development of strength asymmetries that are characteristic of advanced hip OA appear warranted.

Abbreviations
Add: Adductors; GMax: Gluteus maximus; GMed: Gluteus medius; GMin: Gluteus minimus; Hams: Hamstrings; HHS: Harris hip score; ICC: Intraclass correlation coefficient; JSW: Joint space width; KL: Kellgren-Lawrence; MRI: Magnetic resonance imaging; OA: Osteoarthritis; Quad: Quadricpes; TFL: Tensor fasciae latae

Acknowledgements
The authors wish to thank Dr. Gary Shepherd (Qscan Radiology Clinics), Dr. Peter Mills, and the participants for support with the project.

Funding
Funding was provided by a Griffith University Area of Strategic Investment Grant in Chronic Disease Prevention for participant anterior-posterior radiographs of the pelvis and hips. AL received a Griffith University Postgraduate Research Scholarship and a Griffith University International Postgraduate Research Scholarship.

Authors' contributions
AL, MC, BB and RB conceived the design of this study. AL and MC acquired the data. LD, AL, RB carried out the analysis and interpretation of the data. LD, AL and RB drafted the article. All authors revised the manuscript for intellectual content and approved the final version.

Competing interests
Laura Diamond is an editorial board member for BMC Musculoskeletal Disorders. The other authors declare that they have no competing interests.

Author details
[1]Menzies Health Institute Queensland, School of Allied Health Sciences, Griffith University, Gold Coast, QLD 4222, Australia. [2]Pontifical Catholic University (PUCRS), Porto Alegre, Brazil. [3]University of Rio dos Sinos (UNISINOS), São Leopoldo, Brazil. [4]Australian Catholic University, Brisbane, QLD 4014, Australia. [5]Centre of Clinical Research Excellence in Spinal Pain, Injury & Health, School of Health & Rehabilitation Sciences, The University of Queensland, Brisbane, QLD, Australia.

References
1. DiBonaventura M, Gupta S, McDonald M, Sadosky A. Evaluating the health and economic impact of osteoarthritis pain in the workforce: results from the National Health and wellness survey. BMC Musculoskelet Disord. 2011;12:83.
2. Lane NE. Osteoarthritis of the hip. N Engl J Med. 2007;357:1413–21.
3. Eitzen I, Fernandes L, Kallerud H, Nordsletten L, Knarr B, Risberg MA. Gait characteristics, symptoms, and function in persons with hip osteoarthritis: a longitudinal study with 6 to 7 years of follow-up. J Orthop Sports Phys Ther. 2015;45:539–49.
4. Constantinou M, Barrett R, Brown M, Mills P. Spatial-temporal gait characteristics in individuals with hip osteoarthritis: a systematic literature review and meta-analysis. J Orthop Sports Phys Ther. 2014;44:291–7.
5. Castaño-Betancourt MC, Rivadeneira F, Bierma-Zeinstra S, Kerkhof HJM, Hofman A, Uitterlinden AG, Van Meurs JBJ. Bone parameters across different types of hip osteoarthritis and their relationship to osteoporotic fracture risk. Arthritis Rheum. 2013;65:693–700.
6. Arnold CM, Faulkner RA. The effect of aquatic exercise and education on lowering fall risk in older adults with hip osteoarthritis. J Aging Phys Act. 2010;18:245–60.
7. Bennell KL, Hinman R. Exercise as a treatment for osteoarthritis. Curr Opin Rheumatol. 2005;17:634–40.
8. Lane NE, Buckwalter JA. Exercise and osteoarthritis. Curr Opin Rheumatol. 1999;11:413–6.
9. McNair PJ, Simmonds MA, Boocock MG, Larmer PJ. Exercise therapy for the management of osteoarthritis of the hip joint: a systematic review. Arthritis Res Ther. 2009;11:1–9.
10. Puett DW, Griffin MR. Published trials of nonmedicinal and noninvasive therapies for hip and knee osteoarthritis. Ann Intern Med. 1994;121:133–40.
11. Tilden HM, Reicherter AE, Reicherter F. Use of an aquatics program for older adults with osteoarthritis from clinic to the community. Top Geriatr Rehabil. 2010;26:128–39.
12. Arokoski MH, Arokoski JP, Haara M, Kankaanpaa M, Vesterinen M, Niemitukia LH, Helminen HJ. Hip muscle strength and muscle cross sectional area in men with and without hip osteoarthritis. J Rheumatol. 2002;29:2185–95.
13. Madsen OR, Brot C, Petersen MM, Sorensen OH. Body composition and muscle strength in women scheduled for a knee or hip replacement. A comparative study of two groups of osteoarthritic women. J Clin Rheumatol. 1997;16:39–44.
14. Rasch A, Bystrom AH, Dalen N, Berg HE. Reduced muscle radiological density, cross-sectional area, and strength of major hip and knee muscles in 22 patients with hip osteoarthritis. Acta Orthop. 2007;78:505–10.
15. Rasch A, Dalen N, Berg HE. Muscle strength, gait, and balance in 20 patients with hip osteoarthritis followed for 2 years after THA. Acta Orthop. 2010;81:183–8.
16. Reardon K, Galea M, Dennett X, Choong P, Byrne E. Quadriceps muscle wasting persists 5 months after total hip arthroplasty for osteoarthritis of the hip: a pilot study. Intern Med J. 2001;31:7–14.
17. Rossi MD, Brown LE, Whitehurst MA. Assessment of hip extensor and flexor strength two months after unilateral total hip arthroplasty. J Strength Cond Res. 2006;20:262–7.
18. Suetta C, Aagaard P, Rosted A, Jakobsen AK, Duus B, Kjaer M, Magnusson SP. Training-induced changes in muscle CSA, muscle strength, EMG, and rate of force development in elderly subjects after long-term unilateral disuse. J Appl Physiol. 2004;97:1954–61.
19. Suetta C, Andersen JL, Dalgas U, Berget J, Koskinen S, Aagaard P, Magnusson SP, Kjaer M. Resistance training induces qualitative changes in muscle morphology, muscle architecture, and muscle function in elderly postoperative patients. J Appl Physiol. 2008;105:180–6.
20. Grimaldi A, Richardson C, Durbridge G, Donnelly W, Darnell R, Hides J. The association between degenerative hip joint pathology and size of the gluteus maximus and tensor fascia lata muscles. Man Ther. 2009;14:611–7.
21. Rasch A, Bystrom AH, Dalen N, Martinez-Carranza N, Berg HE. Persisting muscle atrophy two years after replacement of the hip. J Bone Joint Surg. 2009;91:583–8.
22. Suetta C, Aagaard P, Magnusson SP, Andersen LL, Sipila S, Rosted A, Jakobsen AK, Duus B, Kjaer M. Muscle size, neuromuscular activation, and rapid force characteristics in elderly men and women: effects of unilateral long-term disuse due to hip-osteoarthritis. J Appl Physiol. 2007;102:942–8.
23. Zhang W, Nuki G, Moskowitz RW, Abramson S, Altman RD, Arden NK, Bierma-Zeinstra S, Brandt KD, Croft P, Doherty M, et al. OARSI recommendations for the management of hip and knee osteoarthritis: part III: changes in evidence following systematic cumulative update of research published through January 2009. Osteoarthr Cartil. 2010;18:476–99.
24. Svege I, Fernandes L, Nordsletten L, Holm I, Risberg MA. Long-term effect of exercise therapy and patient education on impairments and activity limitations in people with hip osteoarthritis: secondary outcome analysis of a randomized clinical trial. Phys Ther. 2016;96:818–27.
25. French HP, Cusack T, Brennan A, Caffrey A, Conroy R, Cuddy V, FitzGerald OM, Fitzpatrick M, Gilsenan C, Kane D, et al. Exercise and manual physiotherapy arthritis research trial (EMPART) for osteoarthritis of the hip: a multicenter randomized controlled trial. Arch Phys Med Rehabil. 2013;94:302–14.
26. Loureiro A, Mills PM, Barrett RS. Muscle weakness in hip osteoarthritis: a systematic review. Arthritis Care Res. 2013;65:340–52.
27. Zacharias A, Pizzari T, English DJ, Kapakoulakis T, Green RA. Hip abductor muscle volume in hip osteoarthritis and matched controls. Osteoarthr Cartil. 2016;24:1727–35.
28. Grimaldi A, Richardson C, Stanton W, Durbridge G, Donnelly W, Hides J. The association between degenerative hip joint pathology and size of the gluteus medius, gluteus minimus and piriformis muscles. Man Ther. 2009;14:605–10.
29. Roos EM, Herzog W, Block JA, Bennell KL. Muscle weakness, afferent sensory dysfunction and exercise in knee osteoarthritis. Nat Rev Rheumatol. 2011;7:57–63.
30. Mahomed NN, Arndt DC, McGrory BJ, Harris WH. The Harris hip score: comparison of patient self-report with surgeon assessment. J Arthroplast. 2001;16:575–80.
31. Kellgren JH, Lawrence JS. Radiological assessment of rheumatoid arthritis. Ann Rheum Dis. 1957;16:485–93.
32. Auleley GR, Giraudeau B, Dougados M, Ravaud P. Radiographic assessment of hip osteoarthritis progression: impact of reading procedures for longitudinal studies. Ann Rheum Dis. 2000;59:422–7.
33. Altman RD, Gold GE. Atlas of individual radiographic features in osteoarthritis, revised. Osteoarthr Cartil. 2007;15(Suppl A):A1–56.
34. Constantinou M, Loureiro A, Carty C, Mills P, Barrett R. Hip joint mechanics during walking in individuals with mild-to-moderate hip osteoarthritis. Gait Posture. 2017;53:162–7.
35. Von Elm E, Altman DG, Egger M, Pocock SJ, Gøtzsche PC, Vandenbroucke JP. The strengthening the reporting of observational studies in epidemiology (STROBE) statement: guidelines for reporting observational studies. Prev Med. 2007;45:247–51.

36. Carty CP, Barrett RS, Cronin NJ, Lichtwark GA, Mills PM. Lower limb muscle weakness predicts use of a multiple- versus single-step strategy to recover from forward loss of balance in older adults. J Gerontol A Biol Sci Med Sci. 2012;67:1246–52.

37. Kellis E, Baltzopoulos V. Gravitational moment correction in isokinetic dynamometry using anthropometric data. Med Sci Sports Exerc. 1996; 28:900–7.

38. Dempster WT. Space requirements of the seated operator: geometrical, kinematic, and mechanical aspects of the body, with special reference to the limbs. 1955.

39. Klausmeier V, Lugade V, Jewett BA, Collis DK, Chou LS. Is there faster recovery with an anterior or anterolateral THA? A pilot study. Clin Orthop Relat Res. 2010;468:533–41.

40. Konrath JM, Vertullo CJ, Kennedy BA, Bush HS, Barrett RS, Lloyd DG. Morphologic characteristics and strength of the hamstring muscles remain altered at 2 years after use of a hamstring tendon graft in anterior cruciate ligament reconstruction. Am J Sports Med. 2016;44:2589–98.

41. Brosseau L, Wells GA, Pugh AG, Smith CAM, Rahman P, Gallardo ICA, Toupin-April K, Loew L, De Angelis G, Cavallo S. Ottawa panel evidence-based clinical practice guidelines for therapeutic exercise in the management of hip osteoarthritis. Clin Rehabil. 2016;30:935–46.

42. Kim C, Linsenmeyer KD, Vlad SC, Guermazi A, Clancy MM, Niu J, Felson DT. Prevalence of radiographic and symptomatic hip osteoarthritis in an urban United States community: the Framingham osteoarthritis study. Arthritis Rheumatol. 2014;66:3013–7.

43. Bender R, Lange S. Adjusting for multiple testing--when and how? J Clin Epidemiol. 2001;54:343–9.

44. Perneger TV. What's wrong with Bonferroni adjustments. BMJ. 1998;316: 1236–8.

45. Saxby DJ, Lloyd DG. Osteoarthritis year in review 2016: mechanics. Osteoarthr Cartil. 2017;25:190–8.

5

A new acute scaphoid fracture assessment method: a reliability study of the 'long axis' measurement

Benjamin J. F. Dean[1,2]* , Nicholas D. Riley[2], Earl Robert McCulloch[2], Jennifer C. E. Lane[1,2], Amy Beth Touzell[3] and Alastair J. Graham[4]

Abstract

Background: The aim of this study was to assess the inter observer and intra observer reliability of acute scaphoid fracture classification methods including a novel 'long axis' measurement, a simple method which we have developed with the aim of improving agreement when describing acute fractures.

Methods: We identified sixty patients with acute scaphoid fractures at two centres who had been investigated with both plain radiographs and a CT (Computed Tomography) scan within 4 weeks of injury. The fractures were assessed by three observers at each centre using three commonly used classification systems and the 'long axis' method.

Results: Inter observer reliability: based on X-rays the 'long axis' measurement demonstrated substantial agreement (Intraclass Correlation Coefficient (ICC) =0.76) and was significantly more reliable than the Mayo ($p < 0.01$), the most reliable of the established classification systems with moderate levels of agreement (kappa = 0.56). Intra observer reliability: the long axis measurement demonstrated almost perfect agreement whether based on X-ray (ICC = 0.905) or CT (ICC = 0.900).

Conclusions: This study describes a novel pragmatic 'long axis' method for the assessment of acute scaphoid fractures which demonstrates substantial inter and intra observer reliability. The 'long axis' measurement has clear potential benefits over traditional classification systems which should be explored in future clinical research.

Keywords: Scaphoid, Fracture, Classification, Acute, Non-union

Background

Scaphoid fractures represent around 2–3% of all fractures and around 10% of all fractures in the hand, while the younger population is more typically affected although fractures do occur in the elderly [1]. Fractures of the mid-portion of the scaphoid, the so-called 'waist', are the most common [1]. The existing evidence suggests that the risk non-union is considerably higher for more proximal fractures [2]. Despite large numbers of publications on outcomes of scaphoid fracture management there are large inconsistencies in the published data. Combining these data groups is notoriously difficult for a number of reasons including variable demographics, inconsistent definitions of fracture type, and inconsistent methodology for defining outcome. There is particular interest in the behaviour of proximal pole fractures but no consensus on how this subgroup should be defined. This method could be used to give more reliable and reproducible descriptions of fracture type.

A number of classification systems have been described, with the most widely used being the Herbert, Russe and Mayo methods. However the reliability of these tools has been shown to be rather limited [3]. Despite the frequently-discussed distinction between proximal pole and waist fractures, there is no published reliable method of distinguishing between the two. The Mayo classification system divides the scaphoid into proximal, middle and

* Correspondence: bendean1979@gmail.com
[1]Nuffield Department of Orthopaedics, Rheumatology and Musculoskeletal Sciences (NDORMS), University of Oxford, Botnar Research Centre, Windmill road, Oxford OX3 7LD, UK
[2]Nuffield Orthopaedic Centre, Windmill road, Oxford OX3 7LD, UK
Full list of author information is available at the end of the article

distal third fractures, as well as distal tubercle and distal intra-articular fractures. Russe divided fractures into those with horizontal oblique, transverse or vertical oblique fracture lines [4]. The Herbert system divides acute fractures into either stable (Type A) and unstable (Type B), with various subdivisions with these types [5]. No study has described a method for determining precisely the location or the size of the proximal pole. For example the SWIFFT study protocol defines a proximal pole fracture as involving the 'proximal fifth' but does not describe how one can reliably determine when a fracture involves the proximal fifth [6]. This makes it difficult to compare studies and particularly difficult to perform meta-analysis on data from published cohorts. While the anatomical and radiological definition of proximal pole, waist and distal pole fractures is likely to remain contentious, looking at a more continuous measure of fracture site may give more clarity.

The primary aim of this study was to assess the reliability of acute scaphoid fracture assessment metrics including the new 'long axis' measurement. The secondary aims were to compare the reliability of this new method with three established classification systems, and to compare the reliability of each of these methods when using plain radiographs and CT. The null hypothesis was that there would be no difference in reliability between the older methods and the new 'long axis' measurement.

Methods

Using local surgical databases we retrospectively identified sixty patients with acute scaphoid fractures across two centres that had been investigated with both plain radiographs and a CT scan within 4 weeks of injury. We excluded non acute scaphoid fractures as well as those associated with acute carpal dislocation. All injuries were sustained from the beginning of 2013 to the end of 2016.

The patient demographics were recorded. Two senior surgical trainees and an experienced hand surgeon analysed the plain radiographs and CT scans in each centre. The observers were briefed on recent literature which describes the long axis passing from the proximal point through the centre of the waist to the most distal point, with the most distal point being very close to the centre of the tubercle just radial to its apex [7, 8].

The Classification according to Russe, Herbert and Mayo systems were recorded. In addition the observers recorded the long axis length of the scaphoid, the distance at which the fracture line crossed the long axis, distance at which the proximal fracture line crossed a line perpendicular to long axis on ulnar border, distance at which fracture line crossed a line perpendicular to long axis on radial border, presence of a sagittal plane deformity, presence of a coronal plane deformity, presence of significant fragmentation and the scapholunate angle. The presence of coronal/sagittal

deformity or significant comminution was a subjective observer-based decision, i.e. the observer made a subjective decision as to whether any coronal or sagittal deformity and whether comminution was present in binary terms, no quantifiable metric was used.

The classification and characteristics were recorded separately at different times for both plain radiographs and CT scans. The long axis length of scaphoid was measured from the most proximal ulnar corner of the scaphoid to the centre of the scaphoid tubercle distally (distal point (dp)) (Figs. 1 and 2).

The radiographs were analysed pragmatically with the specific (long axis/radial/ulnar) measurements taken from what was deemed the best long axis view by each observer. The CT scans were analysed using InSight PACS (Insignia medical systems, UK) and the scaphoid orientated to obtain the best long axis view in the opinion of the observer for the specific measurements in this plane. The fracture position was measured using the

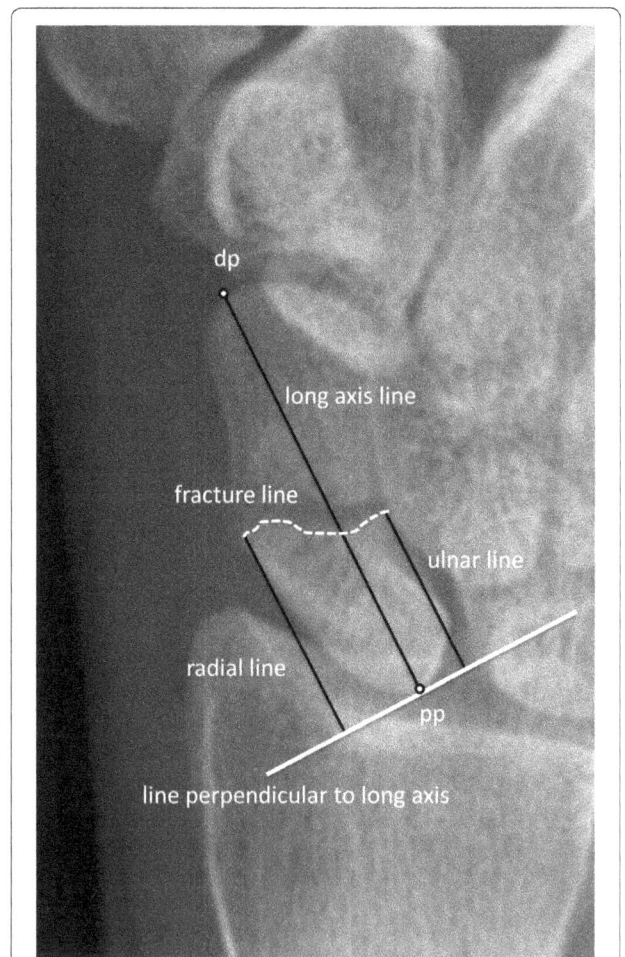

Fig. 1 Plain radiograph with the key points relating to 'long axis' measurement marked. Detailed legend - a scaphoid fracture with the distal point (dp), proximal point (pp), the long axis line, the fracture line, a line perpendicular to the long axis, and the radial and ulnar lines

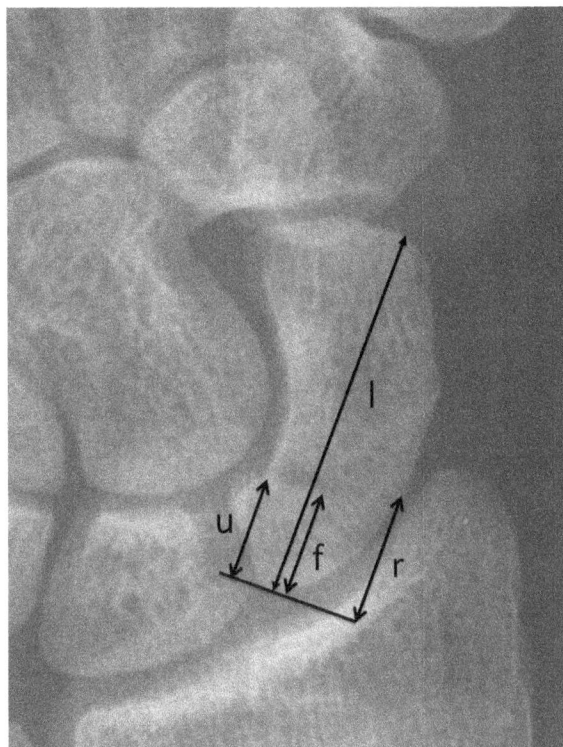

Fig. 2 Plain radiograph of a scaphoid fracture demonstrating the measurements made. Detailed legend - the long axis (l) and the distance along the long axis to the fracture site are shown (f, fracture distance), while the ulnar (u) and radial (r) distances to the fracture site are also shown. Note (f) is measured along (l) but for ease of demonstrating the methodology (f) has been moved just adjacent to (l). In this example the long axis measurement is f/l which equals 0.28

mid-sagittal coronal image. One observer at each centre repeated the X-ray and CT based assessments six months later to test intra-observer reliability.

Statistics

Statistical analysis was carried using SPSS version 24 for Windows (IBM Corp). Data was normally distributed unless otherwise stated. Results are expressed as mean (SD) unless otherwise stated. Inter-observer reliability was determined for ordinal data using Cohen's Kappa and for continuous data using the Intraclass Correlation Coefficient (ICC). ICCs were denoted as the single measures (average measures). Statistical significance was set at a level of $p < 0.05$. The interpretation of the degree of agreement determined by the Kappa and ICC is generally graded as slight (0.01–0.2), fair (0.21–0.40), moderate (0.41–0.60), substantial (0.61–0.80) and almost perfect (> 0.81) [9]. When calculating the ICC for more than two observers the ICC was re-calculated; whereas for the Kappa statistic a mean was used when an overall value was calculated for more than two observers. We did not carry out a formal power calculation, as this is not

standard practice for reliability studies [10]; however our sample size and number of observers was comparable with the best practice described within the literature [11].

Results

Patient demographics

Table 1 depicts the basic patient demographics including age, sex and the times from injury to imaging. The mean patient age was close to 30 years and a large majority of patients were male in both centres. All imaging was carried out within a month of injury.

Inter-observer reliability of X-ray based results

Table 2 and Appendix 1 show the inter observer reliability of the all X-ray based assessments. The Mayo classification system was the most reliable of the established classification systems with moderate agreement (kappa = 0.566), with the Herbert and Russe systems demonstrating fair and slight agreement respectively. The long axis measurement demonstrated substantial agreement (ICC = 0.758) and was more reliable than the ulnar and radial measurements. The degree of agreement of measuring sagittal plain deformity was poor (ICC = 0), while the degree of agreement for coronal plain deformity; comminution and scapholunate angle was moderate. The reliability of the 'long axis' measurement versus established classification systems is shown in Fig. 3, with the 'long axis' measurment demonstrating significantly greater reliability than the established methods.

Inter-observer reliability of CT based results

Table 3 and Appendix 2 show the reliability of each tool when using CT. Just as with plain radiographs the Mayo classification system was the most reliable of the established classification systems with moderate agreement (kappa = 0.542), with the Herbert and Russe systems demonstrating fair and slight agreement respectively. Long axis measurement demonstrated substantial agreement (ICC = 0.701); measuring using the radial or ulnar border of the scaphoid was less reliable than the central axis. Reliability was lower for CT measurements than those made based on X-rays. However the reliability of assessment of sagittal deformity (ICC = 0.201) and comminution (ICC = 0.525) was better on CT than on plain radiographs.

Table 1 Patient demographics and injury details

	Centre 1	Centre 2
Patient number	30	30
Age	31.4 (11.3)	29 (13.9)
Sex	27 M/3 F	25 M/5 F
Median time from injury to Xrays in days (IQR)	0 (0–7)	0 (0–5)
Median time from injury to CT in days (IQR)	6.5 (5–13)	12.5 (6.5–21)

Table 2 Inter observer reliability of the X-ray based measurements

System	Centre 1	Centre 2	Overall mean
Russe	0.131	0.120	0.126
Herbert	0.345	0.386	0.366
Mayo	0.609	0.522	0.566
Long axis	0.732	0.784	0.758
Sagittal deformity	−0.02	0.0167	0.00
Coronal deformity	0.425	0.438	0.432
Comminution	0.410	0.529	0.470
Scapholunate angle	0.389	0.580	0.485

Table 3 Inter observer reliability of the CT based measurements

System	Centre 1	Centre 2	Overall mean
Russe	0.085	0.055	0.070
Herbert	0.389	0.308	0.348
Mayo	0.531	0.553	0.542
Long axis	0.715	0.686	0.701
Sagittal deformity	0.210	0.192	0.201
Coronal deformity	0.212	0.240	0.226
Comminution	0.328	0.722	0.525

Relationship between X-ray and CT based results

The degree of agreement between the X-ray and CT based assessments are shown in Table 4 and Appendix 3. The Mayo demonstrated substantial agreement (kappa = 0.791) compared to the moderate agreement of the Herbert (kappa = 0.591) and the fair agreement of the Russe (0.217). The long axis measurement demonstrated moderate agreement (ICC = 0.571).

Intra-observer reliability of X-ray and CT based results

The data describing the inter-observer reliability is shown in Table 5 and Appendix 4. As regards X-ray based assessment, the Mayo classification system showed the highest inter-observer reliability of the established classification

systems with almost perfect agreement (kappa = 0.824), with the Herbert and Russe systems both demonstrating substantial agreement. The long axis measurement demonstrated almost perfect agreement whether based on X-ray (ICC = 0.895) or CT (ICC = 0.889).

Discussion

A simple 'long axis' measurement of the relative distance of the fracture site along the long axis of the scaphoid demonstrates a substantial level of inter observer reliability which is significantly better than other scaphoid classification systems. We found The Mayo to be the most reliable of among popular scaphoid classification systems with a moderate level of inter observer reliability. The new 'long axis' metric can be reliably measured on both X-ray and CT, while its other significant advantage over other classification systems is that it provides a way of quantifying fracture position with significant potential benefits for use in clinical research.

Our results are consistent with previous work in this area showing limited reliability of traditional methods [3, 12, 13]. Desai et al. demonstrated that the Russe and Herbert systems had fair levels of agreement, similar to the level of reliability shown in this study [12], while assessments of fracture level, comminution and displacement showed moderate inter- and intra-observer reproducibility [12]. Bhat et al. demonstrated that measures such as the intra-scaphoid angles (sagittal

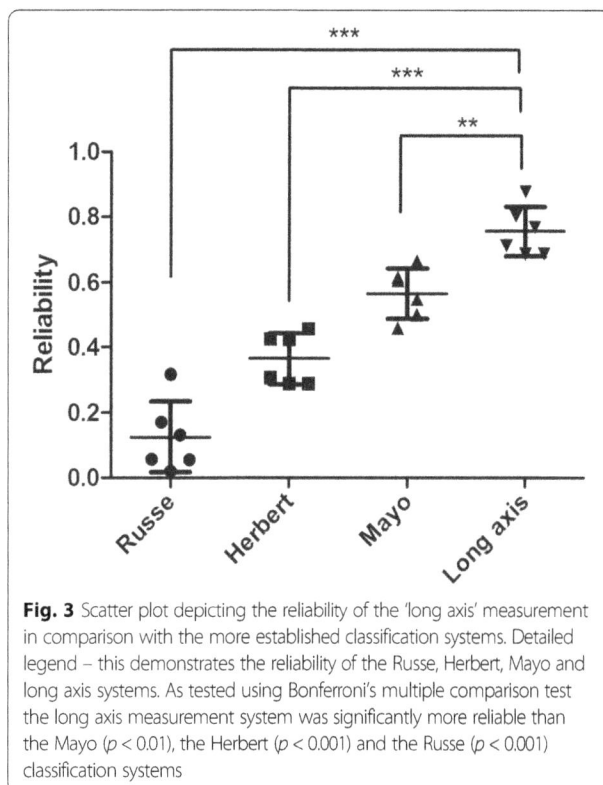

Fig. 3 Scatter plot depicting the reliability of the 'long axis' measurement in comparison with the more established classification systems. Detailed legend – this demonstrates the reliability of the Russe, Herbert, Mayo and long axis systems. As tested using Bonferroni's multiple comparison test the long axis measurement system was significantly more reliable than the Mayo ($p < 0.01$), the Herbert ($p < 0.001$) and the Russe ($p < 0.001$) classification systems

Table 4 The degree of agreement between X-ray and CT based measurements

System	Centre 1	Centre 2	Overall mean
Russe	0.027	0.407	0.217
Herbert	0.506	0.676	0.591
Mayo	0.778	0.799	0.788
Long axis	0.594	0.548	0.571
Sagittal deformity	0.251	0.274	0.262
Coronal deformity	0.339	0.355	0.347
Comminution	0.436	0.325	0.381

Table 5 Intra observer reliability of the X-ray and CT based measurements: the 'long axis' measurement versus established classification systems.

System	Xray	CT
Russe	0.583	0.550
Herbert	0.694	0.839
Mayo	0.824	0.855
Long axis	0.895	0.889

and coronal), the height-to-length ratio and the dorsal scaphoid cortical angle have poor reproducibility [13]. To our knowledge no system for quantifying how relatively proximal or distal an acute fracture has either been created or assessed for reliability, although a method with demonstrable reliability has previously been described relating to scaphoid non-unions [14]. We found that assessing the position of the fracture in relation to the long axis was reliable when measuring from plain radiographs and CT scans. While the use of CT scans is important when measuring union [6] they are not uniformly used in treatment planning initially and it is useful to have a valid measure of fracture position based on plain radiographs alone. This method can be used to allow analysis of a more continuous measure of fracture site and outcome, or alternatively as a tool to allocate fractures into categories such as 'proximal 20%' or 'proximal third'. When publishing raw data for meta-analysis this method might allow research teams to remove and reassign category boundaries. It is also likely that with greater standardisation of methodology the data will become more reliable [10]. It is important to note that this study is one of reliability and not validity. It is not possible to state whether the new 'long axis' measurement is 'better' than any other method, this study has simply shown that it is more reliable. Certainly, future research is necessary to demonstrate that the 'long axis' measurement is of real clinical meaning, for example in predicting the likelihood of scaphoid fracture union.

Strengths and limitations

This study was pragmatic in terms of how the 'long axis' measurement should be performed and yet reliability was high. We would therefore expect reliability of the 'long axis' method to be applicable to other centres. There was a range in the level of experience of the observers taking part in the study. We feel that a variable level of seniority and experience gives more generalisable results which easily translate into clinical practice more realistically; any method of assessing acute scaphoid fractures should

be simple to use and not require extensive levels of experience. The slightly poorer reliability of the long axis measurement on CT versus X-ray may be related to the freedom of the instructions given to the observers in terms of how to perform this calculation; it may be that future attempts to calculate a long axis measurement on CT need to be more specific and detailed in terms of precisely how observers should go about this.

The most important strength of this study is that the 'long axis' method enables the quantification of fracture position. A limitation of the long axis measurement is that it does not describe any information regarding the obliquity of the fracture in any plane, therefore fractures that are particularly oblique to the long axis in the coronal plan may extend deceptively proximally and this will not be communicated by using the central long axis measurement in isolation. It would be possible to calculate the approximate obliquity of the fracture plane using the long axis, radial and ulnar measurements; this is a feasible area for future research. There are also options of using three dimensional CT reconstructions define the fracture plane in multiple dimensions, relative to the long axis.

Conclusions

This study describes a novel pragmatic 'long axis' method for the quantification of acute scaphoid fractures which demonstrates substantial inter and intra observer reliability. The 'long axis' method offers benefits over traditional classification in terms of reliability, allocation of fractures to anatomical subgroups, and contributing to future debate on the definition and implications of proximal pole injuries.

Clinical relevance

- The most widely used acute scaphoid classification systems are not particularly reliable and do not quantify the approximate fracture location
- A simple 'long axis' measurement of the relative distance of the fracture site along the long axis of the scaphoid demonstrates significantly better inter observer reliability than the widely used classification systems
- This novel 'long axis' metric can be reliably measured on both plain radiographs and CT, while it provides a way of reliably quantifying fracture position which has significant potential uses in future clinical research

Appendix 1

Table 6 Xray based reliability

	Centre 1				Centre 2				Overall mean
	1 vs 2	1 vs 3	2 vs 3	Mean	1 vs 2	1 vs 3	2 vs 3	Mean	
Russe reliability (Kappa)	0.317	0.021	0.056	0.131	0.171	0.058	0.132	0.120	0.126
Herbert reliability (kappa)	0.289	0.289	0.457	0.345	0.424	0.426	0.308	0.386	0.366
Mayo reliability (kappa)	0.665	0.615	0.548	0.609	0.607	0.459	0.500	0.522	0.566
Central distance reliability (ICC)	0.713(0.832)	0.803(0.891)	0.687(0.815)	0.732(0.891)	0.688(0.815)	0.768(0.869)	0.878(0.935)	0.784(0.916)	0.758(0.904)
Ulnar distance reliability(ICC)	0.657(0.793)	0.857(0.923)	0.650(0.788)	0.709(0.880)	0.664(0.798)	0.359(0.528)	0.765(0.867)	0.590 (0.812)	0.650(0.846)
Radial distance reliability(ICC)	0.656(0.792)	0.785(0.880)	0.708(0.829)	0.716(0.883)	0.581(0.735)	0.600(0.750)	0.385(0.556)	0.523(0.767)	0.620(0.825)
Sagittal deformity reliability(kappa)	−0.119	0.118	−0.05	−0.02	−0.061	0.048	0.063	0.0167	0.00
Coronal deformity reliability(kappa)	0.333	0.250	0.692	0.425	0.659	0.328	0.328	0.438	0.432
Comminution deformity reliability(kappa)	0.268	0.514	0.447	0.410	0.561	0.615	0.412	0.529	0.470
SL angle reliabilityICC)	0.331(0.498)	0.422(0.594	0.435(0.607)	0.389(0.656)	0.688(0.815)	0.449(0.620)	0.629(0.773)	0.580(0.806)	0.485(0.731)

Appendix 2

Table 7 CT based reliability

	Centre 1				Centre 2				Overall mean
	1 vs 2	1 vs 3	2 vs 3	Mean	1 vs 2	1 vs 3	2 vs 3	Mean	
Russe reliability(Kappa)	0.00	0.253	0.00	0.084	0.066	0.056	0.156	0.055	0.070
Herbert reliability(kappa)	0.464	0.389	0.314	0.389	0.271	0.425	0.227	0.308	0.348
Mayo reliability(kappa)	0.562	0.568	0.463	0.531	0.717	0.462	0.481	0.553	0.542
Central distance reliability(ICC)	0.748(0.856)	0.687(0.814)	0.701(0.825)	0.715(0.883)	0.636(0.717)	0.569(0.725)	0.600(0.750)	0.686(0.867)	0.701(0.875)
Ulnar distance reliability(ICC)	0.667(0.800)	0.664(0.798)	0.476(0.645)	0.598(0.817)	0.400(0.572)	0.359(0.528)	0.178(0.302)	0.307(0.571)	0.453(0.694)
Radial distance reliability(ICC)	0.650(0.788)	0.717(0.835)	0.569(0.725)	0.644(0.844)	0.455(0.625)	0.596(0.747)	0.224(0.366)	0.437(0.699)	0.541(0.772)
Sagittal deformity reliability(kappa)	0.400	0.067	0.163	0.21	0.366	0.098	0.112	0.192	0.201
Coronal deformity reliability(kappa)	0.268	0.118	0.250	0.212	0.420	0.189	0.112	0.240	0.226
Comminution deformity reliability(kappa)	0.279	0.279	0.426	0.328	0.684	0.815	0.667	0.722	0.525

Appendix 3

Table 8 Xray versus CT reliability

	Centre 1				Centre 2				Overall mean
	1	2	3	Mean	1	2	3	Mean	
Russe reliability(Kappa)	0.00	0.00	0.082	0.027	0.054	0.224	0.944	0.407	0.217
Herbert reliability(kappa)	0.705	0.412	0.402	0.506	0.544	0.586	0.898	0.676	0.591
Mayo reliability(kappa)	0.918	0.627	0.790	0.778	0.904	0.804	0.688	0.799	0.788
Central distance reliability(ICC)	0.724(0.840)	0.464(0.634)	0.593(0.744)	0.594(0.739)	0.767(0.868)	0.427(0.599)	0.451(0.621)	0.548(0.696)	0.571(0.718)
Ulnar distance reliability(ICC)	0.826(0.905)	0.349(0.517)	0.573(0.728)	0.583(0.717)	0.449(0.620)	0.465(0.635)	0.161(0.278)	0.358(0.511)	0.471(0.614)
Radial distance reliability(ICC)	0.719(0.837)	0.467(0.637)	0.784(0.879)	0.657(0.784)	0.751(0.858)	0.393(0.565)	0.271(0.427)	0.472(0.617)	0.565(0.700)
Sagittal deformity reliability(kappa)	0.267	0.217	0.270	0.251	0.405	0.05	0.366	0.274	0.262
Coronal deformity reliability(kappa)	0.634	0.333	0.050	0.339	0.189	0.772	0.105	0.355	0.347
Comminution deformity reliability(kappa)	0.298	0.585	0.426	0.436	0.815	0.615	0.359	0.325	0.381

Appendix 4

Table 9 Inter observer reliability for X-ray and CT based assessments

	Observer 1		Observer 2		Mean	
	X-ray	CT	X-ray	CT	X-ray	CT
Russe reliability(Kappa)	0.628	0.679	0.538	0.420	0.583	0.550
Herbert reliability(kappa)	0.749	0.850	0.639	0.828	0.694	0.839
Mayo reliability(kappa)	0.831	0.838	0.817	0.871	0.824	0.855
Central distance reliability(ICC)	0.905(0.950)	0.900(0.948)	0.884(0.938)	0.878(0.935)	0.895(0.944)	0.889(0.946)
Ulnar distance reliability(ICC)	0.820(0.901)	0.920(0.958)	0.568(0.725)	0.839(0.912)	0.694(0.813)	0.807(0.890)
Radial distance reliability(ICC)	0.822(0.902)	0.931(0.964)	0.850(0.919)	0.755(0.860)	0.836(0.911)	0.843(0.912)
Sagittal deformity reliability(kappa)	0.765	0.891	0.612	0.636	0.689	0.764
Coronal deformity reliability(kappa)	0.818	0.826	0.433	0.622	0.626	0.724
Comminution deformity reliability(kappa)	0.774	0.840	0.689	0.944	0.732	0.892

Abbreviations
CT: Computed tomography; ICC: Intraclass Correlation Coefficient

Acknowledgements
We would like to thanks all the staff at both Oxford University Hospitals and Buckinghamshire Health who have helped in any way in the carrying out of this work.

Funding
This research received no specific grant from any funding agency in the public, commercial or not-for-profit sectors.

Authors' contributions
BJFD, AG, and NR contributed to study conception and design, data collection and analysis, drafting of the article and critical revision of the article. EM, JL, and AT contributed to data collection and analysis, and the critical revision of the article. All authors read and approved the final manuscript.

Competing interests
No benefits in any form have been received or will be received from a commercial party related directly or indirectly to the subject of this article. The authors declare that they have no competing interests.

Author details
[1]Nuffield Department of Orthopaedics, Rheumatology and Musculoskeletal Sciences (NDORMS), University of Oxford, Botnar Research Centre, Windmill road, Oxford OX3 7LD, UK. [2]Nuffield Orthopaedic Centre, Windmill road, Oxford OX3 7LD, UK. [3]Frankston Hospital, Frankston, VIC, Australia. [4]Buckinghamshire Hospitals NHS Trust, High Wycombe Hospital, High Wycombe, Amersham HP11 2TT, UK.

References
1. Duckworth AD, Jenkins PJ, Aitken SA, Clement ND, Court-Brown CM, McQueen MM. Scaphoid fracture epidemiology. J Trauma Acute Care Surg. 2012;72(2):E41–5.
2. Eastley N, Singh H, Dias JJ, Taub N. Union rates after proximal scaphoid fractures; meta-analyses and review of available evidence. J Hand Surg European Vol. 2013;38(8):888–97.
3. Ten Berg PW, Drijkoningen T, Strackee SD, Buijze GA. Classifications of acute scaphoid fractures: a systematic literature review. J Wrist Surg. 2016;5(2):152–9.
4. Russe O. Fracture of the carpal navicular. Diagnosis, non-operative treatment, and operative treatment. J Bone Joint Surg Amer Vol. 1960;42-A:759–68.
5. Herbert TJ, Fisher WE. Management of the fractured scaphoid using a new bone screw. J Bone Joint Surg Br. 1984;66(1):114–23.
6. Dias J, Brealey S, Choudhary S, et al. Scaphoid waist internal fixation for fractures trial (SWIFFT) protocol: a pragmatic multi-Centre randomised controlled trial of cast treatment versus surgical fixation for the treatment of bi-cortical, minimally displaced fractures of the scaphoid waist in adults. BMC Musculoskelet Disord. 2016;17:248.
7. Heaton DJ, Trumble T, Rhodes D. Determination of the central Axis of the scaphoid. J Wrist Surg. 2015;4(3):214–20.
8. Guo Y, Tian GL. The length and position of the long axis of the scaphoid measured by analysis of three-dimensional reconstructions of computed tomography images. J Hand Surg Eur Vol. 2010;36(2):98–101.
9. Viera AJ, Garrett JM. Understanding interobserver agreement: the kappa statistic. Fam Med. 2005;37(5):360–3.
10. Tawonsawatruk T, Hamilton DF, Simpson AH. Validation of the use of radiographic fracture-healing scores in a small animal model. J Orthop Res. 2014;32(9):1117–9.
11. Walter SD, Eliasziw M, Donner A. Sample size and optimal designs for reliability studies. Stat Med. 1998;17(1):101–10.
12. Desai VV, Davis TR, Barton NJ. The prognostic value and reproducibility of the radiological features of the fractured scaphoid. J Hand Surg. 1999;24(5):586–90.
13. Bhat M, McCarthy M, Davis TR, Oni JA, Dawson S. MRI and plain radiography in the assessment of displaced fractures of the waist of the carpal scaphoid. J Bone Joint Surg Am. 2004;86(5):705–13.
14. Trail I, Stanley D. The Scaphoid edited by Slutsky, D. 1st edition. 2010;Chapter 6.

Incidence of calcaneal apophysitis in Northwest Istanbul

Ceylan H. H.[1*] [iD] and Caypinar B.[2]

Abstract

Background: Calcaneal apophysitis is a common clinical entity affecting children and adolescents. It is also known as Sever's disease. Heel pain without a recent trauma is the primary manifestation. There are limited studies on the incidence of this disease. In this study, we aimed to report the regional incidence in Istanbul.

Methods: This retrospective audit of health records of all paediatric patients aged 6–17 years between January 1, 2014, and December 15, 2017 was undertaken. During this period, data were extracted from health records that recorded calcaneal apophysitis as the primary diagnosis.

Results: The 4-year incidence of calcaneal apophysitis was found to be 0.35% (74 of 20,967 paediatric patients). It commonly affected males, and bilateral cases were more common than unilateral cases. There were more admissions during the spring season, which may indicate a possible association with physical activity.

Conclusion: Although calcaneal apophysitis is a relatively common paediatric foot problem, due to its benign course and spontaneous healing capacity, most physicians are not interested in this topic. However, increased awareness of this diagnosis is important for reducing the rates of unnecessary radiological examinations and orthopaedic referrals. With increased knowledge, most cases may be diagnosed at the family physician level, which may decrease the economic burden on the health system. Incidence reports from various countries and regions may be published in the future.

Keywords: Sever's disease, Calcaneal apophysitis, Heel pain

Background

Calcaneal apophysitis, or Sever's disease, is a common entity among paediatric and adolescent patients who present to a physician with heel pain [1–11]. This disorder is an overuse syndrome and was first identified by James Warren Sever in 1912 [12]. The basic pathology is repetitive microtrauma that induces calcaneal apophysis damage [7, 13, 14]. Although various mechanisms have been discussed in the literature, there is not a single mechanism explaining this pathology in all cases. The clinical manifestation is typically characterised by pain that can be localised by palpation to the posteroinferior region of the calcaneus. The medial-lateral squeeze test may be helpful for clinical diagnosis. The symptoms are exacerbated by sports that require extreme physical activity [1, 5–7, 11, 13, 15, 16]. Although the symptoms are usually associated with physical activity, resting pain can also be observed in advanced cases. Different studies have shown the considerable impact of calcaneal apophysitis on health-related quality of life [9, 17].

Calcaneal apophysitis tends to occur between the ages of 8 and 13 years in girls and between the ages of 11 and 15 years in boys [7]. Its incidence among all musculoskeletal injuries has been reported to be between 2 and 16%, [1] but is believed to be even higher in the active paediatric population [1, 5–7, 11, 15, 16]. Calcaneal apophysitis has a benign course, and treatment is conservative. Resting, applying ice, stretching, strengthening the calf muscles, using heel-elevating supports or orthoses and taking anti-inflammatory drugs largely solve the problem [1, 2, 7, 10, 13, 18–21]. Fixation with a resting plaster has been reported for rare, persistent cases [6, 13]. Although the disease usually has a benign course, it sometimes requires extended treatment or causes an active athlete to stay away from the field for a period of

* Correspondence: drhhc@yahoo.com
[1]Lutfiye Nuri Burat Devlet Hastanesi, 50.Yil Mah., 2107 Sok, 34256 Sultangazi, Istanbul, Turkey
Full list of author information is available at the end of the article

time [7, 14]. Anamnesis and physical examination are sufficient for diagnosis [1, 3, 7, 8, 10–12, 22, 23]. Magnetic resonance imaging is recommended for ruling out fracture, tumour, or infection in suspicious cases [24].

Increased knowledge of calcaneal apophysitis and its incidence will help physicians diagnose the disease with anamnesis and examination and help reduce the need for further radiological evaluations, which are harmful to patients. In this study, we aimed to determine the incidence of calcaneal apophysitis by examining the data on paediatric patients with heel pain who were admitted to our hospital located in Northwest Istanbul, which has a higher birth-rate and larger paediatric population than most regional hospitals of Turkey.

Methods

Paediatric patients who were admitted to our outpatient clinic with heel pain over 4 years (between January 1, 2014, to December 15, 2017) and diagnosed with calcaneal apophysitis were included in the study.

The records of all patients who were admitted to our outpatient clinic within these 4 years and aged between 6 and 17 years at the time of initial admission were obtained from the database records. Both orthopaedic surgeons had a standard approach to paediatric heel pain cases, which included a detailed anamnesis and physical examination. In addition to the detailed anamnesis, the heel squeeze test was applied for all children bilaterally and recorded in the patient's initial visit. The anamnesis records were scanned for the terms 'heel' and 'Sever'. All accessed files were transferred to a table sheet, and content verification was conducted on individual records separately by two orthopaedic surgeons. At first, all trauma cases were excluded. Second, files without a diagnosis of calcaneal apophysitis or those including an anamnesis record that differed from the manifestation of calcaneal apophysitis were excluded. Among the remaining files, patients with missing or incomplete anamnesis data ($n = 12$) or patients whose diagnosis of calcaneal apophysitis seemed suspicious ($n = 5$) were also excluded. In all, a total of 74 patients were identified. The patients' age, sex, affected side, admission month, and symptom duration before admission were noted.

Results

During this four-year period, a total of 20,967 paediatric patients aged 6 to 17 years were admitted to our hospital for various complaints. Only 91 of them had a complaint of isolated calcaneal tenderness without a history of recent trauma. Among these 91 children, 74 were identified to have a diagnosis of calcaneal apophysitis.

The anamnesis records revealed that the distribution of patients who had a diagnosis of calcaneal apophysitis changed each year. The case distribution in the last 4

years was noted: there were 23 cases in 2014, 19 in 2015, 11 in 2016, and 21 in 2017 (Table 1). Of the 74 patients diagnosed with calcaneal apophysitis, 59 were male, and 15 were female. The mean age of our patient group was 10.77 (6.87–15.73) years. The average age was 11.14 (8.04–15.73) years for boys and 9.28 (6.87–13.20) years for girls at the time of each admission. Of the 74 patients, symptoms were bilateral in 46 (62.16%) patients and unilateral in the rest. The average time between the onset of complaints and admission to the outpatient clinic was 12.7 (min 2-max 108) weeks. The patient with the longest period of complaints was a girl who was 11 years old at the time of admission.

At first, ibuprofen treatment was initiated in all patients. The daily dose was divided into two and suggested to be given every 12 h. Additionally, stretching exercises were described to the families, and they were asked to monitor the child's practice at home. All patients were called for follow-up after 2 weeks of treatment. Among the 69 patients who were reached for follow-up, the treatment was found to be effective. The exception was a 9-year-old boy. An MRI examination was obtained to exclude other possible pathologies but revealed no additional pathology except oedema of the calcaneal apophysis. The patient underwent non-weight-bearing mobilisation with a custom-made ankle orthosis for 4 weeks. Then, due to residual pain and dissatisfaction, passive stretching exercises for 2 weeks under a physiotherapist's supervision were attempted. Although the patient still reported some residual pain in the eighth week after the treatment was completed, his family declared that the symptoms were significantly relieved compared to those at the first admission. X-ray examination was performed for all of our patients upon request of their families.

The 4-year incidence of calcaneal apophysitis was found to be 0.35% (74 of 20,967). Calcaneal apophysitis commonly affected males, and bilateral involvement was more common than unilateral involvement. We observed that there were more admissions during the spring season (Fig. 1). This finding indicates a possible association of the disease with physical activity.

Table 1 Distribution of cases for each year

Year	Diagnosis of Sever's disease (n)	Total number of admissions aged 6–17 years (n)	Incidence (%)
2014	23	5111	0.45
2015	19	4819	0.39
2016	11	4519	0.24
2017	21	6518	0.32
Overall	74	20,967	0.35

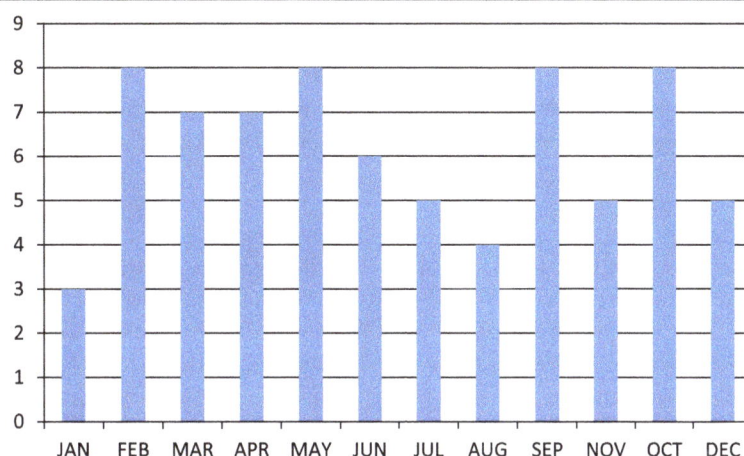

Fig. 1 Distribution of all calcaneal apophysitis cases upon admission

Discussion

In this study, we aimed to determine the incidence of calcaneal apophysitis in the general paediatric population from records at our hospital. Due to the higher birth-rate and higher paediatric patient admission rates at our hospital than at most regional hospitals of Turkey, the reported data are able to reflect the actual disease incidence in the general population. The large sample size is an advantage of our study, as it reduces the risk of detecting coincidentally high incidences. The overall 4-year incidence of calcaneal apophysitis was found to be 0.35% in our cohort. Boys were affected more often than girls, and bilateral presentation was dominant.

Although calcaneal apophysitis is common in paediatric patients with heel pain, there are limited studies on the incidence and prevalence of the disease in the general population [11]. Sports trauma clinics have reported higher incidences, but these data were considered insufficient for reflecting the overall incidence [20]. Orava reported the 6-years incidence of calcaneal apophysitis to be 22.7% [16]. These previous studies focused primarily on patient cohorts, which may be considered an overuse group and may be biased when representing the actual incidence of calcaneal apophysitis [11]. In a study by Wiegerinck et al. in the Netherlands, the authors evaluated general paediatric population data over three consecutive years, they calculated the annual incidence rate and then calculate the mean over the 3 years, and reported the 3-years incidence of calcaneal apophysitis to be 0.37%, which is similar to our findings [11]. In the same study, the authors reported the disease's annual incidence in 2010 to be 0.49% based on physicians' records [11]. However, it was also emphasised that this increase in disease incidence may be entirely incidental. Similar to the mentioned study, the annual incidence changed year by year in our cohort, and we found the 4-year

incidence of calcaneal apophysitis in the general population to be approximately 0.35%.

Calcaneal apophysitis was radiologically and clinically identified by Sever in the early twentieth century and was called Sever's disease in the literature [12]. Sever's first definition reported that this disease occurred primarily in inactive and overweight children [12]. Radiological findings related to the disease were also emphasised in this first report. Lewin claimed that this condition was a painful inflammation of the epiphysis and was a result of traction of the epiphysis by the Achilles tendon and plantar fascia in opposite directions [22]. High levels of activity and obesity were identified as risk factors [14, 25]. Apophyseal traction in the insertion side of the Achilles tendon may be related to overuse during the rapid growth period in adolescence [23]. Calcaneal apophysitis has a benign course that is self-limiting in nature [16]. Symptoms typically resolve after fusion of the apophysis and calcaneus [12]. The inflammatory process rarely results in an apophyseal fracture, [26] and no apophyseal fractures were found in our patient group.

Calcaneal apophysitis typically presents in children between the ages of 8 and 15 years [2, 23]. A case of calcaneal apophysitis in a 6 year old was reported in the literature [27]. This condition is 2–3 times more common in males than in females, and the symptoms are bilateral in 60% of cases [4]. In accordance with current knowledge, the age distribution of our patient group is between 6 and 15 years old, and boys were affected more often than were girls. The symptoms were bilateral in 62.16% of patients.

A conservative approach is commonly adopted in the treatment of calcaneal apophysitis. Ice application, stretching, resting and activity modification are treatment methods emphasised in the literature [3, 5, 14, 15, 21]. Studies that reported the positive effects of heel supports, ice application, and stretching used these methods in combination [5, 7, 21]. Similarly, some authors recommended heel supports in addition to restrictions on sports activity [1, 10, 18]. Some authors recommended using arch-supporting devices, which increase the traction effect of the gastrocnemius-soleus complex on pronating deformities of the foot [14]. Heel supports are thought to be effective through decreasing the traction effect of the gastrocnemius-soleus complex on the growing apophysis [28, 29]. The best method for calcaneal apophysitis management is not clear, and definitive evidence of the superiority of these known methods is limited [1, 14]. Wiegerinck et al. compared the wait-and-see, heel raise inlay, and physical therapy methods and could not find a significant difference among these methods [30]. However, the heel support group was more satisfied with the outcomes than the other groups after 6 weeks of treatment. A current prospective randomised study by James et al. showed the positive effect of heel risers over prefabricated orthotics in the early period of the disease [14]. In our patient group, none of the patients were recommended the use of heel or arch supports. Only one resistant case required fixation with an orthosis and non-weight-bearing mobilisation for 4 weeks.

There is limited literature on the efficacy of nonsteroidal anti-inflammatory therapy in the treatment of calcaneal apophysitis. Karahan et al. reported good results with 3 weeks of ibuprofen and topical diclofenac in addition to heel supports and stretching exercises [31]. Oral NSAIDs and short leg fixation plasters [6, 24] and local ketoprofen gel administration were reported in other studies [21]. We prescribed appropriate doses of ibuprofen to all our patients and found it to be a cheap and effective treatment.

Increased calcaneal apophysis density and fragmentation are observed on direct X-ray evaluation in calcaneal apophysitis. However, these findings are not pathognomonic to calcaneal apophysitis and may also be observed in healthy children [1, 3, 7, 8, 10, 16, 23, 24, 27, 31]. While the diagnosis is based on the clinical presentation and anamnesis, direct X-ray may be used to exclude other potential pathologies [24]. Possible reasons for heel pain, such as stress fracture, osteomyelitis, Achilles tendinitis, and calcaneal cysts, should be considered in the differential diagnosis [24]. An MRI examination may be useful for this purpose. In calcaneal apophysitis, MRI findings are limited to bone marrow oedema in most cases, and increased gadolinium uptake may be another finding [24]. In our patient group, we did not use such imaging methods, except in one patient that underwent an MRI scan due to persistent pain. A single lateral calcaneus X-ray image was obtained from all patients for confirmation only.

This study has certain limitations. Due to the retrospective nature of this study, some of the calcaneal apophysitis cases in our hospital database may have been excluded due to the inability to access their records or incomplete anamnesis forms completed during admission. As emphasised in a previous study, 50% of patients with musculoskeletal disorders do not consult a physician for their complaints [32]. Some calcaneal apophysitis patients may go to their local doctor, physical therapist or podiatrist, and some may never be admitted to a hospital despite their complaints and ability to reach the hospital. These patients may have received treatment from their family physicians without a diagnosis. For these reasons, the actual incidence may be higher than that indicated by our study. The second limitation was that X-ray examination was performed upon the request of the families. Because parents are paying for their child's healthcare, and want an X-ray to be taken. X-ray examination is not necessary, and the current literature strongly advises against taking an X-ray for calcaneal apophysitis diagnosis. However, socio-economic conditions forced us to use X-ray examination. Although we could not detect any atypical findings, one of our patients was resistant to medical treatment. We also used non-weight mobilisation based on outdated literature, which was the wrong approach based on current knowledge. Restriction of daily activities is not currently recommended. Another limitation is that there were no available data on the sports or daily activity levels of the children at initial admission. Therefore, these details could not be discussed in our study. A prospective study can record complete patient data and include records from the family physician, podiatrist, and orthopaedic surgeon, thus overcoming these obstacles and allowing a more precise regional incidence to be reported.

Conclusion

Although it is a relatively common paediatric foot problem, due to its benign course and spontaneous healing capacity, most physicians are not interested in calcaneal apophysitis. However, increased awareness of the clinical diagnosis is important for reducing the rates of unnecessary radiological examinations and orthopaedic referrals. Most cases of calcaneal apophysitis can be diagnosed by family and local physicians, which may decrease the economic burden on the health system. Further research on diagnosis and treatment needs to be published for an increased understanding of calcaneal apophysitis. In addition, further research may result in incidence reports from different regions around the world.

Conclusion for families

When to worry? Calcaneal apophysitis is a benign and transient condition that can be easily managed at home and does not require consultation or investigation. Despite its benign course, families should be aware of some clinical signs that may indicate the presence of other heel problems. If the heel pain is constant or occurs at night, if there is erythema or swelling, if the child is unwell, and if the child is between the ages of 7–14 years, consultation with a healthcare practitioner is mandatory.

What to do? If the diagnosis is calcaneal apophysitis, do not worry. It is a transient condition related to your child's bone growth. During this period, rest and ice application may be helpful. Some modifications to sport activities can also be effective. Shoe modification, including heel risers, may be helpful during this period. Medical treatment with basic anti-inflammatory drugs is sufficient in most cases.

Availability of data and materials
The datasets used and analysed in the present study are available from the corresponding author on reasonable request by e-mail (drhhc@yahoo.com).

Authors' contributions
HHC had the initial idea for the present study, collected the data, analysed the data, and wrote the majority of the manuscript. BC helped with study design, writing the manuscript, data analysis and language editing. Both authors have read and approved the final manuscript.

Authors' information
Hasan H. Ceylan, MD; Specialist Orthopaedics and Trauma Surgery; Turkish Board Certified. Currently: Attending surgeon in Lutfiye Nuri Burat State Hospital, Department of Orthopaedic Surgery. 50.yil mah. 2107 sok. Sultangazi, Istanbul, Turkey. Baris Caypinar, MD; Specialist Orthopaedics and Trauma Surgery; Turkish Board Certified. Currently: Consultant Scholar in Gelisim University, Department of Physiotherapy. Avcilar, Istanbul, Turkey.

Competing interests
The authors declare that they have no competing interests.

Author details
[1]Lutfiye Nuri Burat Devlet Hastanesi, 50.Yil Mah., 2107 Sok, 34256 Sultangazi, Istanbul, Turkey. [2]Gelisim University, Istanbul, Turkey.

References
1. Scharfbillig RW, Jones S, Scutter SD. Sever's disease: what does the literature really tell us? J Am Podiatr Med Assoc. 2008;98(3):212–23.
2. Hendrix CL. Calcaneal apophysitis (sever disease). Clin Podiatr Med Surg. 2005;22(1):55–62.
3. Hussain S, Hussain K, Hussain S, Hussain S. Sever's disease: a common cause of paediatric heel pain. BMJ Case Reports. 2013;2013:bcr2013009758. https://doi.org/10.1136/bcr-2013-009758.
4. Krul M, van der Wouden JC, Schellevis FG, van Suijlekom-Smit LW, Koes BW. Foot problems in children presented to the family physician: a comparison between 1987 and 2001. Fam Pract. 2009;26(3):174–9.
5. Kvist M, Heinonem O. Calcaneal apophysitis (Sever's disease)—a common cause of heel pain in young athletes. Scand J Med Sci Sports. 1991;1(4):235–8.
6. Madden CC, Mellion MB. Sever's disease and other causes of heel pain in adolescents. Am Fam Physician. 1996;54(6):1995–2000.
7. Micheli LJ, Ireland ML. Prevention and management of calcaneal apophysitis in children: an overuse syndrome. J Pediatr Orthop. 1987;7(1):34–8.
8. Rachel JN, Williams JB, Sawyer JR, Warner WC, Kelly DM. Is radiographic evaluation necessary in children with a clinical diagnosis of calcaneal apophysitis (sever disease)? J Pediatr Orthop. 2011;31(5):548–50.
9. Scharfbillig RW, Jones S, Scutter S. Sever's disease--does it effect quality of life? Foot (Edinburgh, Scotland). 2009;19(1):36–43.
10. Weiner DS, Morscher M, Dicintio MS. Calcaneal apophysitis: simple diagnosis, simpler treatment. J Fam Pract. 2007;56(5):352–5.
11. Wiegerinck JI, Yntema C, Brouwer HJ, Struijs PA. Incidence of calcaneal apophysitis in the general population. Eur J Pediatr. 2014;173(5):677–9.
12. Sever J. Apophysis of os calcis. NY State J Med. 1912;95:1025.
13. James AM, Williams CM, Haines TP. Heel raises versus prefabricated orthoses in the treatment of posterior heel pain associated with calcaneal apophysitis (Sever's disease): a randomised control trial. J Foot Ankle Res. 2010;3:3.
14. James AM, Williams CM, Haines TP. Effectiveness of footwear and foot orthoses for calcaneal apophysitis: a 12-month factorial randomised trial. Br J Sports Med. 2016;50(20):1268–75.
15. Leri JP. Heel pain in a young adolescent baseball player. J Chiropr Med. 2004;3(2):66–8.
16. Orava S, Virtanen K. Osteochondroses in athletes. Br J Sports Med. 1982;16(3):161–8.
17. James AM, Williams CM, Haines TP. Health related quality of life of children with calcaneal apophysitis: child & parent perceptions. Health Qual Life Outcomes. 2016;14:95.
18. Perhamre S, Lundin F, Norlin R, Klässbo M. Sever's injury; treat it with a heel cup: a randomized, crossover study with two insole alternatives. Scand J Med Sci Sports. 2011;21(6):e42-7. https://doi.org/10.1111/j.1600-0838.2010.01140.x. Epub 2010 Jul 29.
19. Hunt GC, Stowell T, Alnwick GM, Evans S. Arch taping as a symptomatic treatment in patients with Sever's disease: a multiple case series. Foot. 2007;17(4):178–83.
20. James AM, Williams CM, Haines TP. Effectiveness of interventions in reducing pain and maintaining physical activity in children and adolescents with calcaneal apophysitis (Sever's disease): a systematic review. J Foot Ankle Res. 2013;6(1):16.
21. White RL. Ketoprofen gel as an adjunct to physical therapist management of a child with Sever disease. Phys Ther. 2006;86(3):424-33.
22. Lewin P. Apophysitis of the os calcis. Surg Gynecol Obstet. 1926;41:578.
23. Ogden JA, Ganey TM, Hill JD, Jaakkola JI. Sever's injury: a stress fracture of the immature calcaneal metaphysis. J Pediatr Orthop. 2004;24(5):488–92.
24. Lawrence DA, Rolen MF, Morshed KA, Moukaddam H. MRI of heel pain. AJR Am J Roentgenol. 2013;200(4):845–55.
25. McKenzie DC, Taunton JE, Clement DB, Smart GW, McNicol KL. Calcaneal epiphysitis in adolescent athletes. Can J Appl Sport Sci. 1981;6(3):123–5.
26. Lee KT, Young KW, Park YU, Park SY, Kim KC. Neglected Sever's disease as a cause of calcaneal apophyseal avulsion fracture: case report. Foot Ankle Int. 2010;31(8):725–8.
27. Volpon JB, de Carvalho FG. Calcaneal apophysitis: a quantitative radiographic evaluation of the secondary ossification center. Arch Orthop Trauma Surg. 2002;122(6):338–41.
28. Micheli LJ, Fehlandt AF Jr. Overuse injuries to tendons and apophyses in children and adolescents. Clin Sports Med. 1992;11(4):713–26.
29. Peck DM. Apophyseal injuries in the young athlete. Am Fam Physician. 1995;51(8):1891–5. 1897-1898
30. Wiegerinck JI, Zwiers R, Sierevelt IN, van Weert HC, van Dijk CN, Struijs PA. Treatment of calcaneal Apophysitis: wait and see versus orthotic device versus physical therapy: a pragmatic therapeutic randomized clinical trial. J Pediatr Orthop. 2016;36(2):152–7.
31. Karahan YA, Salbaş E, Tekin L, Yaşar O, Küçük A. Sever Hastalığı: Çocuklarda topuk ağrısının önemli bir nedeni; Olgu Sunumu. Turk J Osteoporos/Turk Osteoporoz Dergisi. 2014;20(2):86-8. https://doi.org/10.4274/tod.04695.
32. Picavet H, Schouten J. Musculoskeletal pain in the Netherlands: prevalences, consequences and risk groups, the DMC 3-study. Pain. 2003;102(1):167–78.

7

Up-regulated expression of E2F2 is necessary for p16INK4a-induced cartilage injury

Xinnan Bao[1] and Xinyu Hu[2]*

Abstract

Background: Cartilage degradation would result in osteoarthritis (OA). p16INK4awas found in some age-related diseases. In this study, we aimed to determine the role of p16INK4a during OA and to investigate the underlying mechanisms.

Methods: Enzyme-linked immunosorbent assay (ELISA) was performed to test the activity of senescence-associated secretory phenotype (SASP). Real-time PCR (RT-PCR) and Western blot were used to determine the expressions of target genes.

Results: The increased expressions of p16INK4a and E2F2 were accompanied with cartilage degradation induced by IL-1β. Over-expression of p16INK4a enhanced the secretion of SASP markers (TGFβ, IL-6, IL-8, IL-1α, MMP3 and MMP13), reduced the expression of type II procollagen (COL2A1).Thus, the over-expression of p16INK4a lead to cartilage injury. Moreover, we found that the expression of E2F2 was enhanced in p16INK4a over-expression group, and that cartilage injury caused by p16INK4a was alleviated by depleting E2F2.

Conclusions: p16INK4a was up-regulated during the cartilage injury in OA. p16INK4a promoted cartilage injury by increasing the expression of E2F2. Thus, this study extends the molecular regulation network for understanding pathological progression of OA, and provides potential therapeutic target for OA.

Keywords: p16INK4a, E2F2, Senescence-associated secretory phenotype (SASP), Osteoarthritis (OA)

Background

Osteoarthritis (OA) is one of the most common chronic diseases among aged population [1, 2]. Various factors, for example, abnormal joint development, joint injury, overweight, inherent factor and aging, contribute to the pathophysiology of OA [3, 4]. Although OA and aging are not inter-related, the onset and progression of the former is closely related to the later [5]. During the process of aging, senescence-associated secretory phenotype (SASP), which includes growth factors (such as TNF-β), pro-inflammatory cytokines (such as IL-6, IL-8, IL-1α) and matrix remodeling regulatory metalloproteases (such as MMP1 and MMP13) [6], expressed highly. SASP is able to induce inflammation that may lead to low-grade chronic inflammation and invovled in degenerative disorders including OA [7–10]. Viewed from the molecular perspective, OA is an outcome of cartilage degradation. The hallmark event in OA is the extracellular matrix degradation of articular cartilage [11]. Type II procollagen (COL2A1) helps maintain skeletal structure of cartilage [12]. The degradation of COL2A1 in cartilage matrix is critical in initiating cartilage degradation. So far, OA remains difficult to be treated, and the treatment strategies are largely restricted to symptom management [13]. Thus, preventing destruction of COL2A1 and the secretion of SASP may be helpful to delay the progression of OA.

The transcript of p16INK4a derives from alternative splicing of *INK4a/ARF* [14]. By binding to CDK4 and CDK6 and repressing phosphorylation of pRb, p16INK4a is well known as a cell cycle regulator [15]. Moreover, the increased expression of p16INK4a is often accompanied

* Correspondence: xinyuhu_33yhx@163.com
[2]Orthopedic Trauma Department, The First People's Hospital of Changzhou, No.185 Juqian Street, Changzhou, Jiangsu Province 213003, China
Full list of author information is available at the end of the article

with cell senescence [16, 17].In addition, dysregulation of p16INK4a is common among human cancers [14, 18]. Researchers suggested that p16INK4a may participate in tumor cell escape from senescence [19, 20]. E2F2 is also a transcription factor that belongs to E2F family. Similar to p16INK4a, E2F2 takes part in cell cycle regulation [21, 22]. It has been reported that E2Fs could be released from pRb and could promote the G1/S. In addition, E2F2 can also maintain quiescence by repressing cell cycle regulators [21]. Researchers have proved that the transfection of E2F decoy oligodeoxynucleotides was helpful in preventing the generation of MMP-1, IL-1β and IL-6 [23]. As an apparent increase of E2F2 has been observed by researchers in rheumatoid arthritis (RA) synovial tissues [24], thus, it can be speculated that p16INK4a and E2F2 may participate in the progression of OA.

The aim of this study was to investigate the potential roles of p16INK4a and E2F2 in OA and to examine possible relations between p16INK4a and E2F2 in OA. The current study would expand the current understanding on pathophysiology of OA and provide promising drug target candidates for treating OA.

Methods

Cell culture

Human chondrocytes (#4650, ScienCell, USA) were cryopreserved at P0 and delivered frozen. The cells were cultured in DMEM/F-12 (Gibco, USA) containing 10% FBS at 37 °C. The medium was supplemented with 100 U/ml and penicillin/streptomycin. As previously described [25–27], recombinant IL-1β (R&D Systems) (10 ng/ml) was used to induce cartilage injury for 48 h. Experiments were performed independently for at least 3 times.

Cell transfection

The cells (1.0×10^5 cells per well) were seeded into 24-well plate. Prior to transfection, the cells have been starved overnight. pCMV-HA vector was a gift from Christopher A Walsh (Addgene plasmid #32530), pCMV-p16 INK4A was a gift from Bob Weinberg, (Addgene plasmid # 10916) and pCMV-HA-E2F2 was a gift from KristianHelin (Addgene plasmid # 24226) [28, 29]. The E2F2 siRNA (MBS8214676) and siRNA negative control (MBS8241404) were purchased from MyBio Source. The plasmid was transfected into the cells using Lipo 3000 Reagent (Life Science, USA). After being transfected for 6 h, the cells were maintained in fresh medium supplemented with 10% FBS and then prepared for the subsequent experiments.

Cell proliferation assay

Cells (4000 cells/well) were plated into 24-well tissue culture plates (Corning Inc., Corning, NY). Cell proliferation

was determined by using sulphonatedtetrazolium salt, and 4-[3-(4-iodophenyl)-2-(4-nitrophenyl)-2H-5-tetrazolio]-1 and 3-benzene disulphonate (WST-1) cell counting kits (Beyotime, China), following the manufactory's instructions. The OD at 450 nm was read using a microplate reader (Biorad, USA).

Enzyme-linked immunosorbent (ELISA) assay

The cells were harvested and centrifuged at 3000 g at 4 °C for 10 min. Following the manufacturer's protocol, the levels of SASP markers TGFβ, IL-6, IL-8, IL-1α, MMP3 and MMP13 in the collected supernatants were examined using ELISA kits (R&D Systems). The absorbance was read at 405 nm using a microplate reader (Bio-rad, USA).

Real-time PCR

Total RNA was isolated from cells using Trizol regent (Life Science) following the manufacturer'sprotocol. cDNA was reversed from total RNA using PrimeScript™ II 1st Strand cDNA Synthesis Kit (Takara, Japan). Amplification of the target genes from cDNA was performed using SYBR Green real-time PCR Master Mix (ToYoBo, Japan) under the conditions as follows: at 95 °C for 10 s, 40 cycles at 95 °C for 5 s and at 60 °C for 30 s. The primers used for RT-PCR were as follows:

p16INK4a sense: 5'- GCGGG GAGCAGCATGGAGC-3';
p16INK4a anti-sense: 5'- CCGAATAGTTACG GTCG-3';
E2F2 sense:5'-CCTTGGAGGCTACTGACAGC-3';
E2F2antisense: 5'-CCACAGGTAGTCGTCCTGGT-3';
Col II sense: 5'-CAATCCAGCAAACGTTCCCA-3';
Col II antisense: 5'-CAGGCGTAGGAAGGTCATCT-3';
Cdc6 sense: 5'- CAGCTGTTGAACTTCCCACC-3';
Cdc6 antisense: 5'- GCTCTCCTGCAAACATCCAG-3';
MCM6 sense: 5'-CCGAAATCCAGTTTGTGCCA-3';
MCM6 antisense: 5'-TGCTAAGCTTGGAGACGTCA-3';
β-actin sense: 5'-CTAAGGCCAACCGTGAAAAG-3';
β-actin antisense: 5'-AACACAGCCTGGATGGCTAC-3'.

Western blot

The cells were collected using cell lysissolution (Sigma) and denatured at 100 °C for 5 min. The protein concentrations were tested using bicinchoninic acid (BCA) Protein Assay Kit (Pierce, USA). Dodecyl sulphate polyacrylamide gel (SDS-PAGE) electrophoresis was performed to separate the proteins. Next, the proteins were transblotted onto nitrocellulose membranes (Amersham, USA). Primary antibodies were added after the membranes have been blocked with 5% not-fat milk. Then, the membranes were maintained at 4 °C overnight. Primary antibodies were as follows: anti-Col2A1 (1:8000, ab34712,abcam), anti-E2F2 (1:1000, ab65222), anti-p16INK4a (1:5000,ab108349) and anti-β-actin (ab8226,1:5000). Secondary antibodies (abcam) were incubated at room temperature for 2 h. The blot bands were developed with Enhanced chemiluminescence (Amersham).The density of bands was quantified using Quantity one 4.6.2.

Statistics

Data were shown as mean ± Standard Deviation (SD). Student's t test or one-way analysis of variance (ANOVA) following Dunett's post hoc tests was used to compare result differences. $P < 0.05$ was considered as statistically significant.

Results

p16INK4a and E2F2 were up-regulated in Interleukin (IL)-1β- induced cartilage injury

Interleukin (IL)-1β, an important proinflammatory cytokine, contributes to the degradation of Col2A1 during OA [30, 31]. According to previous studies [32, 33], we detected the expressions of Col2A1, p16INK4a and E2F2 in the presence of 1, 5, 10 ng/ml IL-1β. We found that the expression of Col2A1 was decreased by IL-1β, while the expression of p16INK4a and E2F2 was increased by IL-1β. The effect of IL-1β was strongest at the 10 ng/ml (Fig. 1a-b). Thus, we selected 10 ng/ml IL-1β to treat the chondrocytes. In addition, the expression of E2F1 remains stable under the treatment of IL-1β (Fig. 1c). As shown in Fig. 2a, the secretion of SASP markers, which included TGFβ, IL-6, IL-8, IL-1α, MMP3 and MMP13 was induced by the treatment of 10 ng/ml IL-1β.

The effect of p16INK4a over-expression on cartilage injury

p16INK4a has been recognized as a senescent contributor in various tissues [34]. The expression of SASP markers was determined in order to investigate the role of p16INK4a in cartilage injury. The results showed that over-expression of p16INK4a enhanced the secretion of TGFβ, IL-6, IL-8, IL-1α, MMP3 and MMP13 (Fig. 3a), and that the expression of Col2A1 was also reduced by over-expression of p16INK4a. Interestingly, the expression of E2F2 was higher in p16INK4a group than that in control group (Fig. 3b-c).

E2F2 was necessary for the cartilage injury caused by over-expression of p16INK4a

The effect of E2F2 on cartilage injury was examined in order to further study the potential relation between p16INK4a and E2F2. As shown in Fig. 4, compared to control group, the over-expressions of both p16INK4a and E2F2 reduced the expression of Col2A1, which was then increased by the depletion of E2F2. Moreover, the expression of Col2A1 was found to be lower in p16INK4a + si-E2F2 group than that in p16INK4a group. Nevertheless, the expression of Col2A1 was slightly reduced in p16INK4a + E2F2 group, compared to that in p16INK4a group. Furthermore, results from ELISA showed that secretion of SASP markers (TGFβ, IL-6, IL-8, IL-1α, MMP3 and MMP13) was increased in

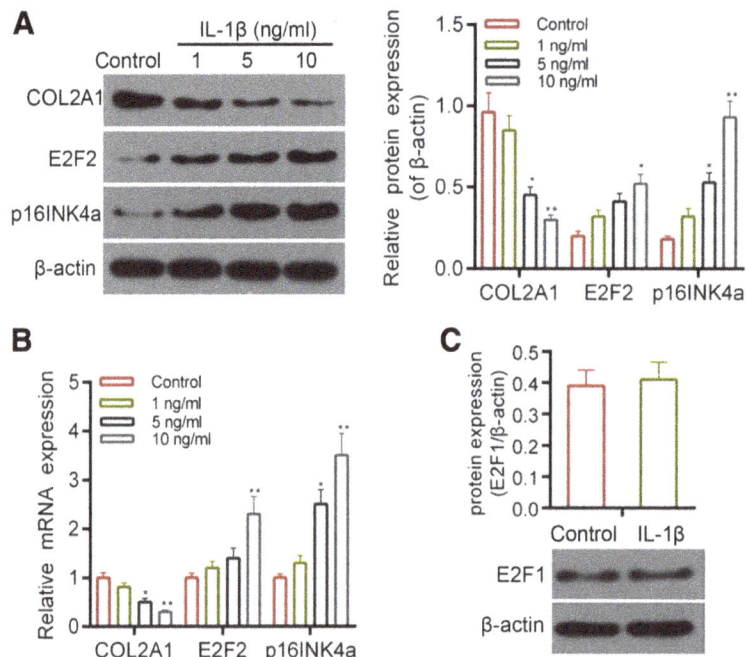

Fig. 1 (**a**) Western blot assay for the expression of Col2A1, p16INK4a and E2F2. (**b**) Real-time PCR (RT-PCR) for the expression of Col2A1, p16INK4a and E2F2. (**c**) Western blot assay for the expression of E2F2 in the cells treated with 10 ng/ml IL-1β.*$P < 0.05$,**$P < 0.01$ vs. control. Data are shown as mean ± SD, $n = 4$

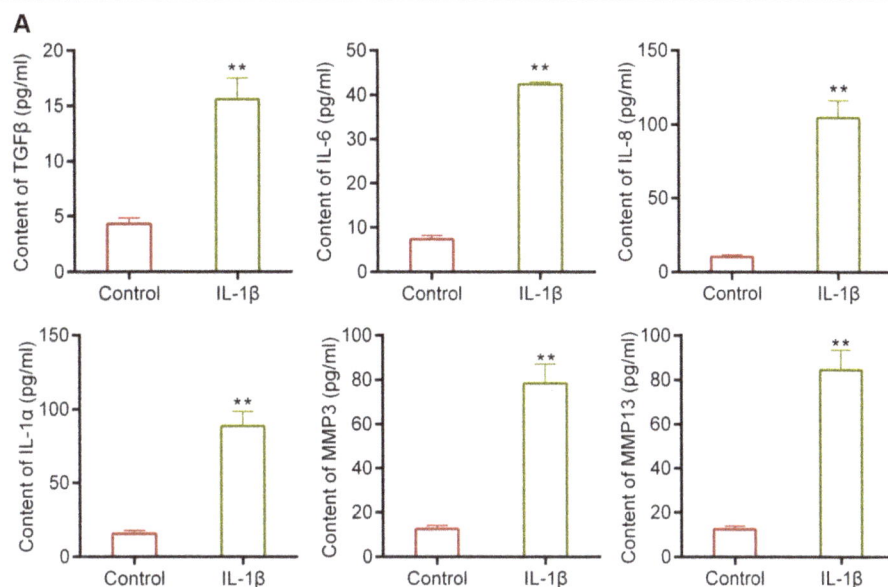

Fig. 2 (**a**) Determination of the secretion of SASP markers, including TGFβ, IL-6, IL-8, IL-1α, MMP3 and MMP13, using ELISA assay. **P < 0.01 vs. control. IL-1β, cells were treated with IL-1β. Data were shown as mean ± SD, n = 5

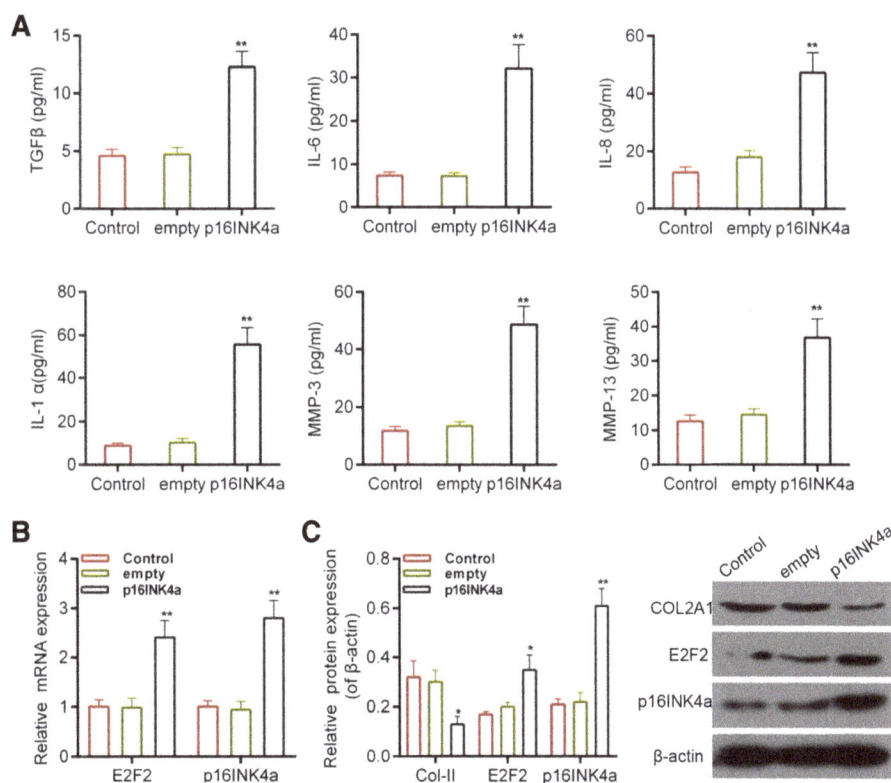

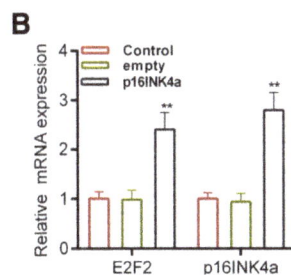

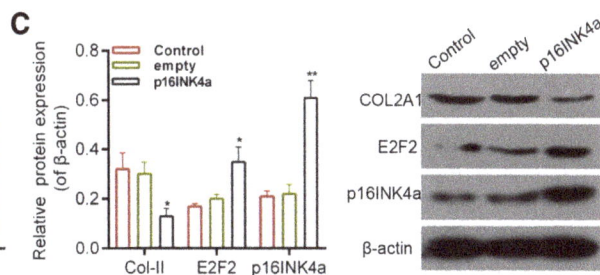

Fig. 3 (**a**) ELISA assay for the secretion of SASP markers after the over-expression of p16INK4a. (**b**) RT-PCR for detecting the expressions of Col2A1, p16INK4a and E2F2. (**c**) The expressions of Col2A1, p16INK4a and E2F2 by Western blot assay. *P < 0.05 and **P < 0.01 vs. empty. Empty, cells were transfected with over-expression empty vector; p16INK4a, cells were transfected with p16INK4a over-expression vector. Data were shown as mean ± SD, n = 5

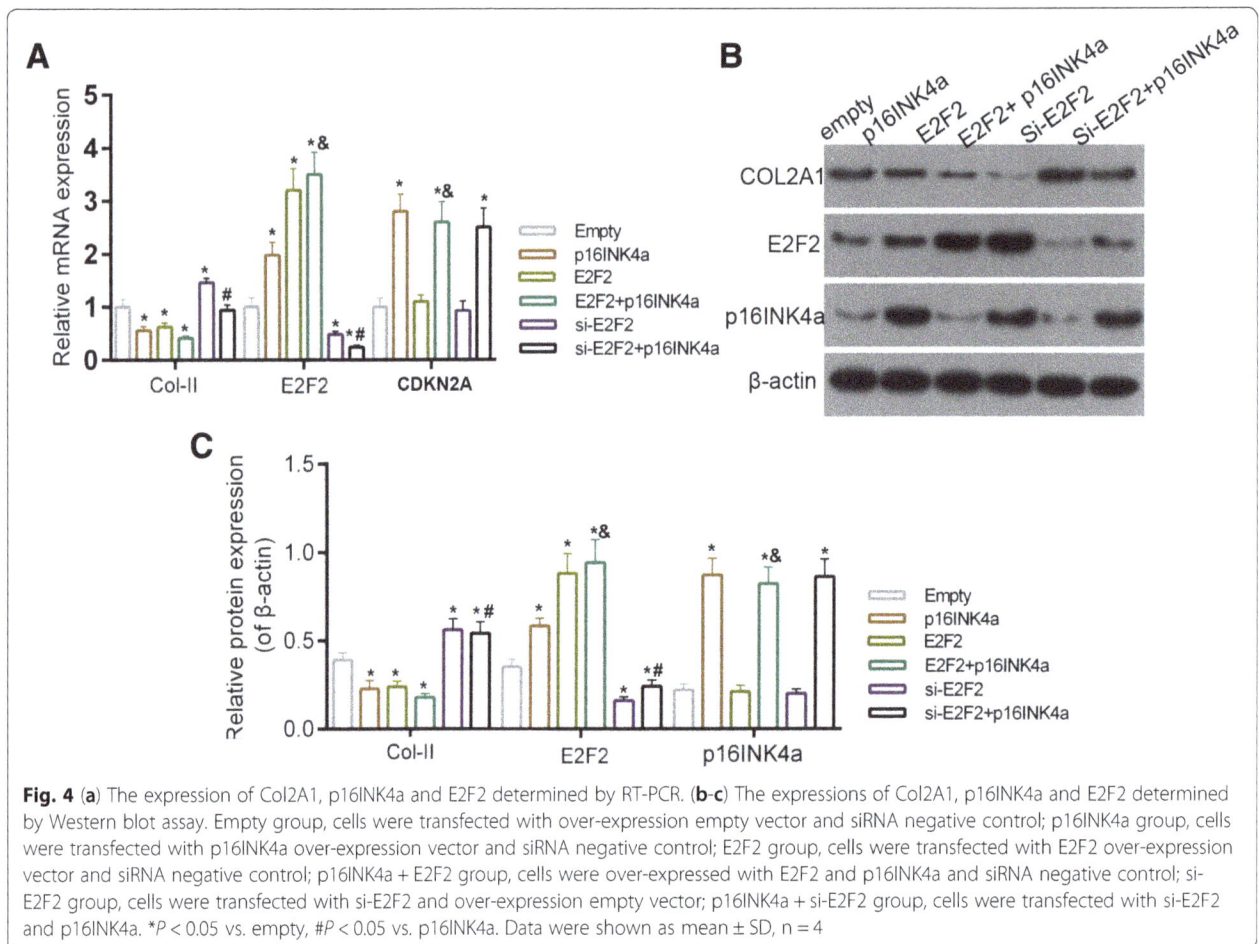

Fig. 4 (**a**) The expression of Col2A1, p16INK4a and E2F2 determined by RT-PCR. (**b-c**) The expressions of Col2A1, p16INK4a and E2F2 determined by Western blot assay. Empty group, cells were transfected with over-expression empty vector and siRNA negative control; p16INK4a group, cells were transfected with p16INK4a over-expression vector and siRNA negative control; E2F2 group, cells were transfected with E2F2 over-expression vector and siRNA negative control; p16INK4a + E2F2 group, cells were over-expressed with E2F2 and p16INK4a and siRNA negative control; si-E2F2 group, cells were transfected with si-E2F2 and over-expression empty vector; p16INK4a + si-E2F2 group, cells were transfected with si-E2F2 and p16INK4a. *$P < 0.05$ vs. empty, #$P < 0.05$ vs. p16INK4a. Data were shown as mean ± SD, $n = 4$

p16INK4a and E2F2 groups, while such a secretion was repressed in si-E2F2 group. Moreover, compared to that in p16INK4a group, the secretion of SASP markers was inhibited in p16INK4a + si-E2F2 group (Fig. 5).

The effect of p16INK4a over-expression on cell proliferation of chondrocytes

Cell proliferation was determined by using the WST-1 cell counting kit. We found that transfection of p16INK4a or E2F2 resulted in a significant inhibition of cell proliferation. The down-regulation of E2F2 was observed to recover the proliferation of cells that have been transfected with p16INK4a (Fig. 6a). In addition, the mRNA expression of cell cycle-specific genes was detected, and the data showed that transfection of p16INK4a or E2F2 inhibited the expressions of CDC6 and MCM6, and that the down-regulation of E2F2 rescued the expressions of CDC6 and MCM6 in the cells that have been transfected with p16INK4a (Fig. 6b).

Discussion

Tissue deconstruction is a consequence of aging. The integrity and function loss in senescent cells are caused by chronic inflammation and remodel of extracellular matrix [35, 36]. OA is a degenerative disease accompanied with progressive cartilage degradation. Aging is one of the most significant risk factors in OA [1, 2]. Although the mechanisms underlies OA awaits to be fully understood, the cartilage integrity is believed to be affected by inflammatory cytokines and matrix remodeling.

In this study, based on a previous study [37], IL-1β was used to induce the cartilage degradation so as to establish a model of OA. The secretion of SASP markers TGFβ, IL-6, IL-8, IL-1α, MMP3 and MMP13 was found to be increased in response to IL-1β treatment. Moreover, the expression of Col2A1, an index of cartilage degradation [38], was reduced in IL-1β group in comparison to that in control group. p16INK4a is realted to age-related diseases [39]. As expected, the expression of p16INK4a was strongly induced by IL-1β. Consistent to our results, a previous study has also pointed out that SASP was exhibited in p16INK4a-positive cells [36]. A study has also reported that expression of p16INK4a was a biomarker of chondrocyte aging and was correlated with several SASP transcripts even though the loss of p16 did not affect the expression of SASP in mouse

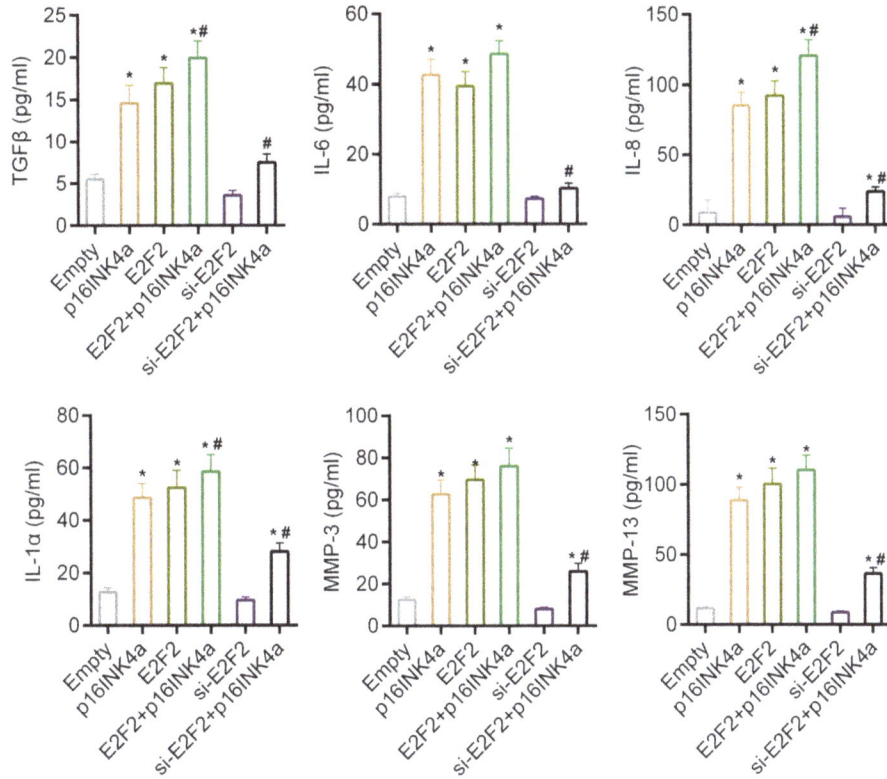

Fig. 5 ELISA assay for SASP markers. Empty group, cells were transfected with over-expression empty vector and siRNA negative control. p16INK4a group, E2F2 indicated the over-expressions of p16INK4a and E2F2 respectively. Si-E2F2 indicated the depletion of E2F2. *P < 0.05 vs. empty. #P < 0.05, vs. p16INK4a. Data were shown as mean ± SD, n = 5

[40].These results revealed that the expression of p16INK4a was positively related to the secretion of SASP during cartilage injury. However, SASP can also be restrained by p16INK4a under some conditions [41]. The different effect of p16INK4a on SASP may be caused by different cell contexts. In addition, as a transcription factor, E2F2 was increased in RA synovial tissues [24]. Thus, we determined the expression of E2F2 in IL-1β-treated cells, and found a higher expression of E2F2 in IL-1β group in comparison to that in control group. As a family member of E2F2, E2F1 may have an overlapping function with E2F2.

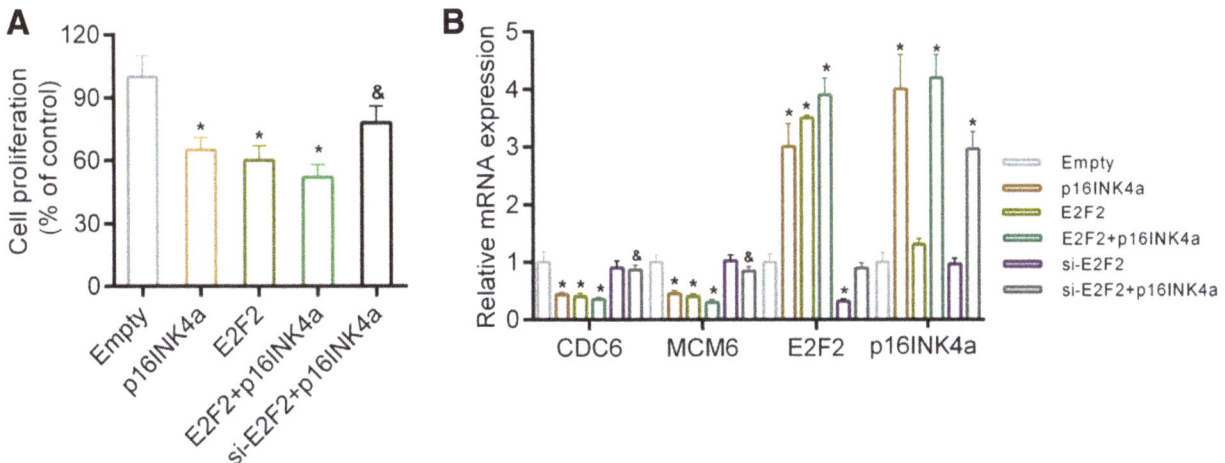

Fig. 6 (a) Cell proliferation was detected by WST-1 cell counting kit. *P < 0.05 vs. control. Data were shown as mean ± SD, n = 5. (b) The expressions of CDC6, MCM6, p16INK4a and E2F2 determined by RT-PCR. Data were shown as mean ± SD, n = 4.*P < 0.05 vs. empty.&P < 0.05, vs. p16INK4a

Nevertheless, the expression of E2F1 was not affected by IL-1β.

It has been proved that p16INK4a was able to inhibit cell cycle by targeting CDK4/6, and therefore maintaining the activity of retinoblastoma (pRb) that could control cell fate decision of chondrocytes [42–44]. E2F family members can be released from pocket protein members (retinoblastoma, p107 and p130) and can promote the G1/S progression [45, 46]. The effect of p16INK4a over-expression was examined in this study. Our results showed that secretion of SASP was promoted by over-expressing p16INK4a. Furthermore, the expressions of Col2A1 and E2F2 were higher in p16INK4a group in comparison to those in control. Taken together, the cartilage injury was expanded by over-expressing p16INK4a. In addition, the increased expression level of E2F2 may exacerbate cartilage injury. Consistently, some recent studies pointed that E2F2 functioned as a repressor of transcription and an inhibitor of cell proliferation in some cell context [47, 48]. Therefore, it is possible that E2F2 may interact with other proteins or factors functioning as a negative transcriptional regulator [49].

Subsequent investigations were performed to further determine whether E2F2 was necessary for cartilage injury caused by p16INK4a. Our results indicated that cartilage injury was induced by over-expressing p16INK4a and E2F2, by increasing the secretion of SASP markers and by repressing the expression of Col2A1. Moreover, we detected the expressions of cell cycle specific genes (CDC6 and MCM6). CDC6 is essential for the assembly of MCM complex in DNA replication and that MCM complex assembly is necessary for cells to enter S-phase [50].The cell proliferation and the expressions of CDC6 and MCM6 were inhibited by over-expressing p16INK4a or E2F2. The down-regulation of E2F2 in the cells transfected with p16INK4a was observed to recover the cell proliferation and the expressions of CDC6 and MCM6. However, according to previous studies, the peak expressions of CDC6 and MCM6 are in G1/S during DNA replication and are dependent on E2F [51–53]. Thus, it is possible that over-expressing E2F2 might prevent cell cycle progression through competitive inhibition of E2F2 transcriptional activity (though the mechanism underlying such a competitive inhibition was not clear). Taken together, the depletion of E2F2 alleviated cartilage injury caused by p16INK4a, suggesting that E2F2 was necessary for p16INK4a-induced OA progression. Nevertheless, the co-expression of p16INK4a and E2F2 increased the secretion of TGFβ and IL-8 in comparison to over-expressing p16INK4a alone. However, no significant synergistic action of p16INK4a and E2F2 was observed. A previous study has shown that other signals or pathways, for example, p38 MAPK and extracellular signal-regulated kinase (ERK) signaling, also took part in cell senescence [54]. This may be explained by the fact that cartilage degradation is controlled by many other signals and regulators [55, 56]. Therefore, the molecular mechanism of cartilage degradation still remains to be further investigated.

In addition, microRNAs have also been used in diagnosis of OA. For instance, Researchers have proved that p16INK4a could be regulated by miR-24 during matrix remodeling in OA [57]. Therefore, it would be helpful for the diagnosis and molecular treatment of OA to explore the same type of regulators of p16INK4a during OA. Although it can be concluded that E2F2 is a downstream target of p16INK4a, unfortunately, within the scope of this study, we were unable to provide a specific explanation about how p16INK4a regulated E2F2. Thus, it would be interesting to study whether SASP markers and/or Col2A1can be directly regulated by E2F2. It is beneficial to further illustrate the molecular pathological of cartilage degradation during OA.

Conclusions
In summary, this study demonstrated that over-expression of p16INK4a promoted cartilage injury. Over-expression of p16INK4a increased the secretion of SASP markers and reduced the expression of Col2A1. Moreover, the expression of E2F2 was necessary for p16INK4a-induced cartilage injury. Overall, this study determined the role of p16INK4a/E2F2 in OA, and such a result helped provide therapeutic targets for treating OA.

Authors' contributions
Substantial contributions to conception and design: XB. Data acquisition, data analysis and interpretation: XH. Drafting the article or critically revising it for important intellectual content: XH. Final approval of the version to be published: XB, XH.

Competing interests
The authors declare that they have no competing interests.

Author details
Department of Orthopedics, The First People's Hospital of Changzhou, No.185 Juqian Street, Changzhou, Jiangsu Province 213003, China. ²Orthopedic Trauma Department, The First People's Hospital of Changzhou, No.185 Juqian Street, Changzhou, Jiangsu Province 213003, China.

References
1. Yang JH, et al. Osteoarthritis Affects Health-Related Quality of Life in Korean Adults with Chronic Diseases: The Korea National Health and Nutritional Examination Surveys 2009-2013. Korean J Fam Med. 2017;38(6):358–64.
2. Dillon CF, Rasch EK, Gu Q, Hirsch R. Prevalence of knee osteoarthritis in the United States: arthritis data from the third National Health and nutrition examination survey 1991-94. J Rheumatol. 2006;33(11):2271–9.
3. Katz SI. Commentary: setting priorities for research funding at the National Institute of Arthritis and Musculoskeletal and Skin Diseases (NIAMS). J Am Acad Dermatol. 2015;73(3):392–4. https://doi.org/10.1016/j.jaad.2015.06.014.
4. Glyn-Jones S, Palmer AJ, Agricola R, Price AJ, Vincent TL, Weinans H, Carr AJ. Osteoarthritis. Lancet. 2015;386(9991):376–87.

5. Loeser RF. Aging and osteoarthritis: the role of chondrocyte senescence and aging changes in the cartilage matrix. Osteoarthr Cartil. 2009;17(8): 971–9.

6. Rodier F, Campisi J. Four faces of cellular senescence. J Cell Biol. 2011;192(4): 547–56.

7. Kumar M, Seeger W, Voswinckel R. Senescence-associated secretory phenotype and its possible role in chronic obstructive pulmonary disease. Am J Respir Cell Mol Biol. 2014;51(3):323–33.

8. Zhu Y, Armstrong JL, Tchkonia T, Kirkland JL. Cellular senescence and the senescent secretory phenotype in age-related chronic diseases. Curr Opin Clin Nutr Metab Care. 2014;17(4):324–8.

9. Campisi J, Andersen JK, Kapahi P, Melov S. Cellular senescence: a link between cancer and age-related degenerative disease? Semin Cancer Biol. 2011;21(6):354–9.

10. Onat A, Can G. Enhanced proinflammatory state and autoimmune activation: a breakthrough to understanding chronic diseases. Curr Pharm Des. 2014;20(4): 575–84.

11. Aigner T, Rose J, Martin J, Buckwalter J. Aging theories of primary osteoarthritis: from epidemiology to molecular biology. Rejuvenation Res. 2004;7(2):134–45.

12. Gao Y, Liu S, Huang J, Guo W, Chen J, Zhang L, Zhao B, Peng J, Wang A, Wang Y, et al. The ECM-cell interaction of cartilage extracellular matrix on chondrocytes. Biomed Res Int. 2014;648459(10):18.

13. Ni GX, Li Z, Zhou YZ. The role of small leucine-rich proteoglycans in osteoarthritis pathogenesis. Osteoarthr Cartil. 2014;22(7):896–903.

14. Sharpless NE, DePinho RA. The INK4A/ARF locus and its two gene products. Curr Opin Genet Dev. 1999;9(1):22–30.

15. Hayward RL, Smyth JF. Editorial comment on 'A senescence program controlled by p53 and p16INK4a contributes to the outcome of cancer therapy' by Schmitt et al. Eur J Cancer. 2002;38(17):2207–9.

16. Robles SJ, Adami GR. Agents that cause DNA double strand breaks lead to p16INK4a enrichment and the premature senescence of normal fibroblasts. Oncogene. 1998;16(9):1113–23.

17. Serrano M, Lin AW, McCurrach ME, Beach D, Lowe SW. Oncogenic ras provokes premature cell senescence associated with accumulation of p53 and p16INK4a. Cell. 1997;88(5):593–602.

18. Stott FJ, Bates S, James MC, McConnell BB, Starborg M, Brookes S, Palmero I, Ryan K, Hara E, Vousden KH, et al. The alternative product from the human CDKN2A locus, p14(ARF), participates in a regulatory feedback loop with p53 and MDM2. EMBO J. 1998;17(17):5001–14.

19. Ohtani N, Yamakoshi K, Takahashi A, Hara E. The p16INK4a-RB pathway: molecular link between cellular senescence and tumor suppression. J Med Investig. 2004;51(3–4):146–53.

20. Oruetxebarria I, Venturini F, Kekarainen T, Houweling A, Zuijderduijn LM, Mohd-Sarip A, Vries RG, Hoeben RC, Verrijzer CP. P16INK4a is required for hSNF5 chromatin remodeler-induced cellular senescence in malignant rhabdoid tumor cells. J Biol Chem. 2004;279(5):3807–16.

21. Infante A, Laresgoiti U, Fernández-Rueda J, Fullaondo A, Galán J, Díaz-Uriarte R, Malumbres M, Field SJ, Zubiaga AM. E2F represses cell cycle regulators to maintain quiescence. Cell Cycle. 2008;7(24):3915–27.

22. Chen Q, Hung FC, Fromm L, Overbeek PA. Induction of cell cycle entry and cell death in postmitotic lens fiber cells by overexpression of E2F1 or E2F2. Invest Ophthalmol Vis Sci. 2000;41(13):4223.

23. Tomita T, Kunugiza Y, Tomita N, Takano H, Morishita R, Kaneda Y, Yoshikawa H. E2F decoy oligodeoxynucleotide ameliorates cartilage invasion by infiltrating synovium derived from rheumatoid arthritis. Int J Mol Med. 2006; 18(2):257–65.

24. Chang X, Yue L, Liu W, Wang Y, Wang L, Xu B, Pan J, Yan X. CD38 and E2F transcription factor 2 have uniquely increased expression in rheumatoid arthritis synovial tissues. Clin Exp Immunol. 2014;176(2):222–31.

25. Montaseri A, Busch F, Mobasheri A, Buhrmann C, Aldinger C, Rad JS, Shakibaei M. IGF-1 and PDGF-bb suppress IL-1β-induced cartilage degradation through down-regulation of NF-κB signaling: involvement of Src/PI-3K/AKT pathway. PLoS One. 2011;6(12):e28663.

26. Chen CT, Park S, Bhargava M, Torzilli PA. Inhibitory Effect of Mechanical Load on IL-1 Induced Cartilage Degradation Is Mediated by Interferon-Gamma and IL-1 Receptor 1. In: ASME 2008 Summer Bioengineering Conference; 2008. p. 713–4.

27. Wang J, Chen L, Jin S, Lin J, Zheng H, Zhang H, Fan H, He F, Ma S, Li Q. Altered expression of microRNA-98 in IL-1β-induced cartilage degradation and its role in chondrocyte apoptosis. Mol Med Rep. 2017;16(3):3208–16.

28. Lukas J, Petersen BO, Holm K, Bartek J, Helin K. Deregulated expression of E2F family members induces S-phase entry and overcomes p16INK4A-mediated growth suppression. Mol Cell Biol. 1996;16(3):1047–57.

29. Medema RH, Herrera RE, Lam F, Weinberg RA. Growth suppression by p16ink4 requires functional retinoblastoma protein. Proc Natl Acad Sci U S A. 1995;92(14):6289–93.

30. Li Z, Meng D, Li G, Xu J, Tian K, Li Y. Celecoxib combined with Diacerein effectively alleviates osteoarthritis in rats via regulating JNK and p38MAPK signaling pathways. Inflammation. 2015;38(4):1563–72.

31. Mabey T, Honsawek S. Cytokines as biochemical markers for knee osteoarthritis. World J Orthop. 2015;6(1):95–105.

32. Legendre F, Baugé C, Roche R, Saurel AS, Pujol JP. Chondroitin sulfate modulation of matrix and inflammatory gene expression in IL-1beta-stimulated chondrocytes--study in hypoxic alginate bead cultures. Osteoarthritis Cartilage. 2008;16(1):105.

33. Yuan Y, Zhang GQ, Chai W, Ni M, Xu C, Chen JY. Silencing of microRNA-138-5p promotes IL-1β-induced cartilage degradation in human chondrocytes by targeting FOXC1:miR-138 promotes cartilage degradation. Bone Joint Res. 2016;5(10):523.

34. Zindy F, Quelle DE, Roussel MF, Sherr CJ. Expression of the p16INK4a tumor suppressor versus other INK4 family members during mouse development and aging. Oncogene. 1997;15(2):203–11.

35. Ba TH, et al. Chronic autoimmune-mediated inflammation: a senescent immune response to injury. Drug Discovery Today. 2013;18(7-8):372–9.

36. Coppe JP, Desprez PY, Krtolica A, Campisi J. The senescence-associated secretory phenotype: the dark side of tumor suppression. Annu Rev Pathol. 2010;5:99–118.

37. van de Loo FA, Joosten LA, van Lent PL, Arntz OJ, van den Berg WB. Role of interleukin-1, tumor necrosis factor alpha, and interleukin-6 in cartilage proteoglycan metabolism and destruction. Effect of in situ blocking in murine antigen- and zymosan-induced arthritis. Arthritis Rheum. 1995; 38(2):164–72.

38. Christgau S, Garnero P, Fledelius C, Moniz C, Ensig M, Gineyts E, Rosenquist C, Qvist P. Collagen type II C-telopeptide fragments as an index of cartilage degradation. Bone. 2001;29(3):209.

39. Baker DJ, Wijshake T, Tchkonia T, LeBrasseur NK, Childs BG, van de Sluis B, Kirkland JL, van Deursen JM. Clearance of p16Ink4a-positive senescent cells delays ageing-associated disorders. Nature. 2011; 479(7372):232–6.

40. Diekman BO, Sessions GA, Collins JA, Knecht AK, Strum SL, Mitin NK, Carlson CS, Loeser RF, Sharpless NE. Expression of p16INK4a is a biomarker of chondrocyte aging but does not cause osteoarthritis. Aging Cell. 2018; 17(4):e12771.

41. Coppé JP, Rodier F, Patil CK, Freund A, Desprez PY, Campisi J. Tumor suppressor and aging biomarker p16INK4a induces cellular senescence without the associated inflammatory secretory phenotype. J Biol Chem. 2011;286(42):36396–403.

42. Miller JP, Yeh N, Vidal A, Koff A. Interweaving the cell cycle machinery with cell differentiation. Cell Cycle. 2007;6(23):2932–8.

43. LuValle P, Beier F. Cell cycle control in growth plate chondrocytes. Front Biosci. 2000;1(5):D493–503.

44. Yeh N, Miller JP, Gaur T, Capellini TD, Nikolich-Zugich J, de la Hoz C, Selleri L, Bromage TG, van Wijnen AJ, Stein GS, et al. Cooperation between p27 and p107 during endochondral ossification suggests a genetic pathway controlled by p27 and p130. Mol Cell Biol. 2007;27(14):5161–71.

45. Johnson DG, Cress WD, Jakoi L, Nevins JR. Oncogenic capacity of the E2F1 gene. Proc Natl Acad Sci U S A. 1994;91(26):12823–7.

46. Zacksenhaus E, Jiang Z, Phillips RA, Gallie BL. Dual mechanisms of repression of E2F1 activity by the retinoblastoma gene product. EMBO J. 1996;15(21): 5917–27.

47. Pusapati RV, Weaks RL, Rounbehler RJ, Mcarthur MJ, Johnson DG. E2F2 suppresses Myc-induced proliferation and tumorigenesis. Mol Carcinog. 2010;49(2):152–6.

48. Chen D, Chen Y, Forrest D, Bremner R. E2f2 induces cone photoreceptor apoptosis independent of E2f1 and E2f3. Cell Death Differ. 2013;20(7): 931–40.

49. Laresgoiti U, Apraiz A, Olea M, Mitxelena J, Osinalde N, Rodriguez JA, Fullaondo A, Zubiaga AM. E2F2 and CREB cooperatively regulate transcriptional activity of cell cycle genes. Nucleic Acids Res. 2013; 41(22):10185–98.

50. Cook JG, Park CH, Burke TW, Leone G, Degregori J, Engel A, Nevins JR. Analysis of Cdc6 function in the assembly of mammalian prereplication complexes. Proc Natl Acad Sci U S A. 2002;99(3):1347–52.

51. Hateboer G, Wobst A, Petersen BO, Le CL, Vigo E, Sardet C, Helin K. Cell cycle-regulated expression of mammalian CDC6 is dependent on E2F. Mol Cell Biol. 1998;18(11):6679–97.

52. Borlado LR, Méndez J. CDC6: from DNA replication to cell cycle checkpoints and oncogenesis. Carcinogenesis. 2008;29(2):237–43.

53. Ohtani K, Iwanaga R, Nakamura M, Ikeda M, Yabuta N, Tsuruga H, Nojima H. Cell growth-regulated expression of mammalian MCM5 and MCM6 genes mediated by the transcription factor E2F. Oncogene. 1999;18(14):2299–309.

54. Hasasna HE, et al. Rhus coriaria induces senescence and autophagic cell death in breast cancer cells through a mechanism involving p38 and ERK1/2 activation. Scientific Reports. 2015;5.

55. Buckland J. Osteoarthritis: epigenetic clues into the molecular basis of OA. Nat Rev Rheumatol. 2014;10(7):383.

56. Hashimoto M, Nakasa T, Hikata T, Asahara H. Molecular network of cartilage homeostasis and osteoarthritis. Med Res Rev. 2008;28(3):464–81.

57. Philipot D, Guerit D, Platano D, Chuchana P, Olivotto E, Espinoza F, Dorandeu A, Pers YM, Piette J, Borzi RM, et al. p16INK4a and its regulator miR-24 link senescence and chondrocyte terminal differentiation-associated matrix remodeling in osteoarthritis. Arthritis Res Ther. 2014;16(1):p. R58.

8

Phospholipase C signaling activated by parathyroid hormone mediates the rapid osteoclastogenesis in the fracture healing of orchiectomized mice

Wei Li[1†], Liang Yuan[1†], Guojun Tong[1], Youhua He[1], Yue Meng[1], Song Hao[1], Jianting Chen[1], Jun Guo[2], Richard Bringhurst[2] and Dehong Yang[1*]

Abstract

Background: The age-related osteoporosis is an increasing risk severely threatening the live quality of aged people. Human parathyroid hormone (hPTH) is applied to the therapy of osteoporosis successfully, however, the mechanism, especially the signaling pathway activated in the healing fracture by PTH is still unknown.

Methods: The once daily injections of hPTH(1–34) and GR (1–34) (the PLC deficient analog) into the orchiectomized male mice with bone fracture, were started at the second day after fracture and lasted for 4 weeks. To explore the role of phospholipase C signaling in the androgen-deficient fracture healing, the fracture healing were evaluated via radiography, micro-CT, biomechanics testing, serum biochemistry, bone marrow cell culture and gene expression quantification.

Results: After two weeks of fracture, both peptides significantly increased bone mineral density (BMD), bone mass content (BMC) and bone volume (BV/TV) in the healing area. However, compared to hPTH(1–34), GR(1–34) induced more woven bones, the higher BMC and BMD, as well as the less serum TRAP and osteoclasts. After four weeks of treatment, the effects of hPTH(1–34) on fracture healing showed no difference to those of GR(1–34). Consistently, GR(1–34) induced the similar osteogenesis but less osteoclastogenesis under the ex vivo condition immediately after administration compared to hPTH(1–34), which was verified by the weaker activation of RANKL, NFATC1, TRAP and Cathepsin K in GR(1–34) treatment.

Conclusion: These results indicated that the PLC signaling activated by the intermittent injection of hPTH(1–34) leads to the bone resorption by rapidly activating the osteoclastogenesis in the fracture healing zone.

Keywords: Parathyroid hormone, Fracture healing, Phopholipase C, Osteoporosis, Osteoclastogenesis

Background

Previous studies showed that both the osteoporosis-related morbidity and mortality in men actually were higher than those in women in later life [1, 2]. The increased risk of fractures is closely associated with the decline of testosterone production, which causes a high turnover bone loss from cancellous bone sites [1, 3, 4]. However, supplement of androgen or testosterone replacement therapy takes a high risk of causing complications in circulating, urinary and endocrine systems [5–7]. By far, the most reliable bone-forming medicine for male osteoporosis without triggering severe complications is human parathyroid hormone (hPTH) [2], a key factor regulating the systemic metabolism of calcium and phosphate [8]. Animal studies demonstrate that hPTH promotes bone volume [9], fracture healing [10–12] and spinal bone fusion [13]. In practice, the intermittently subcutaneous injection of hPTH successfully ameliorates the osteoporosis and

* Correspondence: smu_yangdehong2018@163.com

[†]Wei Li and Liang Yuan contributed equally to this work.

[1]Department of Spinal Surgery, Nanfang Hospital, Southern Medical University, Guangzhou 510515, China

Full list of author information is available at the end of the article

osteoporotic fracture in human [14–18]. Although PTH is secreted as a peptide with 84 amino acids, the 34 amino acids at the amino-terminus, namely the PTH(1–34) possesses the entire activity of the full length PTH [19], which has been proved in the animal fracture models of tibial and other bones [20, 21]. However, if the effect of PTH on the entire bone is identical or different to that on the fracture site is still in debated, because the intermittently subcutaneous injection of hPTH (1–34) enhances the bone mineral density (BMD) and bone formation in callus, as well as several osteogenic markers in serum [22–25]. In contrast, the prolonged exposure to PTH leads to bone resorption, as opposed of bone formation in the intermittent exposure [19, 26].

Both PTH and PTH(1–34) work through the type I PTH receptor (PTHR1) to activate several G protein coupled signaling cascades, including cyclic adenosine monophosphate (cAMP)/protein kinase A (PKA), phospholipase C (PLC)/protein kinase C (PKC) and PLC-independent/PKC [19, 26, 27]. Since the activation of each pathway has been mapped to the different domains within hPTH(1–34), the ligand analogs of hPTH(1–34) specific for a certain pathway were developed by mutating the key amino acid residues within hPTH(1–34) [19], which provides a powerful tool to analysis the functional of a specific signaling during bone formation and resorption. Combining these analogs with the genetically modified mice, the effects of the different signaling pathways induced by hPTH on osteoblastogenesis, osteoclastogenesis and bone metabolism have been widely investigated [9, 28, 29]. The analog of hPTH(1–34) which combines the mutations of $Ser^1 \rightarrow Gly^1$ and $Glu^{19} \rightarrow Arg^{19}$ into hPTH (1–34), namely the GR(1–34), is able to accumulate cAMP as hPTH(1–34) does, but unable to activate PLC even at a high concentration [26].

As reported previously, the cAMP/PKA mediates the beneficial effects of hPTH on fracture healing [9]. Our recent study and recent unpublished data revealed that the PKA-dependent PKC contributed to the effects of cAMP/PKA on bone formation [27], and the 29–34 amino acids of hPTH [hPTH(29–34)] triggers PLC-independent/PKC signaling [26]. These findings indicate that the PLC signaling associated with PTH are much more compound than expected. Thus, to clarify if the PLC signaling involved in the controversial functions of PTH administration would shed novel light on bone metabolism and osteoporosis treatment. In this study, the orchiectomized (ORX) male mice were employed as the model of androgen-related osteoporosis. By comparing the effects between the intermittently administrated hPTH(1–34) and GR(1–34), we explore that the role of PLC signaling performed in the fracture site of the ORX male mice.

Methods
Animals
One hundred and forty-seven C57BL/6 J male mice of seven-week-old were purchased from and acclimatized for 1 week before orchiectomy at the Laboratory Animal Center of Southern Medical University (Guangzhou, China). The animal research protocol was approved by the Animal Care and Use Committee of Southern Medical University. All applicable Southern Medical University guidelines for the care and use of animals were followed. All procedures performed in studies involving animals were in accordance with the ethical standards of the Southern Medical University.

Orchiectomy and bone fracture model
Mice were anesthetized using the MATRX VMR small animal anesthesia machine (model VMR; USA) with continuous inhalation of 2% isoflurane mixed with oxygen. The sham treated animals underwent skin and scrotum incision without the testis removal, while the ORX mice had both testes entirely removed as previously described [2]. One week after surgery, a cross-sectional fracture was generated in the mid-shaft of the right femur by inserting a pin (0.45 mm in diameter) into the marrow cavity from the distal end and then, penetrating through the mid shaft of the femur. An incision was made in the middle region of the right thigh to expose the mid-shaft of the femur into the intermuscle space. A complete fracture was made by cutting the shaft of the femur, where the intramedullary pin was remained to stabilize the fracture ends [12].

Administration of hPTH(1–34) and the analog GR(1–34)
hPTH(1–34) and GR(1–34) were synthesized at GL Biochem (Shanghai, China). The preparation for administration followed the protocol as described before [9]. Both peptides were injected at the 40 μg/kg subcutaneously once daily for 5 days in every week [30]. The same volume of vehicle (0.05 ml) was administrated into control group. The body weight, serum testosterone, and the bone quantity and quality in the fracture area were measured after the 2 and 4 weeks of injection.

Biochemical assays
Half of one milliliter of blood was collected from the animals after general anesthesia, placed at room temperature for 15 min and then, centrifuged at 4000 rpm to obtain the serum. Enzyme-linked immunosorbent assay (ELISA) kits were applied to detect the levels of serum testosterone (Boster Biological Technology CO. Ltd., Wuhan, China), tartrated-resistant acid phsphatase (TRAP) (Cusabio, Wuhan, China), N-terminal propeptide of type I collagen (P1NP) and C-terminal collagen-type I fragments (CTX) (Immunodiagnostic Systems, Fountain Hills, AZ). Alkaline phosphatase (ALP) was detected with a colorimetric

kinetic determination kit by following the manufacturer's instructions (Byotime, Beijing, China).

Measurement for bone mineral densitometry and bone mineral content

After the mice were sacrificed by carbon dioxide anesthesia and cervical dislocation, the right femur containing the growth of the callus was fixed in 4% paraformaldehyde for 48 h. Then, the soft tissues and intramedullary pin were removed. Bone mineral density (BMD) and bone mineral content (BMC) at the callus were measured by dual-energy X-ray absorptiometry (DEXA) with a densitometer (XR-36, NORLAND Inc., WI, USA). The region of interest (ROI) was a rectangular area (5.4 mm × 3.5 mm) centering on the fracture line, which contained both the newly generated callus tissues and the original bone.

Micro-computed tomography

Micro-Computed tomography (Micro-CT) analysis was conducted by the μCT80 (SCANCO MEDICAL Inc., Switzerland) with the software μCT Evaluation Program V6.5–1 in the specimens after DEXA measurements. Image recording was confined to the callus of the fractured femur. Images of the femur mid-shaft (5.40 mm in length centering on fracture line) were performed using an isotropic voxel (12 μm in size). The grayscale threshold was set up at 220, meaning the values of mineralized tissue are greater than 220. The ROI of measurements was localized to a cylindrical space (5.4 mm in height and 3.5 mm in diameter) focusing at the middle point of fracture line. Three-dimensional (3D) pictures were also reconstructed based on the images from the three spatial dimensions to show the fracture healing. Samples from 12 mice from each group underwent micro-CT scanning and half of these samples were then tested for the biomechanical properties.

Biomechanics testing

Six mice from each group were sacrificed by carbon dioxide anesthesia and cervical dislocation for biomechanics testing. The bone was immersed in PBS for 30 min after the removal of intramedullary pin and surrounding soft tissues, and then, placed between two plates (a span of 8 mm) with the medial and anterior sides facing forward and down, respectively. The bending rigidity of the healing femur was measured on the fourth week after injection by a three-point bending procedure using an Electropuls Test System (E1000; Instron, Inc., Illinois, USA). A central load was applied at the mid-callus with a constant rate of 2 mm/min until failure occurred. The rigidity of the femur was determined from the curve determined by the maximal force and displacement applied on the tested bone.

Histology and histomorphometry

Collected femurs were decalcified in 20% ethylenediaminetetraacetic acid (EDTA) solution for 4 weeks, dehydrated, embedded in paraffin and then, sectioned in 5um for hematoxylin and eosin (HE) staining, Masson's Trichrome staining (Maixin Biotech. Co. Ltd., Fujian, China), TRAP staining (Sigma-Aldrich, 387A-kit, USA), or TRAP immunohistochemical staining (Biosynthesis Biotechnology Co. Ltd., Beijing, China) with the standard protocols or the manufacturer's instructions. 24 images (2 fields per section, 2 sections per sample; for callus formation analysis, magnification is 10; for osteoclasts analysis, magnification is 200) were photographed from 6 mice in each group and analyzed with Image J analysis software. ROI was defined as a rectangular box in the center of healing zone, in which the callus, woven bone and osteoclasts were outlined manually according to the specially stained color with the software.

Ex vivo culture of bone marrow cells

The eight week old male mice were orchiectomized as described above. After one week of the orchiectomy, the mice were sacrificed by carbon dioxide anesthesia and cervical dislocation for femurs dissection and bone marrow collection. The isolated cells were seeded into 24-well plates precoated with collagen type I at 1×10^5 cells/well for the 24 h culture, and then, induced for differentiation as described in the following. The osteogenic medium contained α-MEM supplemented with 10% FBS, 100 U/ml penicillin (Gibco, USA), 100 mg/ml streptomycin (Gibco, USA), 10 mM β-glycerophosphate (Sigma, USA) and 50 μg/m ascorbic acid (Sigma, USA). For osteoclastogenic induction, the cells were cultured in generic (α-MEM supplemented with 10% FBS, 100 U/ml penicillin, and 100 mg/ml streptomycin).

Histochemistry

The treatment of hPTH(1–34) (10 nM) and GR(1–34) (10 nM) were followed a 4/48 h intermittent cycling plan [31]. In brief, the cells were cultured in the medium supplemented with peptides for 4 h and changed into the fore-mentioned medium without peptide for 44 h prior to the next treatment. At the 14th days of culture, ALP and mineralized nodules were examined by histochemical staining. The cells were fixed with 4% paraformaldehyde for 30 min, gently rinsed with PBS and stained for ALP with BCIP/NBT Alkaline Phosphatase Color Development Kit (Beyotime Institute of Biotechnology, Haimen, China), or for mineralized nodule demonstration with 1% Alizarin Red S solution (Sigma, St Louis, MO, USA) for 30 min at room temperature. ALP activity was measured by incubating cell lysates (extracted with 0.2% TritonX-100) in ALP substrate buffer containing the soluble substrate p-nitrophenyl phosphate. The quantification was performed based on the absorbance at 520 nm (Jiancheng Bioengineering Institute, Nanjing, China). To determine the calcium content of the cultures, cells were washed in Ca^{2+}- and Mg^{2+}-free PBS and then, incubated for 3 h in 0.2 ml of 0.6 N HCl. Extracted calcium was then measured spectrophotometrically at 610 nm after the reaction with methylthymol blue (Jiancheng Bioengineering Institute, Nanjing, China). TRAP staining was performed after the 7 days of treatment by using a TRAP staining kit. 10 microscopic fields (10 × 10) were randomly selected for the TRAP positive cells counting. The percentages of TRAP positive cells to total cells were calculated for quantification.

Real-time PCR

Bone marrow stromal cells were isolated and plated into 6 well plates at 4×10^6 cells/cm^2 as described above. After 48 h cultured in the generic medium, cells were subjected to hPTH(1–34) (10 nM), hPTH(1–34) (10 nM) combined with 1 μmol/L U73122 (PLC inhibitor, Abcam, United Kingdom) or GR(1–34) (10 nM). Total RNA was isolated after 4 h later by using RNeasy Mini Kit (Takara BIO, Dalian, China). Expressions of Receptor Activator of Nuclear Factor κ B (RANK) and its ligand (RANKL), osteoprotegrin (OPG), nuclear factor of activated T cells (NFATC) 1, TRAP, Cathepsin K were measured by two-step real-time RT-PCR. Briefly, the first strand of cDNA was synthesized according to the manufacturer's instructions using a PrimeScript® RT reagent Kit (Takara BIO, Dalian, China). For each gene, two specific PCR primers (RANK/fw, 5′- ACCTCCAGTCAGCAAGA AGT-3′, RANK/re, 5′-TCACAGCCCTCAGAATCCAC-3′; RANKL/fw, 5′-AGCCGAGACTACGGCAAGTA-3′, RANKL/re, 5′-GCGCTCGAAAGTACAGGAAC-3′; OPG/ fw, 5′-ACCTCACCACAGAGCAGCTT-3′, OPG/re, 5′-TT GTGAAGCTGTGCAGGAAC-3′; NFATC1/fw, 5′- CCGT TGCTTCCAGAAAATAACA-3′, NFATC1/re, 5′-TGTGG GATGTGAACTCGGAA-3′; TRAP/fw, 5′-TCCTGGCTC AAAAAGCAGTT-3′;TRAP/re, 5′-ACATAGCCCACACC GTTCTC-3′; Cathepsin K/fw, 5′-CTGAAGATGCTTTCC CATATGTGGG-3′, Cathepsin K/re 5′- GCAGGCGTT GTTCTTATTCCGAGC-3′, GAPDH/fw, 5′-TGTCGTGG AGTCTACTGGTG-3′; GAPDH/re, 5′-GC ATTGCTGAC AATCTTGAG-3′) were designed and synthesized by Life Technologies (Shanghai, China). The PCR reactions (94 °C, 20 s; 60 °C, 20 s; 72 °C, 20 s) were performed on an GeneAmp® PCR System 9700 (Applied Biosystems, CA, USA) using a SYBR® Premix EX Tap™ (Takara BIO, Dalian, China). Gene expression was normalized to that of GAPDH and then expressed as fold over control.

Statistical analysis

All statistical analyses were conducted using SPSS version 13.0 (SPSS Inc., Chicago, IL). The results are presented as means ± standard error of the mean (SEM). The significance of differences in BMDs, BMCs, the values of three-point bend testing and CT between treatment groups was analyzed by analysis of variance (ANOVA) with Bonferroni's test for post hoc analysis.

Results

Generation of the orchiectomized model for fracture healing

Compared to the sham-operated mice, the serum testosterone in the orchiectomized mice began to decrease from the third week on until to the end of fifth week after ORX (Additional file 1: Figure S1A). Less trebacular bone and thinner cortical bone were detected in the growth plate of the tibia at the third and fifth week after ORX (Additional file 1: Figure S1B). Although the post-surgery bone volume [BV/TV (%)] was similar to that in the sham animals at the third week after ORX ($p > 0.05$), it was reduced dramatically at the fifth week after ORX compared to the sham animals, reflecting that the loss of bone volume was associated with the decreased testosterone (Additional file 2: Figure S1C).

To address the influence of the decreased testosterone on fracture healing, 3D reconstructions of the healing fracture after 2 weeks of fracture were performed and indicated that both the bone mass and bone volume in the fracture area were significantly decreased in ORX mice (Additional file 2: Figure S2A, B), which was coincided with the slow healing and bone shape recovery in the ORX mice after 4 weeks of fracture (Additional file 2: Figure S2A). Since the fracture healing was greatly retarded in ORX mice compared to the sham group (Additional file 2: Figure S2B), the ORX mice was an ideal model to study bone repairing during androgen deficient osteoporosis.

The stronger healing effect of GR(1–34) during the early fracture in ORX mice

According to the 3D BMD and BV/TV (%) from micro-CT and the 2D BMD and BMC from DEXA, the bone callus was formed in hPTH(1–34), GR(1–34) and control groups after 2 week of fracture, but there were more bone tissues in the hPTH(1–34) and GR(1–34) treated animals than that of the vehicle controls ($N = 12$ in each group; Fig. 1a, *left panel*). Micro-CT scanning revealed that after 4 weeks of fracture, the cortical bones in the ORX mice treated with hPTH(1–34) or GR(1–34) were continuously aligned and the bone callus absorbed, indicating a completely recovered bone fracture. In contrast, the cortical bone treated with vehicle control was discontinuous and the bone callus was still prominent ($N = 12$ in each group; Fig. 1a, *right panel*). The BMD of the fracture treated with hPTH(1–34) and GR(1–34) were significantly higher than that of mice treated with the vehicle control after two weeks of fracture (Fig. 1b).

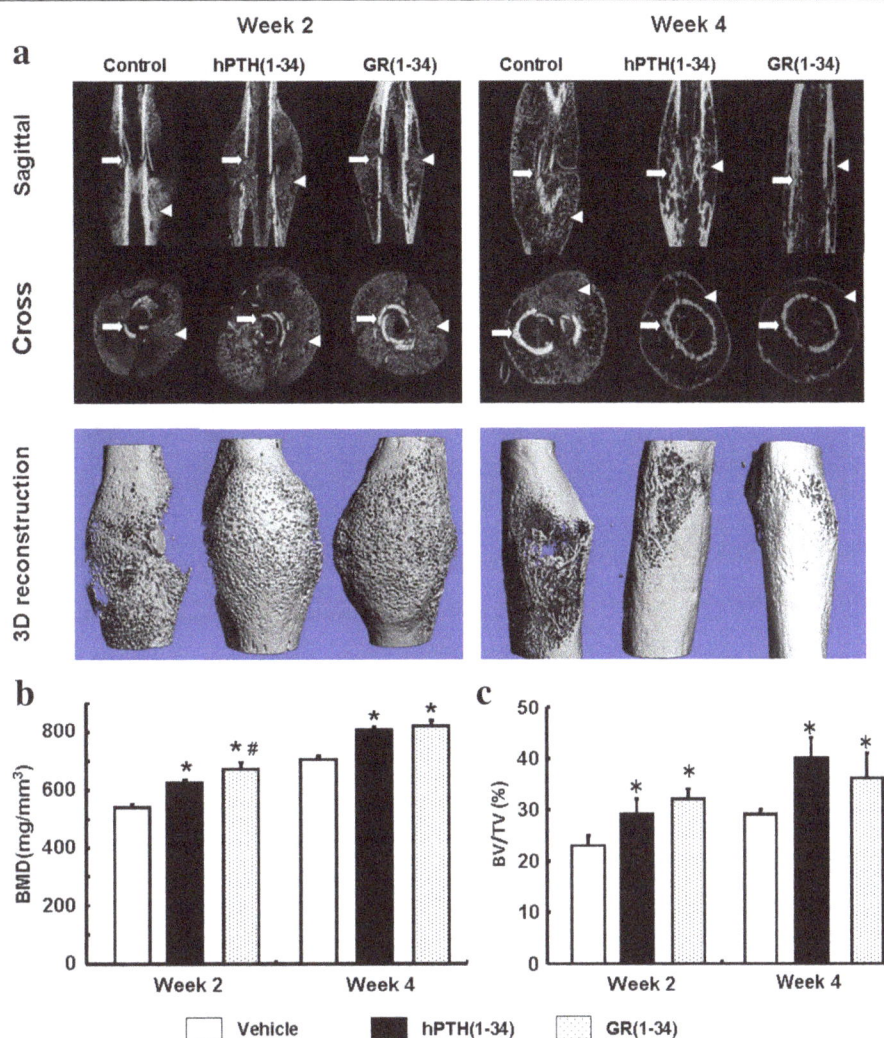

Fig. 1 The effects of hPTH(1–34) and GR(1–34) on bone fracture healing in ORX mice. **a** The 2D and 3D images from micro-CT scanning at 2 weeks (*left panel*) and 4 weeks (*right panel*) after peptide injection showed the cortical bone (white arrows) and cancellous bone (triangles) in the fracture region. **b** The statistical analysis on BMD from micro-CT scanning. **c** The statistical analysis on bone volume [BV/TV (%)] from micro-CT scanning. [Each group contained 12 cases; *$P < 0.05$ for hPTH(1–34) &GR(1–34) vs. vehicle; #$P < 0.05$ for hPTH(1–34) vs. GR(1–34)]

Moreover, GR(1–34) exhibited a greater enhancement on 3D BMD than hPTH(1–34) (Fig. 1b). In addition to BMD, hPTH(1–34) and GR(1–34) also significantly increased the BV/TV (%) compared to the vehicle control (Fig. 1c), though the effect on BV/TV (%) of hPTH(1–34) was similar to that of GR(1–34) (Fig. 1c). Further investigations disclosed that after 4 weeks of fracture, the increasing BMD and BV/TV (%) of the healing sites in the hPTH(1–34) and GR(1–34) groups were both evidently greater than those in vehicle treated mice (Fig. 1b). Even the difference of BMD between the hPTH(1–34) and GR(1–34) treated mice after 2 weeks of fracture was diminished after 4 weeks of fracture (Fig. 1b). Consistent with the outcomes of 3D micro-CT reconstruction, the plain X-ray images confirmed that the well aligned cortical bone in the fracture ends (Fig. 2a). DEXA confirmed that

hPTH(1–34) and GR(1–34) treatments significantly increased BMD and BMC after 2 weeks of fracture (Fig. 2b), as well as the greater BMC in GR(1–34) group compared with the hPTH(1–34) group (Fig. 2c). Similarly, the BMD and BMC of hPTH(1–34) were close to those of GR(1–34) treated mice after 4 weeks of fracture (Fig. 2b, c). In summary, the treatments with either hPTH(1–34) or GR(1–34) could increase the rate of bone healing, while the GR(1–34) appeared to have a greater enhancement on the early fracture healing than hPTH(1–34).

The biomechanical characteristics in the fractured bone of ORX mice

Since the the bone is too soft to endure the mechanical analyses before the fourth week of fracture, the bending force and rigidity of the femurs from the hPTH(1–34)

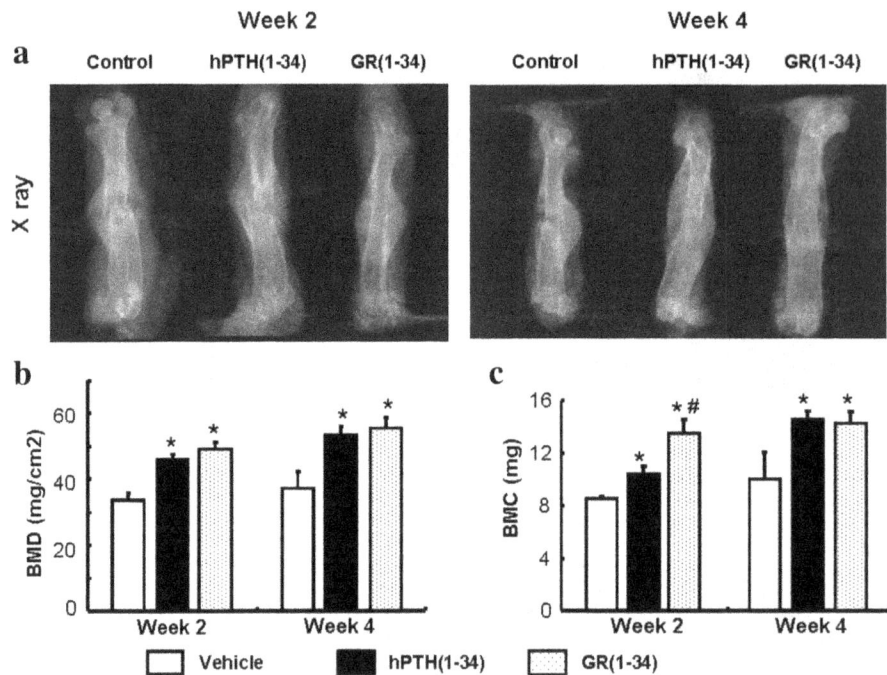

Fig. 2 Bone mineral density and bone mass content in the fracture area measured with DEXA. **a** The plain X-ray images for femur alignment at the 2nd (*left panel*) and 4th week (*right panel*) after peptide injection. **b** The statistical analysis on BMD from DEXA. **c** The statistical analysis on bone volume [BV/TV (%)] from DEXA. [Each group contained 12 cases; *$P < 0.05$ for hPTH(1–34) &GR(1–34) vs. vehicle; #$P < 0.05$ for hPTH(1–34) vs. GR(1–34)]

and GR(1–34) treated and vehicle control mice was compared at the fourth week after fracture. The healing femurs from both the hPTH(1–34) and GR(1–34) treated mice were able to sustain a much greater force (Fig. 3a) and exhibited an increased bending rigidity (Fig. 3b). However, there was no significant difference in the measured biomechaniccal characteristics between the femurs of mice treated with GR(1–34) and hPTH(1–34).

The difference in bone metabolism markers between the hPTH(1–34) and GR(1–34) treated ORX mice

The serum levels of P1NP, CTX and TRAP in both the hPTH(1–34) and GR(1–34) groups remarkably increased at the second week and returned normal as control at the fourth week after fracture (Fig. 4a, b, d). Interestingly, the ALP levels in both the hPTH(1–34) and GR(1–34) groups kept higher than control from the second to the fourth week after fracture (Fig. 4c). Moreover,

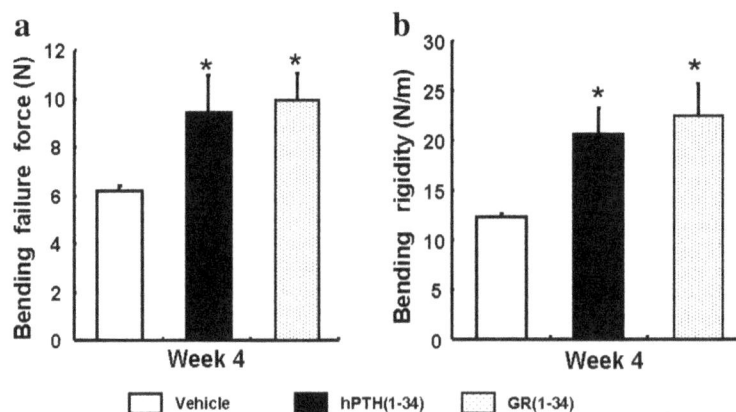

Fig. 3 Mechanical characteristics of the fractured bone in ORX mice. After 4 weeks of peptide or vehicle administration, the bending failure force (**a**) and Bending rigidity (**b**) were measured in the ORX mice for statistical analyses. [Each group contained 6 cases; *$P < 0.05$ for hPTH(1–34) &GR(1–34) vs. vehicle]

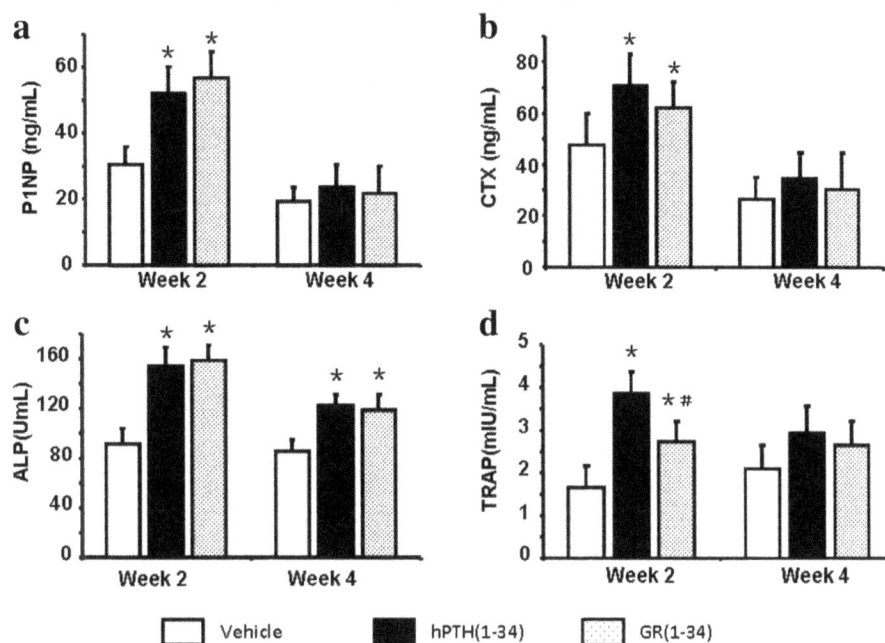

Fig. 4 The serum levels of bone metabolic markers at 2 and 4 weeks after peptide administration in fractured ORX mice. Serum levels of P1NP (**a**), CTX (**b**), ALP (**c**) and TRAP (**d**) at the 2nd and 4th week after peptide administration were measured and present in a statistical summary. [Each group contained 12 cases; *$P < 0.05$ for hPTH(1–34) &GR(1–34) vs. vehicle; #$P < 0.05$ for hPTH(1–34) vs. GR(1–34)]

hPTH(1–34) only induced a higher TRAP level than GR(1–34) at the second week after fracture (Fig. 4d).

The quicker callus transformation and osteoclastogenesis in hPTH(1–34) treated fracture healing

Since GR(1–34) increased more BMD than hPTH(1–34) in the first two weeks after fracture, the histological features in the healing areas at the two weeks after fracture were analyzed to clarify the early healing process. Although no significant difference was found among the callus sizes of the three groups (Fig. 5a, b), the amounts of bony callus were significantly increased in both peptide-injecting groups, especially in the GR(1–34) mice compared with the vehicle group (Fig. 5a, c). Both the hPTH(1–34) and GR(1–34) treatments induced more osteoclasts around the woven bones, but the number and size of the osteoclasts in the hPTH(1–34) group were also more and larger than those in GR(1–34) group (Fig. 5a, d, e).

The quicker induction of TRAP positive cells by hPTH(1–34) in the bone marrow cells of ORX mice

The bone marrow cells isolated from the femurs of ORX mice were applied in the in vitro exploration of the soteoblastogenesis and osteoclastogenesis during the fracture healing of the androgen-deficient osteoporosis. After 2 weeks of the intermittent administration, both hPTH(1–34) and GR(1–34) could induce the ALP activity and calcium deposition at the similar intensity (Fig. 6a, b). On the other and, the intermittent treatments of both

hPTH(1–34) and GR(1–34) significantly increased TRAP$^+$ cells in bone marrow cells culture in 7 days. However, less TRAP$^+$ cells were detected in the culture treated by GR(1–34) compared to that by hPTH(1–34). In the hPTH(1–34) group, $10.2 \pm 3.4\%$ of the TRAP$^+$ cells were multinucleated, while only $2.2 \pm 1.3\%$ in GR(1–34) group (Fig. 6c). There was no multinucleated TRAP$^+$ cells found in vehicle treatment.

The quick activation on the osteoclastogenesis-associated genes by hPTH(1–34) in the bone marrow cells of ORX mice

Quantitative PCR revealed that both hPTH(1–34) and GR(1–34) administration increased the transcription of RANK, RANKL and OPG, but only the increase of RANKL expression by hPTH(1–34) was significantly higher than that by GR(1–34) in the bone marrow cells of the ORX mice (Additional file 3: Figure S3). Similarly, the hPTH(1–34) treatment was capable of inducing the robuster transcription of NFATC1, TRAP and Cathepsin K than GR(1–34) (Additional file 3: Figure S3). Surprisingly, the efficient activation of RANKL, NFATC1, TRAP and Cathepsin K expression by hPTH(1–34) could be neutralized by the PLC inhibitor U73122 (Additional file 3: Figure S3).

Discussion

Orchiectomy has been widely used to mimic the osteoporosis in men [3]. The overall bone volume usually reduced to 40–60% of the normal within 6 to 12 weeks

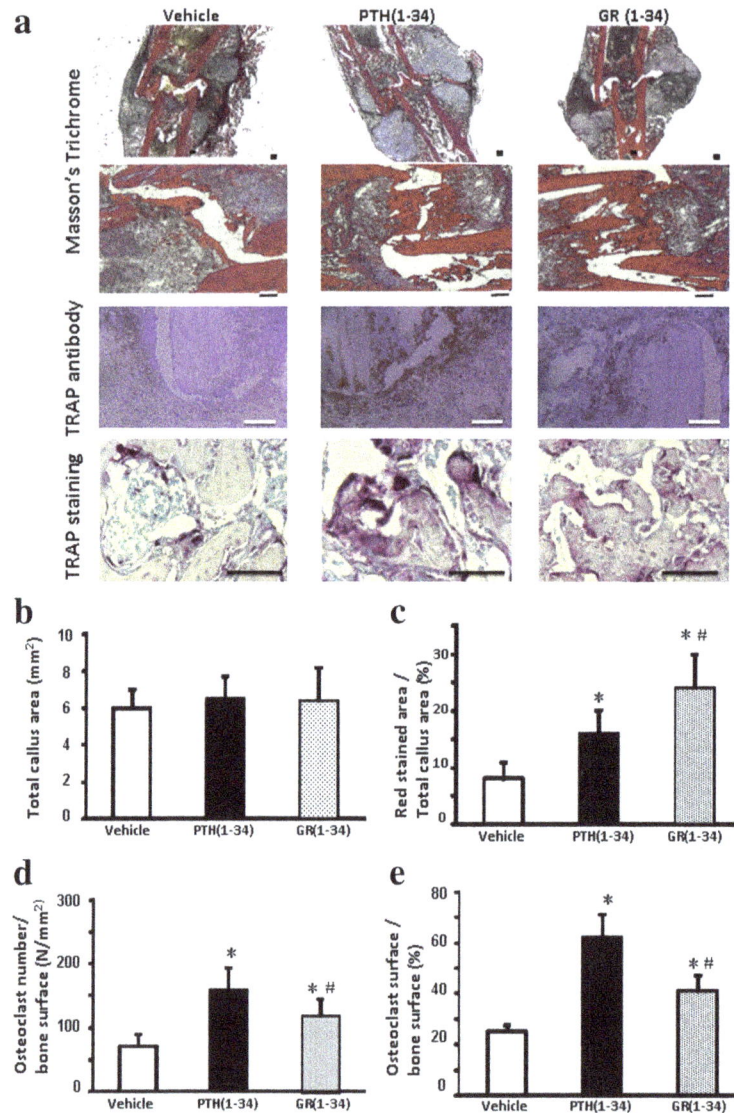

Fig. 5 The effects of hPTH(1–34) and GR(1–34) on callus transformation and osteoclasts formation in the healing area at 2 weeks after fracture. **a** The upper two panels showed the Masson-Goldner Trichrome stain for the cartilage (in blue) and bony (in red) callus formation; the third panel showed the immunohistochemical staining with the monoclonal antibody against TRAP; the bottom panel showed the distribution of osteoclasts on the surface of bone stained by TRAP activity. Histomorphometry of callus (in blue and red) and the proportion of bony callus among total callus were statistically shown in (**b**) and (**c**), respectively. Statistical analyses were shown for the number of osteoclasts per unit area (**d**) and their surface in proportion to bone surface (**e**). [Each group contained 6 cases; scale bar represents 100 μm; *$P < 0.05$ for hPTH(1–34) &GR(1–34) vs. vehicle; #$P < 0.05$ for hPTH(1–34) vs. GR(1–34)]

after orchiectomy in rats [32] and 4 weeks in mice [33], which suggested that the mice used in this study was undergoing a substantial BV loss due to androgen deprivation. Although the nadir testosterone level and its impact on mouse BV in this study were not determined, we indeed found that the weight loss of seminal vesicles and the significantly declined testosterone level after the testis removal (data not shown), which indicated the occurrence of androgen deprivation in the ORX mice. However, we acknowledged that the growth potential of the 8–10 weeks old mice might contribute

to the delayed fracture healing in some extent, because the decline of testosterone was gradual and reached the half of the normal at the fifth week, instead of a rapid decline of testosterone in the previous report [34]. Even though, the differential effects of hPTH(1–34) and GR(1–34) on the fracture healing in both sham and ORX mice indicated that the consequence of the androgen deprivation in the younger ORX mice were still convincing. Besides the androgen deprivation, the lateral damages in the surrounding tissues, such as blood vessels, muscles and nerves, may also affect the fracture

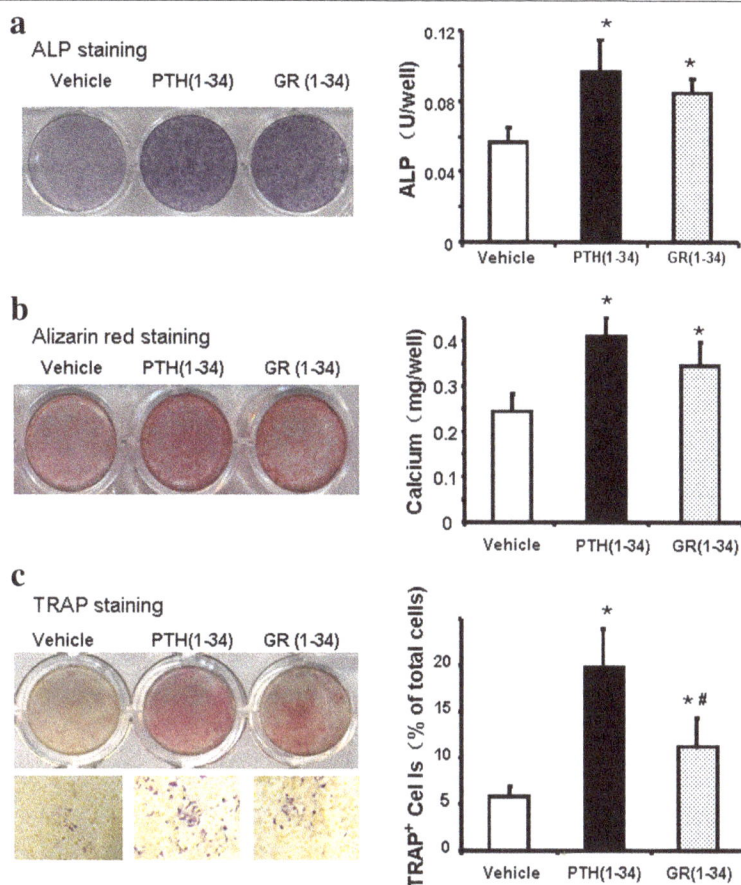

Fig. 6 The effects of hPTH(1–34) and GR(1–34) on osteogenesis and osteoclastogenesis in bone marrow cells of ORX mice. At the 2nd week of administration, ALP activity of the cells in osteogenic medium were stained and measured with a BCIP/NBT Color Development Kit (**a**); the mineralized nodules were stained with Alizarin Red S solution and calcium deposition was quantified spectrophotometrically (**b**). At the 1st week of administration, TRAP staining was performed and the percentage of TRAP+ cells to total cells were counted (**c**). [Three independent experiments were repeated for (**a** & **b**) and six for (**c**); 10 fields at 100 magnitude were randomly selected for TRAP+ cell counting; *$P < 0.05$ for hPTH(1–34) &GR(1–34) vs. vehicle; #$P < 0.05$ for hPTH(1–34) vs. GR(1–34)]

healing in practice. To reduce the influence of later damages on fracture healing as much as possible, the osteotomy model was adopted, as apposed of impacting bone via violence [35]. Although there were still injuries in the soft tissues during the osteotomy, their extent and variations were milder and less than those in the impacting model, which would cause mininal errors in the effects of PTH on fracture healing.

During the early stage, hPTH administration resulted mainly in the newly formed woven bones, especially the bony callus transformation, though the callus sizes were indiscriminate between the treated and untreated animals. At the 4th week after administration, the enhanced bone reconstruction was verified because of the reconnection of cortical bone and the re-absorption of cancellous bone around the fracture. Consistently, the healing bones received peptide treatment exhibited the greater mechanical characteristics than control. As previously reported, it took three weeks for the the normal mice to

recover the strength and stiffness of the fractured femur [36]. However, even at the 4th week after peptide administration, the mechanical index of the fractured femur of ORX mice were still remarkably lower than that of the intact contra-lateral femurs. Therefore, we need to find out the duration required for the complete recovery from bone fracture in ORX mice in the future investigation. Interestingly, the effects of hPTH administration in ORX mice were similar to those in ovariectomized rodents [32], suggesting that the effects of hPTH is associated with sex hormones, but no discrimination between estrogen and androgen.

After 2 weeks of administration, more bone mass (BMC and BMD) and bony callus in fracture healing area of the ORX mice were induced by GR(1–34) compared with hPTH(1–34). The results of serum biochemistry suggested that compared to GR(1–34), the effect of hPTH(1–34) on bone re-absorption was much stronger.

The induction of osteoclasts from the bone marrow cells verified the in vivo consequences. However, both the in vivo and the in vitro experiments revealed that the effects of hPTH(1–34) and GR(1–34) on bone formation and bone resorption in fracture healing showed no significant difference after 4 weeks of administration. Therefore, hPTH(1–34) was suggested to exert a rapid induction of osteoclasts in the fracture healing of ORX mice compared to GR(1–34).

Since GR(1–34) is the analog of hPTH(1–34) and incapable of activating PLC signaling, it is reasonable to speculate that PLC signaling contributed the rapid bone resorption during the fracture healing of ORX mice. PTH was reported to increase osteoclast formation and attachment to bone via both cAMP/PKA and PLC-coupled calcium/PKC pathways in osteoblasts [37, 38]. Although both hPTH(1–34) and GR(1–34) could increase TPAP positive mononucleated and multinucleated cells [39], our study showed that hPTH(1–34) was able to activate both mature and progenitor osteoclasts more quickly, indicated that the rapid osteoclastic commitment and maturation induced by intermittent hPTH(1–34) administration depended on PLC signaling. Since PLC (eg. PLCγ2) was reported to mediate effect of RANKL on osteoclastic differentiation [40], and the inhibitor of PLC signaling decreased the RANK expression in hPTH(1–34) treated group to that in GR(1–34) treated group, it suggested that RANKL could also be a downstream target of PLC signaling. In summary, the intermittently administrated PTH enhances fracture healing of ORX mice, while the PLC signaling activated by PTH mediates a rapid osteogenesis in the healing zone for the bone re-absorption.

Our findings on the role of PLC signaling seems controversial to the work of Guo et al. showing that the deficiency in PLC signaling significantly decreased bone volume and osteoblasts [28]. However, Guo et al. investigated the normal development, while our study focused on an androgen-associated traumatic model. Unlike the mice carrying the mutant PTH receptor, the endogenous PTH can still activate other signaling pathways in the ORX mice receiving PLC-deficient PTH analog. The differential role of PLC in bone development verses bone healing still require to be elucidated. A study on the DSEL mouse reported that DSEL mice displayed a significant decrease in the amount of trebacular bone with little alteration in the cortical bone [29], implying that PLC-dependent and -independent signaling on osteoclastogenesis were not related to PKC signaling [41]. Further study is required to reveal the roles of the PLC-dependent and -independent signaling initiated by PTH in bone resorption, which would benefit the understanding and regulating the balance of bone turnover.

Conclusions

The PLC signaling activated by the intermittent injection of hPTH(1–34) rapidly activates the osteoclastogenesis in the fracture healing zone. This finding provides a novel insight for the effects of hPTH(1–34) on bone resorption, which would benefit the development of the new PTH analog for fracture therapy.

Additional files

Additional file 1: Figure S1. Orchiectomy reduced serum testosterone and trebacular bone volume in male mice. (A) Serum testosterone levels at the third and fifth week. (B) The micro-CT scanning and 3D reconstruction of the trebacular bone of the proximal tibia. (C) Bone volume (BV/TV (%)) was measured at the third and fifth week after the surgery. (There were 12 cases in the sham and ORX groups; *p < 0.05). (TIF 478 kb)

Additional file 2: Figure S2. Retarded fracture healing in ORX mice. (a) The 3D reconstruction of the micro-CT scanning on the fracture region. (b) The bone volume [BV/TV(%)] was measured with micro-CT analysis at the 2nd and 4th week after fracture. (There were 12 cases in the sham and ORX groups; *P < 0.05). (TIF 762 kb)

Additional file 3: Figure S3. The osteoclastogenesis-associated gene expression in the bone marrow cells of ORX mice. After a hours culture with hPTH(1–34), hPTH(1–34) + U73122 and GR(1–34), mRNA was extracted from the bone marrow cells of ORX mice for real-time PCR. [Three independent experiments were repeated for each gene; variables were analyzed using analysis of variance (ANOVA) and Bonferroni's test for post hoc analysis; *P < 0.05 for hPTH(1–34) &GR(1–34) vs. vehicle; #P < 0.05 for hPTH(1–34) vs. GR(1–34)]. (TIF 470 kb)

Abbreviations

ALP: Alkaline phosphatase; BMC: Bone mass content; BMD: Bone mineral density; BV/TV: Bone volume; cAMP: cyclic adenosine monophosphate; CTX: Terminal collagen-type I fragments; DEXA: Dual-energy X-ray absorptiometry; EDTA: Ethylenediaminetetraacetic acid; GR(1–34): Ser^1-> Gly^1 and Glu^{19}-> Arg^{19} into hPTH (1–34); HE: Hematoxylin and eosin; hPTH: Human parathyroid hormone; Micro-CT: Micro-Computed tomography; NFATC: Nuclear factor of activated T cells; OPG: Osteoprotegrin; ORX: Orchiectomized; P1NP: Terminal propeptide of type I collagen; PKA: Protein kinase A; PKC: Protein kinase C; PLC: Phospholipase C; RANK: Receptor Activator of Nuclear Factor κ B; RANKL: Receptor Activator of Nuclear Factor κ B ligand; TRAP: Tartrated-resistant acid phsphatase

Acknowledgements

We would like to express our sincere gratitude to our hospital colleagues, especially the pharmacists, and X-ray technicians who provided technical assistance.

Funding

This work was supported by the National Natural Science Foundation of China (Grant No. 30973061 and 81272043) and the Natural Science Foundation of Guangdong Province (2015A030313256).

Authors' contributions

Designed the research studies: JG, RB, DY. Conducted the experiments: WL, LY. Acquired the data: WL, LY, GT. Data analyses: GT, YH, YM. Provided reagents, technical training for experimental assistants and conducted animal experiments: SH, JC. Manuscript editing: RB, DY. All the authors have read and approved the final submitted manuscript.

Competing interests

The authors declare they have no competing interests.

Author details

[1]Department of Spinal Surgery, Nanfang Hospital, Southern Medical University, Guangzhou 510515, China. [2]Endocrine Unit, Massachusetts General Hospital, Boston, MA 02114, USA.

References

1. Ebeling PR. Androgens and osteoporosis. Curr Opin Endocrinol Diabetes Obes. 2010;17:284–92.
2. Tezval M, Serferaz G, Rack T, Kolios L, Sehmisch S, Schmelz U, et al. Effect of parathyroid hormone on hypogonadism induced bone loss of proximal femur of orchiectomized rat. World J Urol. 2011;29:529–34.
3. Blouin S, Libouban H, Moreau MF, Chappard D. Orchidectomy models of osteoporosis. Methods Mol Biol. 2008;455:125–34.
4. Broulik PD, Broulikova K. Raloxifen prevents bone loss in castrated male mice. Physiol Res. 2007;56:443–7.
5. Daniell HW, Dunn SR, Ferguson DW, Lomas G, Niazi Z, Stratte PT. Progressive osteoporosis during androgen deprivation therapy for prostate cancer. J Urol. 2000;163:181–6.
6. Goldray D, Weisman Y, Jaccard N, Merdler C, Chen J, Matzkin H. Decreased bone density in elderly men treated with the gonadotropin-releasing hormone agonist decapeptyl (D-Trp6-GnRH). J Clin Endoctinol Metab. 1993; 76:288–90.
7. Boonen S, Vanderschueren D, Geusens P, Bouillon R. Age-associated endocrine deficiencies as potential determinants of femoral neck (type II) osteoporotic fracture occurrence in elderly men. Int J Androl. 1997;20:134–43.
8. Lou S, Lv H, Li Z, Tang P, Wang Y. Parathyroid hormone analogues for fracture healing: protocol for a systematic review and meta-analysis of randomised controlled trials. BMJ Open. 2018;8:e019291.
9. Yang D, Singh R, Divieti P, Guo J, Bouxsein ML, Bringhurst FR. Contributions of parathyroid hormone (PTH)/PTH-related peptide receptor signaling pathways to the anabolic effect of PTH on bone. Bone. 2007;40:1453–61.
10. Andreassen TT, Cacciafesta V. Intermittent parathyroid hormone treatment enhances guided bone regeneration in rat calvarial bone defects. J Craniofac Surg. 2004;15:424–7.
11. Mognetti B, Marino S, Barberis A, Martin AS, Bala Y, Di Carlo F, et al. Experimental stimulation of bone healing with teriparatide: histomorphometric and microhardness analysis in a mouse model of closed fracture. Calcif Tissue Int. 2011;89:163–71.
12. Ren Y, Liu B, Feng Y, Shu L, Cao X, Karaplis A, et al. Endogenous PTH deficiency impairs fracture healing and impedes the fracture-healing efficacy of exogenous PTH(1-34). PLoS One. 2011;6:e23060.
13. O'Loughlin PF, Cunningham ME, Bukata SV, Tomin E, Poynton AR, Doty SB, et al. Parathyroid hormone (1-34) augments spinal fusion, fusion mass volume, and fusion mass quality in a rabbit spinal fusion model. Spine (Phila Pa 1976). 2009;34:121–30.
14. Hodsman AB, Hanley DA, Ettinger MP, Bolognese MA, Fox J, Metcalfe AJ, et al. Efficacy and safety of human parathyroid hormone-(1-84) in increasing bone mineral density in postmenopausal osteoporosis. J Clin Endocrinol Metab. 2003;88:5212–20.
15. Marcus R, Wang O, Satterwhite J, Mitlak B. The skeletal response to teriparatide is largely independent of age, initial bone mineral density, and prevalent vertebral fractures in postmenopausal women with osteoporosis. J Bone Miner Res. 2003;18:18–23.
16. McClung MR, San Martin J, Miller PD, Civitelli R, Bandeira F, Omizo M, et al. Opposite bone remodeling effects of teriparatide and alendronate in increasing bone mass. Arch Intern Med. 2005;165:1762–8.
17. Tsuchie H, Miyakoshi N, Kasukawa Y, Nishi T, Abe H, Segawa T, et al. The effect of teriparatide to alleviate pain and to prevent vertebral collapse after fresh osteoporotic vertebral fracture. J Bone Miner Metab. 2016;34:86–91.
18. Zhao Y, Xue R, Shi N, Xue Y, Zong Y, Lin W, et al. Aggravation of spinal cord conpromise following new osteoporotic vertebral comnpression fracture prevented by teriparatide in patients with osteoporotic vertebral conpression fracture prevented by teriparatide in patients with surgical contraindications. Osteoporos Int. 2016;27:3309–17.
19. Swarthout JT, D'Alonzo RC, Selvamurugan N, Partridge NC. Parathyroid hormone -dependent signaling pathways regulating genes in bone cells. Gene. 2002;282:1–17.
20. Brommage R, Hotchkiss CE, Lees CJ, Stancill MW, Hock JM, Jerome CP. Daily treatment with human recombinant parathyroid hormone-(1-34), LY333334, for 1 year increases bone mass in ovariectomized monkeys. J Clin Endocrinol Metab. 1999;84:3757–63.
21. Ellegaard M, Jorgensen NR, Schwarz P. Parathyroid hormone and bone healing. Calcif Tissue Int. 2010;87:1–13.
22. Alkhiary YM, Gerstenfeld LC, Krall E, Westmore M, Sato M, Mitlak BH, et al. Enhancement of experimental fracture-healing by systemic administration of recombinant human parathyroid hormone (PTH 1-34). J Bone Joint Surg Am. 2005;87:731–41.
23. Kaback LA, Soung do Y, Naik A, Geneau G, Schwarz EM, Rosier RN, et al. Teriparatide (1-34 human PTH) regulation of osterix during fracture repair. J Cell Biochem. 2008;105:219–26.
24. Nakajima A, Shimoji N, Shiomi K, Shimizu S, Moriya H, Einhorn TA, et al. Mechanisms for the enhancement of fracture healing in rats treated with intermittent low-dose human parathyroid hormone (1-34). J Bone Miner Res. 2002;17:2038–47.
25. Yang X, Muthukumaran P, DasDe S, Teoh SH, Choi H, Lim SK, et al. Positive alterations of viscoelastic and geometric properties in ovariectomized rat femurs with concurrent administration of ibandronate and PTH. Bone. 2012; 52:308–17.
26. Yang D, Guo J, Divieti P, Bringhurst FR. Parathyroid hormone activates PKC-delta and regulates osteoblastic differentiation via a PLC-independent pathway. Bone. 2006;38:485–96.
27. Tong G, Meng Y, Hao S, Hu S, He Y, Yan W, et al. Parathyroid hormone activates phospholipase C (PLC)-independent protein kinase C signaling pathway via protein kinase a (PKA)-dependent mechanism: a new defined signaling route would induce alternative consideration to previous conceptions. Med Sci Monit. 2017;23:1896–906.
28. Guo J, Chung UI, Kondo H, Bringhurst FR, Kronenberg HM. The PTH/PTHrP receptor can delay chondrocyte hypertrophy in vivo without activating phospholipase C. Dev Cell. 2002;3:183–94.
29. Guo J, Liu M, Yang D, Bouxsein ML, Thomas CC, Schipani E, et al. Phospholipase C signaling via the parathyroid hormone (PTH)/PTH-related peptide receptor is essential for normal bone responses to PTH. Endocrinology. 2010;151:3502–13.
30. Compston J, Cooper A, Cooper C, Gittoes N, Gregson C, Harvey N, et al. UK clinical guideline for the prevention and treatment of osteoporosis. Arch Osteopos. 2017;12:43.
31. Yang D, Guo J, Divieti P, Shioda T, Bringhurst FR. CBP/p300-interacting protein CITED1 modulates parathyroid hormone regulation of osteoblastic differentiation. Endocrinology. 2008;149:1728–35.
32. Gabet Y, Kohavi D, Muller R, Chorev M, Bab I. Intermittently administered parathyroid hormone 1-34 reverses bone loss and structural impairment in orchiectomized adult rats. Osteoporos Int. 2005;16:1436–43.
33. Wu J, Wang XX, Chiba H, Higuchi M, Takasaki M, Ohta A, et al. Combined intervention of exercise and genistein prevented androgen deficiency-induced bone loss in mice. J Appl Physiol. 2003;94:335–3342.
34. Komrakova M, Krischek C, Wicke M, Sehmisch S, Tezval M, Rohrberg M, et al. Influence of intermittent administration of parathyroid hormone on muscle tissue and bone healing in orchiectomized rats or controls. J Endocrinol. 2011;209:9–19.
35. Bonnarens F, Einhorn TA. Production of a standard closed fracture in laboratory animal bone. J Orthop Res. 1984;2:97–101.
36. Uusitalo H, Rantakokko J, Ahonen M, Jamsa T, Tuukkanen J, KaHari V, et al. A metaphyseal defect model of the femur for studies of murine bone healing. Bone. 2001;28:423–9.
37. Huang JC, Sakata T, Pfleger LL, Bencsik M, Halloran BP, Bikle DD, et al. PTH differentially regulates expression of RANKL and OPG. J Bone Miner Res. 2004;19:235–44.
38. Liu BY, Wu PW, Bringhurst FR, Wang JT. Estrogen inhibition of PTH-stimulated osteoclast formation and attachment in vitro: involvement of both PKA and PKC. Endocrinology. 2002;143:627–35.
39. Miyamoto T, Suda T. Differentiation and function of osteoclasts. Keio J Med. 2003;52:1–7.
40. Mao D, Epple H, Uthgenannt B, Novack DV, Faccio R. PLCgamma2 regulates osteoclastogenesis via its interaction with ITAM proteins and GAB2. J Clin Invest. 2006;116:2869–79.
41. Kondo H, Guo J, Bringhurst FR. Cyclic adenosine monophosphate/protein kinase A mediates parathyroid hormone/parathyroid hormone-related protein receptor regulation of osteoclastogenesis and expression of RANKL and osteoprotegerin mRNAs by marrow stromal cells. J Bone Miner Res. 2002;17:1667–79.

9

The clinical effect of an unloader brace on patients with osteoarthritis of the knee, a randomized placebo controlled trial with one year follow up

Hjörtur F. Hjartarson[1,3]* ⬤ and Sören Toksvig-Larsen[2,3]

Abstract

Background: Treatment of patients with knee osteoarthritis is challenging. Unloader braces have been developed with various success. Unloader One® Knee Brace is light, easily-fitted and shown to be effective by the unloading of the affected compartment. The aim of the study was to assess the clinical outcome of the brace vs. a placebo on patients with knee osteoarthritis.

Methods: Initially 150 patients were randomized to receive either the Unloader brace or a control placebo group look-alike brace where the active strips had been removed. The patients were followed up at 6,12,26 and 52 weeks with Knee Society Score (KSS) and Knee injury and Osteoarthritis Outcome Score (KOOS). The reason for dropout was recorded.

Results: A total of 149 patients were included, 74 in the study and 75 in the control group. The mean age was 59.6 vs. 60.2, BMI was 27.5 vs. 26.9, 37% vs. 44% were women in the study vs. control group. Both groups showed improvement in KSS over 52 weeks, with the study group showing higher improvement in mean scores. KSS increased from 64.3 to 84.0 for the study group and from 64.0 to 74.6 for the control group ($p = 0.009$). The study group improved in KSS function from 67.0 to 78.6 ($p < 0.001$) and KOOS for knee related symptoms increased/improved from 64.3 to 72.4 ($p < 0.001$). Activity of daily living increased/improved from 65.3 to 75.2 and Sports/Recreation from 24.6 to 40.2 ($p > 0.001$) whereas the control group did not show significant improvements in any of the scores. The dropout was higher in the control group, 40 vs. 25.

Conclusions: The brace seems to be more effective and better tolerated than the placebo.

Background

Osteoarthritis (OA) is a progressive degenerative joint disease that involves damage to the joint cartilage and changes in the subchondral bone and connective tissue of the joints [1]. Risk factors include obesity, occupation, trauma, excess joint load and hereditary factors [1, 2]. As populations age and obesity increases the burden of knee OA is rising [3]. No cure exists for OA and all current treatments focus on symptom alleviation. Even though there are numerous well-documented treatments available, the treatment of OA of the knee in younger patients as well as older patients with mild to moderate pain still poses a challenge. The current consensus is that non-operative treatment is recommended before surgery, with a combination of pharmacological treatment and non-pharmacological modalities, such as patient education, physical therapy, weight loss, walking aids and braces [4]. In unicompartmental knee OA with valgus/varus misalignment, unloading of the affected compartment has shown to be effective in biomechanical studies [5]. Knee braces unloading the diseased compartment have been shown to be effective in several studies

---
* Correspondence: hjorturfr@gmail.com
[1]Dept of Orthopedics, Landspitali University Hospital, E-4 Fossvogur, 101, Reykjavik, Iceland
[3]Lund University, Lund, Sweden
Full list of author information is available at the end of the article

and are included in many guidelines for the treatment of symptomatic knee OA [6–9]. Many of these studies are limited by having few test subjects or short follow up times. Some studies have failed to show benefit of braces compared to other treatments [10] and a Cochrane review [11] published 2015 states that evidence for the use of braces is inconclusive. In this review osteoarthritis of different types and severities are analyzed. In this study only patients with mild to moderate osteoarthritis (Ahlbäck grade I-II) were included, as we believe this to be the target group for this type of treatment. The aim of this study was to assess the one-year clinical effect of an unloader knee brace compared to a placebo, evaluate compliance and reasons for discontinuing treatment.

Methods

This study was a randomized placebo controlled study in patients with mild to moderate knee OA. All patients included were initially treated in primary care settings, with patient education, physical therapy and analgesic use. Patients visiting our outpatient clinic who met the inclusion criteria were asked to join the study. Some patients were recruited after responding to advertisements in local newspapers and social media. The first patient was included in April 2012 and the last in August 2014. The follow up time was 12 months. An orthopedic surgeon evaluated symptoms and radiographic evidence before inclusion in the study. All patients between 30 to 70 years of age, with knee pain for more than three months, with arthroscopic or radiographic evidence of knee OA (Allbäck or Kellgren-Lawrence grade 1–2) [12], and with BMI < 35 were eligible for the study. Patients who had prior major surgery to the same knee, a history of stroke, neurological or psychiatric problems, patients using opioids or steroids, as well as patients with rheumatoid arthritis, immunological depression or other severe medical problems were excluded.

150 patients were randomized to either a study group or a control group and followed for one year. The study group received an Unloader One® knee brace (Ossur, Iceland, Fig. 1). The Unloader One uses two Dynamic Force Straps (DFS) to impart a force against the lateral side of the knee as the knee extends. The purpose of this force is to reduce the load in the medial knee compartment. The control group received an Unloader One brace, with the DFS removed. The purpose was to create a device that looked like the Unloader One® brace but without its functionality.

Information about age, gender, height, weight and occupation were collected. A study nurse randomized the patients to either of the two groups. An orthopedic technician fitted all the braces and the researchers collecting all the data were blinded. All patients were graded by a physician for Knee Society Score (KSS) [13] and answered

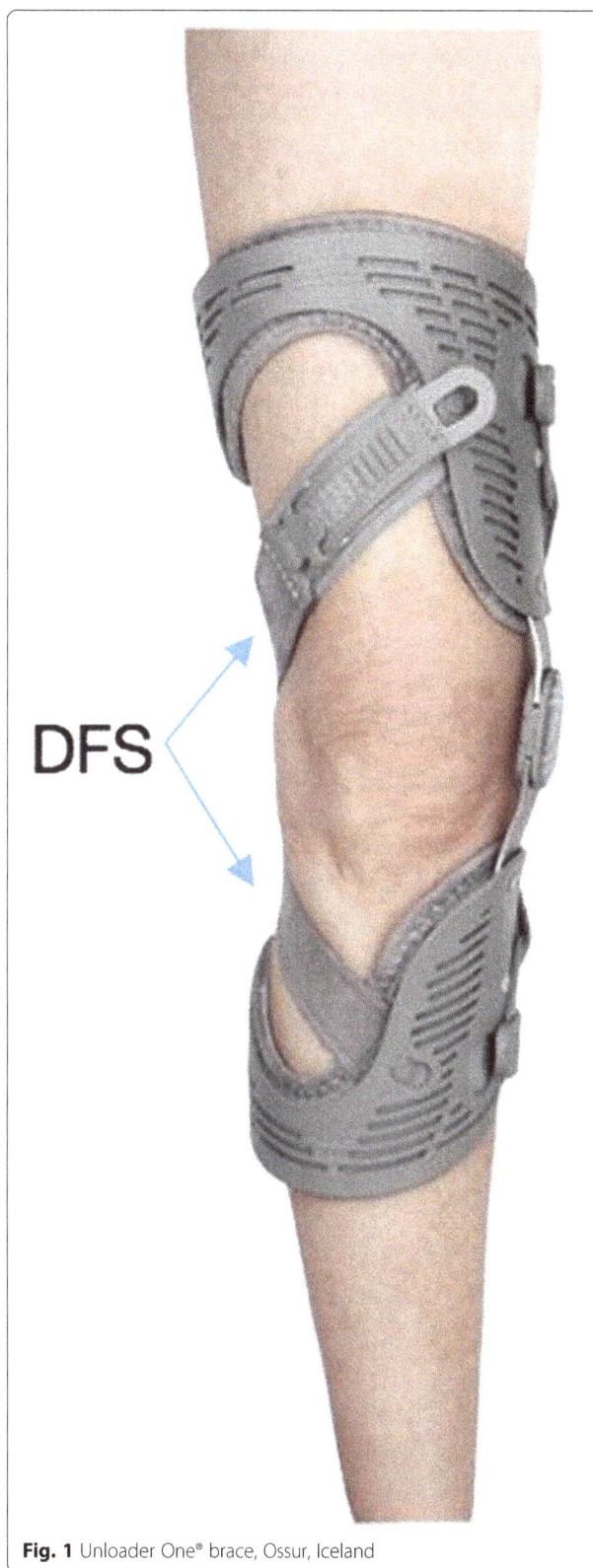

Fig. 1 Unloader One® brace, Ossur, Iceland

self-administered questionnaires; Knee injury and Osteoarthritis Outcome Score (KOOS) [14] before applying the brace at baseline and after 6,12,26 and 52 weeks. The KSS is a mixed outcome score, which is both objective and subjective. The KOOS is a self-administered patient reported outcome measurement questionnaire divided into five subcategories of pain, knee related symptoms, activities of daily living (ADL), sport and recreation (S&R) and quality of life (QoL). When answering the KOOS, patients are asked to consider their experience over the previous week. The results from both of these measurements are presented on a best-to-worst scale from 100 to 0. The KSS Score and function as well as the five subgroups of KOOS were determined as primary endpoints of the study. The reasons for dropout were documented, as well as analgesic use, frequency of doctor visits, absence from work and changes in employment status, which were considered secondary endpoints. Initially an evaluation of the cost of treatment and economic aspects were included as a secondary outcome, but were later discarded due to lack of data. All the patients from the control group that dropped out of the study due to ineffectiveness or mechanical problems were informed that they had a placebo brace and were offered to try out the original brace as one of the treatment options available to them. The treatment is not considered harmful but the placebo treatment may cause delay in treatment.

The data was analyzed and 95% confidence interval was calculated using a mixed model repeated measures analysis of variance. This method uses all available information and includes justifications for baseline imbalance with stratification of randomized confounding factors. An independent statistician analyzed all data presented. Statistical analysis was performed with STATA (StataCorp. 2015. Stata Statistical Software: Release 14. College Station, TX: StataCorp LP.) Power and sample size calculation was done with the PS: Power and Sample Size Calculation program by William D. Dupont and Walton D. Plummer, Jr. version 3,0. 2009 [15].

The results of data collected from KSS and KOOS are presented as estimated marginal mean difference at 6, 12, 24 and 52 weeks and 95% confidence interval.

Results

In total 149 patients answered questionnaires at baseline, 74 in the study group and 75 in the control group. All patients had unilateral medial OA, 80 in the left knee and 68 in the right knee. After 52 weeks 85 patients were still participating in the study, 50 in the study group and 35 in the control group. The reasons for dropout are shown in the flowchart below (Fig. 2). The main reasons for dropout were mechanical problems while using the brace. These problems include problems using the brace while working, sliding off, rubbing, feeling of instability and some patients found the brace to cumbersome to use. Nine patients underwent surgery before the study time was completed, 5 in the study group (3 total knee replacements, 1 total hip replacement, 1 high tibia osteotomy) and 4 in the control group

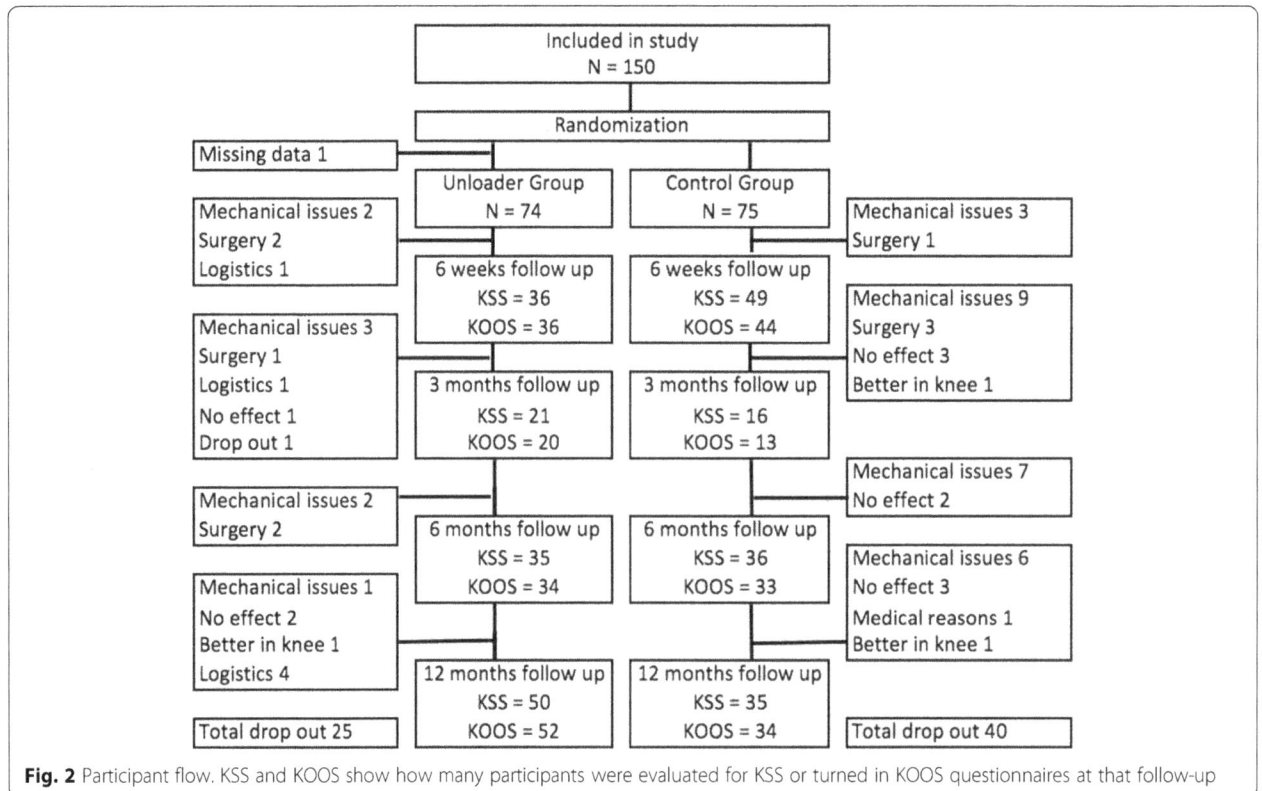

Fig. 2 Participant flow. KSS and KOOS show how many participants were evaluated for KSS or turned in KOOS questionnaires at that follow-up

(2 total knee replacements, 1 high tibia osteotomy and 1 spinal surgery). Some patients chose to discontinue the study due to work or lack of time, but continued to use the unloader brace, and are listed under logistics. Three patients reported silicone reaction or allergy as one of the reason for stop using the brace. One patient was included and given a subject number, but for reasons unknown to us, his data is missing and no record of him being fitted with a brace or called for evaluation. This explains why there are only 149 patients in the study.

Demographics
The baseline demographic and clinical characteristics are shown in Table 1.

Primary endpoints
KSS
Both groups showed an initial decline in KSS at six weeks indicating worsening of symptoms, followed by increase at three months indicating fewer symptoms, which continued until the end of study at twelve months. At six months the study group showed more improvements than the control group and the difference had increased even further at twelve months from 64.3 (95% CI 60.6–68.0) to 84.0 (95% CI 79.5–88.5) compared to 64.0 (95% CI 60.3–67.6) to 74.6 (95% CI 69.3–80.0). The difference at twelve months between the two groups is 9.4 (95% CI 2.4–16.4). (Fig. 3).

KSS function
The study group showed improved function at six weeks, as measured with the KSS functional measurement, with further improvements at 12, 24 and 52 weeks. The study group improved from 67.0 (95% CI 64.0–70.1) to 78.6 (95% CI 74.7–82.5) at 52 weeks, with a difference of 10.6 (95% CI 4.1–17.1). The control group showed slight improvement from 67.1 (95% CI 64.0–70.3) to

70.8 (95% CI 66.2–75.3) with the difference between the groups 7.8 (1.9–13.8) (Fig. 4).

KOOS
The adjusted mean values of the KOOS are listed in Table 2.

KOOS pain On the pain subscale of KOOS, the study group improved from 61.2 (95% CI 58.7–63.7) to 68.9 (95% 66.0–71.8) at 52 weeks, with a difference of 7.7 where a difference of 10 is considered a clinically detectable difference. The control group showed less improvement with a difference between the groups of 5.2 ($p = 0.02$). This difference is not considered clinically important.

KOOS symptoms The study group improved from 64.5 (95% CI 61.8–67.2) to 72.4 (95% CI 74.7–82.5) whereas the control group shows hardly any improvement from baseline. The difference at 52 weeks from baseline for the study group is 7.9 which is slightly less than 10, the clinically detectable cut off mark traditionally used in KOOS scores.

KOOS activities of daily living The sub score for ADL shows an increase in the study group from 65.3 (95% CI 62.9–67.7) to 75.2 (95% CI 72.4–78.0) and a difference of 9.8 ($p < 0.001$) while the control group shows no statistically significant difference from baseline.

KOOS sports and recreation The sub score for sport and recreation increased for the study group during the whole follow-up. The scores for the study group increased from 24.6 (95% CI 21.6–27.6) to 40.2 (95% CI 36.7–43.8) with a difference of 15.7 ($p < 0.001$). The control group did not show much improvement during this time and the difference between the groups at 52 weeks was 12.5 ($p < 0.001$), which is both a clinical and statistical significant difference.

KOOS quality of life The sub score for quality of life did not show much change for either group, the study group increasing from 52.2 (95% CI 49.4–55.0) to 55.7 (95% 52.5–59.0) and the control group actually decreasing from 52.3 (95% CI 49.5–55.1) to 49.5 (95% CI 45.4–53.6). The difference between the groups at 52 weeks was 6.1 ($p = 0.02$) which is not a clinically detectable difference.

Discussions
This exploratory study indicates that pain and function (activity of daily living and sports and recreation) can be improved in comparison to placebo during one-year use of the Unloader brace. The study showed some improvements in primary endpoints except in the KOOS

Table 1 Baseline demographic and clinical characteristics

Baseline characteristics	Study Group	Control Group
Participants	74	75
Age, in years (mean, SD)	59.6 (8.0)	60.3 (6.9)
Female gender	27 (37%)	33 (44%)
BMI (mean, SD)	27.5 (3.0)	26 (3.0)
KOOS Pain (mean, 95% CI)	61.2 (58.7–63.7)	61.1 (58.7–63.6)
KOOS Symtom (mean, 95% CI)	64.6 (61.8–67.2)	64.4 (61.7–67.1)
KOOS ADL (mean, 95% CI)	65.3 (62.9–67.7)	65.1 (62.7–67.5)
KOOS Sport/Rec (mean, 95% CI)	14.6 (21.6–27.6)	25.0 (22.0–28.0)
KOOS QoL (mean, 95% CI)	52.2 (49.4–55.0)	52.3 (49.5–55.1)
KSS Score (mean, 95% CI)	64.3 (60.3–67.6)	64.0 (60.3–67.6)
KSS Function (mean, 95% CI)	67.0 (64.0–70.1)	67.1 (64.0–70.3)

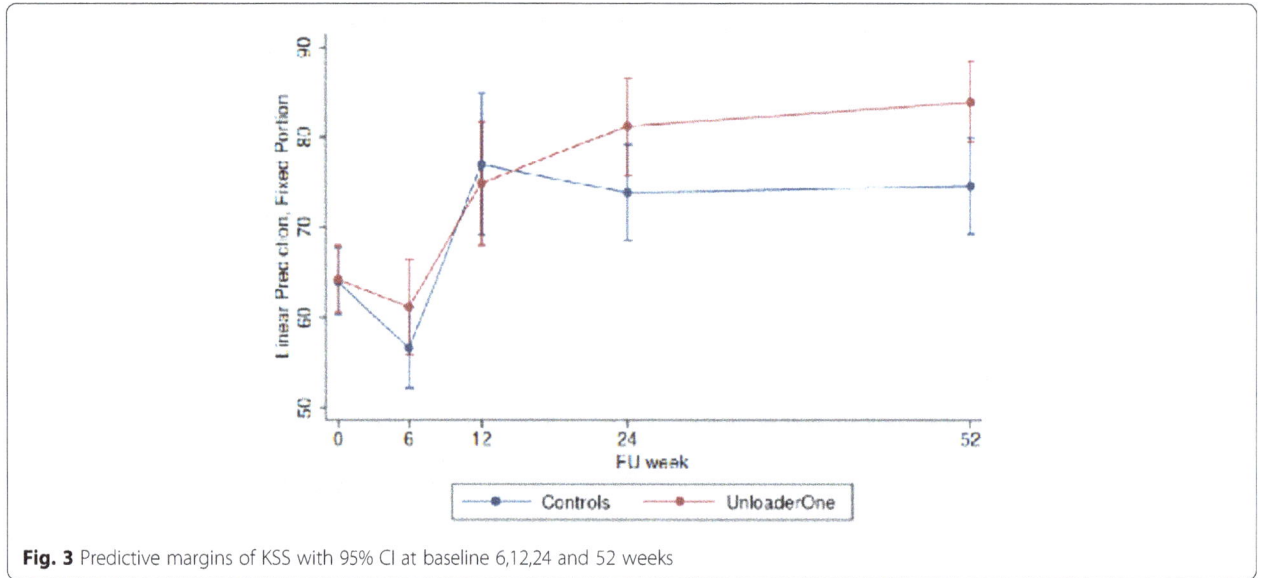

Fig. 3 Predictive margins of KSS with 95% CI at baseline 6,12,24 and 52 weeks

subgroup measuring quality of life at one year follow up. The differences between the groups at 6, 12 and 24 weeks are hard to interpret due to poor return at these intervals. Most patients showed up at some of the follow up appointments i.e. either at six weeks or three months but not both, and some showed up at all appointments. Some subjects stated that they did not have time for all the follow-up visits. Some patients choose not to come to the appointment but sent in the self-administered questionnaires, and others showed up at the appointments but neglected to send in the self-reported questionnaires.

There were more dropouts from the control group than the study group, mostly due to mechanical issues,

such as the brace sliding of the leg or hurting the patient.

It is interesting to note that improvements in KSS score are not evident at the six week follow up and the difference between groups does not become apparent until after six months suggesting that long term follow up is needed to see the difference. Many studies are limited by short follow up times. This also suggests that it may take time for the patients to adjust to the brace in the clinical setting and full results should not be expected immediately.

The high dropout rate in the control group compared to the study group shows in our opinion that the design of the brace matters and supports the theory that

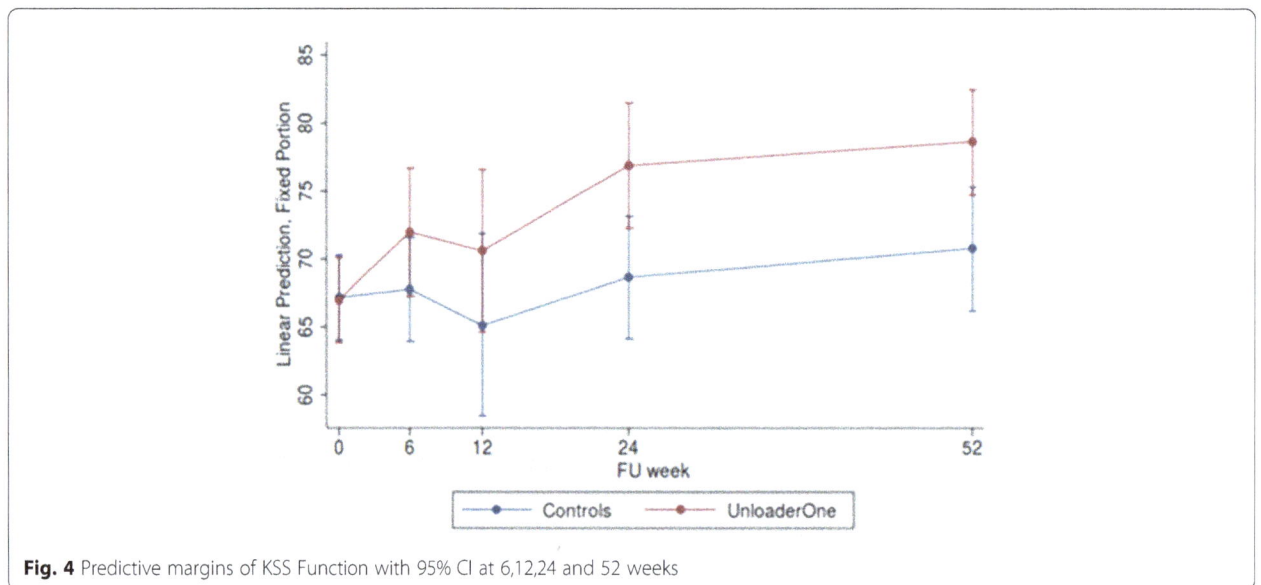

Fig. 4 Predictive margins of KSS Function with 95% CI at 6,12,24 and 52 weeks

Table 2 KOOS change from baseline to week 52, adjusted mean values and 95% confidence intervals

Outcomes	At baseline		At 52 follow up		Change from baseline		Between group
	Unloader	Controls	Unloader	Controls	Unloader	Controls	difference
KOOS Pain	61.2 (58.7, 63.7)	61.1 (58.7, 63.6)	68.9 (66.0, 71.8)	63.7 (60.2, 67.3)	7.7 (4.2, 11.2)	2.6 (1.4, 6.6)	5.2 (0.6, 9.8)
KOOS Symptom	64.5 (61.8, 67.2)	64.4 (61.7, 67.1)	72.4 (69.2, 75.6)	65.4 (61.6, 69.3)	7.9 (4.0, 11.8)	1.0 (−3.4, 5.5)	6.9 (1.9, 11.9)
KOOS ADL	65.3 (62.9, 67.7)	65.1 (62.7, 67.5)	75.2 (72.4, 78.0)	66.9 (63.5, 70.3)	9.8 (6.4, 13.3)	1.8 (−2.1, 5.8)	8.2 (3.8, 12.6)
KOOS Sport/Rec	24.6 (21.6, 27.6)	25.0 (22.0, 28.0)	40.2 (36.7, 43.8)	27.8 (23.4, 32.1)	15.7 (11.3, 20.0)	2.8 (−2.2, 7.8)	12.5 (6.8, 18.1)
KOOS QOL	52.2 (49.4, 55.0)	52.3 (49.5, 55.1)	55.7 (52.4, 59.0)	49.5 (45.4, 53.6)	3.5 (−0.6, 7.6)	−2.7 (−7.5, 2.0)	6.1 (0.9, 11.4)

unloading the affected compartment can relief pain and improve function. With this said, it should be kept in mind that the placebo braces might still have clinical effect as shown in biomechanical studies even though the dynamic tension strap has been removed. This effect might be due to diminished muscular co contractions rather than compartmental unloading as suggested by Ramsey et al. [16].

The KSS questions for pain and function ask patients to remember their experience the previous four weeks and the KOOS questionnaire the previous week. It is a thought for mind if these kinds of outcome scores are appropriate for measuring outcomes for a device that is only used during activity rather than continuous pain relieving effect such as medication or operations. This might explain larger differences between groups in functional scores rather than pain and symptom scores.

There is a clinically and statistically significant improvement in KSS and KSS function for both groups at one year compared with baseline. These results are compatible with previously published studies [17, 18]. There is also difference between groups but it is not statistically significant. For KOOS Pain, symptoms and quality of life there is a slight improvement at one year compared with the baseline for the control group even though it's questionable that this improvement is clinically significant. There is both a clinical and statistical significant improvement in the category of sport and recreation in the study group, with significant difference between the groups at one year follow up.

In the study protocol we had set the economic aspects of brace use as the secondary endpoint. This proved to be more complex than we anticipated and beyond the scope of this article and therefore the secondary endpoint was limited to the dropout rate.

Conclusions

The results of this study reflect our experience in clinical practice, there are many who find braces useful and there are those who don't think that they add anything to their treatment. Further research should be focused on identifying the responders and non-responders of this treatment applying OARSI criteria [19] for responders and to see what if any differentiates these groups.

Abbreviations
ADL: Activities of daily living; BMI: Body max index; KOOS: Knee and Osteoarthritis Outcome Score; KSS: Knee Society Score; OA: Osteoarthritis; OARSI: Osteoarthritis Research Society International; QoL: Quality of life; S&R: Sports and recreation

Acknowledgements
Marie Davidsson and Paul Ipsen for help with administration, Jonas Ranstam for statistics. Saskia Titman for English manuscript editing.

Funding
Össur, Icleand provided braces for this study and departmental research funding.

Authors' contributions
HFH and STL conceived and designed the protocol, collected and analyzed the data, HFH drafted manuscript, HFH and STL proofread manuscript and finalized. All authors read and approved the final manuscript

Competing interests
The authors declare that they have no competing interests. Neither of the authors, nor anyone in their immediate families have any financial ties to Össur.

Author details
[1]Dept of Orthopedics, Landspitali University Hospital, E-4 Fossvogur, 101, Reykjavik, Iceland. [2]Dept of Orthopedics, Hässleholm hospital, Esplanadgatan 19, 281 38 Hässleholm, Sweden. [3]Lund University, Lund, Sweden.

References
1. Bay-Jensen AC, Hoegh-Madsen S, Dam E, Henriksen K, Sondergaard BC, Pastoureau P, Qvist P, Karsdal MA. Which elements are involved in reversible and irreversible cartilage degradation in osteoarthritis? Rheumatol Int. 2010; 30(4):435–42.
2. Neogi T, Zhang Y. Epidemiology of osteoarthritis. Rheum Dis Clin N Am. 2013;39(1):1–19.
3. Woolf AD, Pfleger B. Burden of major musculoskeletal conditions. Bull World Health Organ. 2003;81(9):646–56.
4. Zhang W, Moskowitz RW, Nuki G, Abramson S, Altman RD, Arden N, Bierma-Zeinstra S, Brandt KD, Croft P, Doherty M, et al. OARSI recommendations for the management of hip and knee osteoarthritis, part II: OARSI evidence-based, expert consensus guidelines. Osteoarthr Cartil. 2008;16(2):137–62.
5. Petersen W, Ellermann A, Zantop T, Rembitzki IV, Semsch H, Liebau C, Best R. Biomechanical effect of unloader braces for medial osteoarthritis of the knee: a systematic review (CRD 42015026136). Arch Orthop Trauma Surg. 2016;136(5):649 56.

6.   Rannou F, Poiraudeau S, Beaudreuil J. Role of bracing in the management of knee osteoarthritis. Curr Opin Rheumatol. 2010;22(2):218–22.

7.   Ostrander RV, Leddon CE, Hackel JG, O'Grady CP, Roth CA. Efficacy of unloader bracing in reducing symptoms of knee osteoarthritis. Am J Orthop (Belle Mead NJ). 2016;45(5):306–11.

8.   Brouwer RW, van Raaij TM, Verhaar JA, Coene LN, Bierma-Zeinstra SM. Brace treatment for osteoarthritis of the knee: a prospective randomized multi-Centre trial. Osteoarthr Cartil. 2006;14(8):777–83.

9.   Steadman JR, Briggs KK, Pomeroy SM, Wijdicks CA. Current state of unloading braces for knee osteoarthritis. Knee Surg Sports Traumatol Arthrosc. 2016;24(1):42–50.

10. van Raaij TM, Reijman M, Brouwer RW, Bierma-Zeinstra SM, Verhaar JA. Medial knee osteoarthritis treated by insoles or braces: a randomized trial. Clin Orthop Relat Res. 2010;468(7):1926–32.

11. Duivenvoorden T, Brouwer RW, van Raaij TM, Verhagen AP, Verhaar JA, Bierma-Zeinstra SM: Braces and orthoses for treating osteoarthritis of the knee. Cochrane Database Syst Rev 2015(3):CD004020. https://doi.org/10.1002/14651858.CD004020.pub3.

12. Kellgren JH, Lawrence JS. Radiological assessment of rheumatoid arthritis. Ann Rheum Dis. 1957;16(4):485–93.

13. Insall JN, Dorr LD, Scott RD, Scott WN. Rationale of the knee society clinical rating system. Clin Orthop Relat Res. 1989;(248):13–4.

14. Roos EM, Roos HP, Lohmander LS, Ekdahl C, Beynnon BD. Knee injury and osteoarthritis outcome score (KOOS)--development of a self-administered outcome measure. J Orthop Sports Phys Ther. 1998;28(2):88–96.

15. Dupont WDPW. Power and sample size calculations: a review and computer program. Control Clin Trials. 1990;11:116–28.

16. Ramsey DK, Briem K, Axe MJ, Snyder-Mackler L. A mechanical theory for the effectiveness of bracing for medial compartment osteoarthritis of the knee. J Bone Joint Surg Am. 2007;89(11):2398–407.

17. Kirkley A, Webster-Bogaert S, Litchfield R, Amendola A, MacDonald S, McCalden R, Fowler P. The effect of bracing on varus gonarthrosis. J Bone Joint Surg Am. 1999;81(4):539–48.

18. Sattari S, Ashraf AR. Comparison the effect of 3 point valgus stress knee support and lateral wedge insoles in medial compartment knee osteoarthritis. Iran Red Crescent Med J. 2011;13(9):624–8.

19. Pham T, Van Der Heijde D, Lassere M, Altman RD, Anderson JJ, Bellamy N, Hochberg M, Simon L, Strand V, Woodworth T, et al. Outcome variables for osteoarthritis clinical trials: the OMERACT-OARSI set of responder criteria. J Rheumatol. 2003;30(7):1648–54.

Skull-femoral traction after posterior release for correction of adult severe scoliosis: efficacy and complications

Jun Qiao[1†], Lingyan Xiao[2†], Leilei Xu[1], Zhen Liu[1], Xu Sun[1], Bangping Qian[1], Zezhang Zhu[1*] and Yong Qiu[1]

Abstract

Background: It is a great challenge for spine surgeons to correct severe rigid scoliosis. We developed a three-staged correction (one stage posterior release and screw placement, two stage skull-femoral traction and three stage posterior instrumentation) for adult severe scoliosis. The objective of this study is to investigate safety and efficacy of a three- staged correction for adult severe scoliosis.

Methods: A retrospective review was performed for patients with severe scoliosis receiving three- staged correction (one stage posterior release and screw placement, two stage skull-femoral traction and three stage posterior instrumentation) from June 2001 to October 2014. The inclusion criteria were as follows: [1] age more than 18 years; [2] main curve larger than 90°; [3] a minimum 2-year follow-up. Patients were excluded if they had a history of surgery or anterior release or receiving three column osteotomies.

Results: A total of 63 patients were included (37 female and 26 male), with a mean age of 22.7 years (range: 18–30 years) and follow-up of 42.6 months (range: 24–108 months). The aetiology was congenital in 27 patients, neuromuscular in 18, idiopathic in 11, neurofibromatosis-1 in 4 and Marfan syndrome in 3. The mean traction weight was 28.4 kg (range: 18–32 kg), equal to 57.2% of patients' body weight (range: 42.7–72.3%). The mean traction time was 22.7 days (range: 12–44 days). Postoperative correction rate was 55% (range: 38–78%) for scoliosis and 51% (range: 32–75%) for kyphosis. Contribution of traction to correction was 51% (range: 36–70%) for scoliosis and was 43% (range: 34–55%) for kyphosis.

Conclusions: Three- staged correction (one stage posterior release and screw placement, two stage skull-femoral traction and three stage posterior instrumentation) could effectively correct adult severe scoliosis. The incidence of complications of skull-femoral traction was not low, but transient and could be successfully managed.

Keywords: Adult severe scoliosis, Skull-femoral traction, Complication

Background

It is a great challenge for spine surgeons to correct severe rigid scoliosis and kyphoscoliosis [1]. In addition to large curve, significant pulmonary compromise and neurological deficit would also place patients under risks of surgical complication [2–5]. In the past, multiple forms of traction were employed to increase correction of curve, improve pulmonary function and save neurological function before surgery [6–9]. The development of segmental instrumentation and aggressive osteotomies largely improved correction of severe rigid scoliosis and kyphosis [10–12]. However, traction still has its role in improving pulmonary function and minimizing neurological complications [9, 13, 14]. Moreover, traction could provide wide release of spine that increase flexibility of both primary and secondary curves; whereas, osteotomies could only release a limited range of spine. Halo-gravity traction (HGT) is the most frequently used traction for patients, especially pediatric patients with severe scoliosis or kyphoscoliosis. It could gradually lengthen the height of thoracic spine and rib cage, and enlarge the volume of lungs. Skull-femoral traction was

* Correspondence: zhuzezhang@126.com
†Jun Qiao and Lingyan Xiao contributed equally to this work.
[1]Department of Spine Surgery, the Affiliated Drum Tower Hospital of Nanjing University Medical School, 321 Zhongshan Road, Nanjing, China
Full list of author information is available at the end of the article

a more aggressive form that simultaneously offer caudal and cephalic traction forces. As compared to HGT, skull-femoral traction (SFT) could generate more traction forces [15, 16]. Moreover, the traction time of SFT is shorter than HGT, mostly less than 4 weeks. SFT is more suitable for adult patients, as most pediatric patients could not bear such big traction forces. In this study, we investigated safety and efficacy of a three- staged correction (one stage posterior release and screw placement, two stage skull-femoral traction and three stage posterior instrumentation) for adult severe scoliosis (Fig. 1).

Methods

Patients

A retrospective review was performed for patients with severe scoliosis receiving three- staged correction (one stage posterior release and screw placement, two stage skull-femoral traction and three stage posterior instrumentation) from June 2001 to October 2014. The inclusion criteria were as follows: [1] age more than 18 years; [2] main curve larger than 90°; [3] a minimum 2-year follow-up. Patients were excluded if they had a history of surgery or anterior release or receiving three column osteotomies.

Radiographic analysis

Standing long-cassette antero-posterior (AP) and lateral radiographs of the whole spine were taken before posterior surgery, 10 days after posterior surgery and at final follow-up respectively. Supine antero-posterior (AP) and lateral radiographs were taken before posterior release and screw placement surgery and under traction before posterior instrumentation. Coronal and sagittal curves were measured by Cobb method. Curve flexibility for scoliosis was initially assessed using the supine side bending films in all patients and calculating the percentage of curve correction on these views. Curve flexibility for kyphosis = (Standing kyphosis- supine kyphosis)/ standing kyphosis*100%. Curve correction rate = (initial curve- corrected curve) /initial curve *100%. Contribution of traction to correction = (initial curve-curve after traction)/ (initial curve-postoperative curve) * 100%. CT scans of instrumented levels were performed after first stage surgery to see the positions of pedicle screws.

Posterior release and screw placement

After a midline incision, subcutaneous tissue and subperiosteal was dissected from the spinous processes, laminae and transverse processes. The supra and interspinous ligaments at each level were completely removed. And then, a complete excision of the ligamentum flavum was performed by means of a Kerrison rongeur. The release of this rongeur was extended throughout the ligament, beginning in the midline and proceeding laterally toward both facets. At last, the inferior facet of the superior vertebra was removed, as was much of the superior facet of the inferior vertebra. This release was performed along the instrumented region at each level. Pedicle screws were then

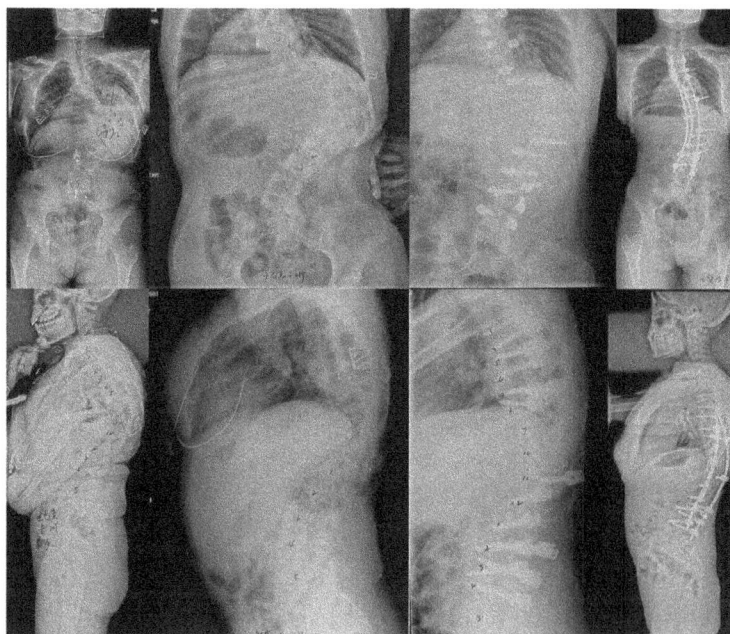

Fig. 1 A 21-year-old female patient with congenital kyphoscoliosis had a scoliosis of 136° and a kyphosis of 85°. Major coronal curve decreased to 100° at side bending radiograph, and kyphosis to 75° at supine radiograph. After 3-week traction, scoliosis was corrected to 75°, and kyphosis to 56°. Postoperative standing radiograph demonstrated scoliosis was corrected to 60°, and kyphosis to 40°

placed by free-hand technique or with the aid of O-arm based navigation system, maintaining the construct density above 70%. Skull-traction was installed after closure of posterior incision.

Traction protocol

Traction was usually started at the second day after posterior surgery with a weight of 2 kg and gradually increased at a rate of 1 to 2 kg per day if patients well tolerated (Fig.3). The maximum traction weight could be 33 to 50% of the whole body weight depending on patients' tolerance. Traction was applied for a minimum of 12 h per day, with the traction weight lessened to 50% in the night. If tolerated, traction could be applied for a maximum of 20 h. In the rest of time, they are allowed out of traction for bathroom privileges and hygiene purposes as well as eating. During the traction, the patient's neurological status was frequently checked. If hyper reflex of the extremities, Babinski sign, paresthesia, dysfunction of cranial nerves or any other neurological compromise were noted, the weight would be immediately reduced. The length of the traction period was mainly determined by the radiographic evidence of curve improvement on weekly radiographs, in addition to clinical evaluation of the patients' pulmonary and neurological function.

Posterior instrumentation

Surgery was performed under traction. Pedicle screws were revised if showed mal-placed at postoperative CT scans. Rod was first placed at concave side of the spine, and then convex side. Satellite rods and segmental correction technique were used if necessary. Correction was gradually achieved with a combination of maneuvers including derotation, translation and the application of cantilever forces. A wake-up test was performed and was positive in all patients.

Statistical analysis of the data was performed using SPSS 17.0 software (SPSS Inc., Chicago, IL, USA). Statistical data were presented as the mean ± standard deviation. The changes of radiographic parameters were compared using paired Student's t test. A Pearson correlation was conducted to assess normally distributed variables. Spearman's rank correlation method was conducted for nonparametric data. Bivariate analyses for correction rates were conducted first, and variables that were significant at $P < 0.05$ or considered relevant to correction rates from a clinical perspective were entered into multivariable linear regression models. Statistical significance was defined as $P < 0.05$.

Results

Patient characteristics

A total of 63 patients were included (37 female and 26 male), with a mean age of 22.7 years (range: 18–30 years) and follow-up of 42.6 months (range: 24–108 months). The aetiology was congenital in 27 patients, neuromuscular in 18, idiopathic in 11, neurofibromatosis-1 in 4 and Marfan syndrome in 3. The mean traction weight was 28.4 kg (range: 18–32 kg), equal to 57.2% of patients' body weight (range: 42.7–72.3%). The mean traction time was 22.7 days (range: 12–44 days).

Radiographic analysis

The average preoperative coronal Cobb angle of main curve was 118.7° (range: 92° -158°) and was 93.1° (range: 70° -139°) for kyphosis. The mean curve flexibility was 18% (range: 0–37%) for scoliosis and 11% (range: 0–22%) for kyphosis. Both coronal and sagittal were continuously reduced under traction. (Fig. 1) Postoperative correction rate was 55% (range: 38–78%) for scoliosis and 51% (range: 32–75%) for kyphosis. Contribution of traction to correction was 51% (range: 36–70%) for scoliosis and was 43% (range: 34–55%) for kyphosis (Fig. 2). Significant difference of curve severity was noted between initial curve and post-traction curve for both coronal and sagittal deformity ($P < 0.05$). The average postoperative coronal Cobb angle of main curve was 57.3° (range: 29° -96°) and 59.6° (range: 29° -102°) at last follow-up. The average postoperative kyphosis was 46.4° (range: 19°- 76°) and 48.1° (range: 20°-78°) at last follow-up. There is no difference between postoperative curve and follow-up curve for both coronal and sagittal deformity ($P < 0.05$). (Table 1).

Factors related to correction rates of traction and correction surgery

Age, preoperative curvature and curve flexibility were correlated to correction rates of traction for scoliosis (age: $r = -0.382$, preoperative curvature: $r = -0.416$, curve flexibility: $r = 0.537$; $P < 0.05$). Age and curve flexibility were correlated to correction rates of traction for kyphosis (age: $r = -0.405$, curve flexibility: $r = 0.493$; $P < 0.05$). Age, correction rates of traction and curve flexibility were correlated to correction rates of surgical correction for scoliosis (age: $r = -0.426$, correction rates of traction: $r = 0.629$, curve flexibility: $r = 0.594$; $P < 0.05$). Age, correction rates of traction and curve flexibility were correlated to correction rates of surgical correction for kyphosis (age: $r = -0.422$, correction rates of traction: $r = 0.568$, curve flexibility: $r = 0.483$; $P < 0.05$). (Table 2).

Multivariable regression analyses found that curve flexibility was related to correction rates of traction for both scoliosis ($r^2 = 0.392$; $P < 0.05$) and kyphosis ($r^2 = 0.375$; $P < 0.05$). Correction rates of traction ($r^2 = 0.421$; $P < 0.05$) and curve flexibility ($r^2 = 0.316$; $P < 0.05$) were related to correction rates of surgery for scoliosis. Correction rates of traction ($r^2 = 0.489$; $P < 0.05$) and curve flexibility ($r^2 = 0.292$; $P < 0.05$) were related to correction rates of surgery for kyphosis.

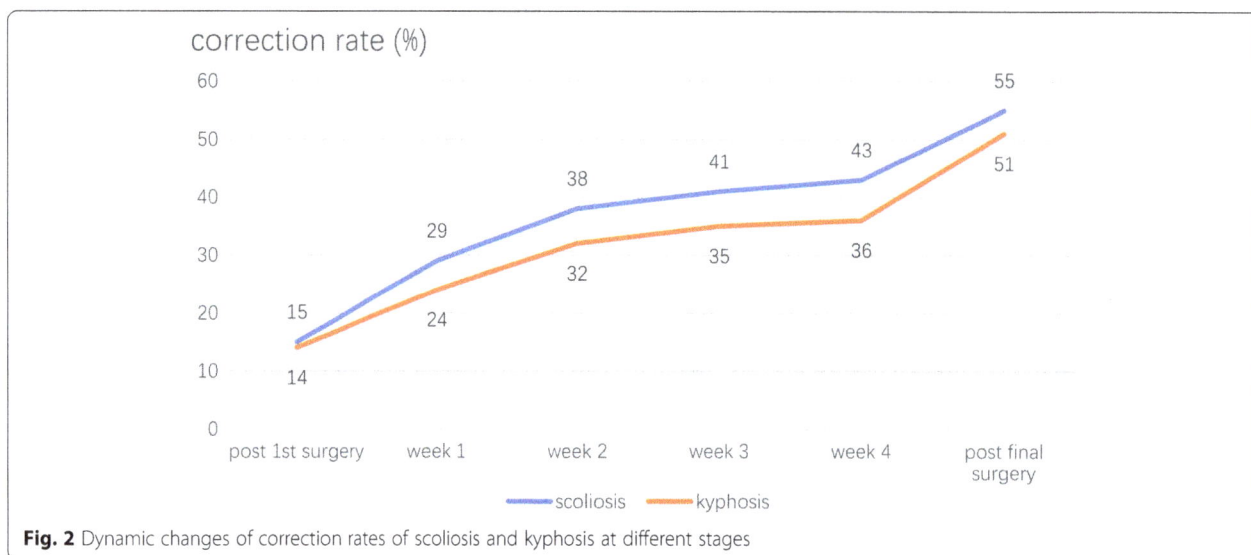

Fig. 2 Dynamic changes of correction rates of scoliosis and kyphosis at different stages

Complications

Surgical complications

In first stage surgery, 17 misplaced screws were observed at 12 patients, and were revised at final surgery. 2 patients developed pleural rupture during last surgery and were sutured operatively. One of the two patients with pleural rupture developed pleural effusion and underwent thoracic close drainage. Neurological deficit was observed at one patient after last surgery. For this patient, the muscle strength of left leg decreased to grade 4 after surgery, and completely recovered at final follow-up. Totally, the incidence of surgical complications was 19.0% for first stage surgery, and 4.8% for final surgery.

Traction complications

Two patients suffered from brachial plexus palsy and one patient femoral nerve palsy. However, complete nerve function restoration was achieved at final follow-up. Transient hematuria occurred in two patients. Gastrointestinal symptoms developed in one patient, and after reducing traction weight, the symptoms relived. Deep vein thrombosis (DVT) developed in two patients, and one patient underwent inferior vena filter placement. Pin infection occurred in two patients, and was controlled by debridement. Totally, the incidence of traction complications was 11.1%.

Table 1 Dynamic changes of curve severity at different stages

	scoliosis	kyphosis
Initial (°)	118.7	93.1
Bending/supine (°)	97.3	83.9
After 1st surgery (°)	99.6	80.1
After traction (°)	67.4	58.2
After final surgery (°)	57.3	46.4
Last follow-up (°)	59.6	48.1

Discussion

Several forms of traction were used for correcting severe scoliosis [2, 8, 15, 17]. Halo-gravity traction (HGT) was the most frequently used traction by using the weight of the body as a counterforce. It can be applied while a patient is in bed or on a wheelchair; thus, allowing patients to be out of bed to socialize and participate in exercise programs [18]. The most significant disadvantage of HGT may be the prolonged hospital stay, which was not accepted by all families. The effect of HGT on curve correction was controversial. Most studies did not support that preoperative-traction would provide superior curve correction to immediate spinal fusion with instrumentation. Seller [19] investigated efficacy of HGT on correction of neuromuscular scoliosis, and found that the surgical correction rates did not differ with or without preop-HGT. Sponseller [20] compared surgical correction of severe spine deformity with preoperative halo traction and without preoperative traction, and found there was no statistically significant difference in main coronal curve correction (62% vs. 59%), operative time, blood loss, and total complication rate (27% vs. 52%) between the two groups. Koller [13] also claimed that HGT should not be expected to significantly improve severe curves without a prior anterior and/or posterior release. However, as compared to increasing curve correction, pulmonary function improvement and recovery of neurological deficit achieved by HGT seems more important. Although no additional curve correction was achieved by HGT, Koller [13] demonstrated that FVC% was improved from 42 ± 20 (14–98) % to 49 ± 20 (19–100) % after HGT in patients with severe and rigid scoliosis and kyphoscoliosis. In their subgroup analysis, five patients with kyphoscoliosis and progressive neurological deficits from a decompensating curve showed

Table 2 Factors related to correction rates of traction and correction surgery

	Scoliosis traction rate		Kyphosis traction rate		Scoliosis correction rate		Kyphosis correction rate	
	r	p	r	p	r	p	r	p
Age	−0.382	0.032[a]	−0.405	0.027[a]	−0.426	0.009[a]	−0.422	0.018[a]
Preoperative scoliosis	−0.416	0.017[a]	–	–	0.218	0.104	–	–
Scoliosis flexibility	0.537	0.006[a]	–	–	0.594	0.002*	–	–
Preoperative kyohisis	–	–	0.176	0.094	–	–	0.228	0.058
Kyphosis flexibility	–	–	0.493	0.017[a]	–	–	0.483	0.021[a]
Scoliosis traction rate	–	–	–	–	0.629	0.002[a]	–	–
Kyphosis traction rate	–	–	–	–	–	–	0.568	0.003[a]

[a]:$p < 0.05$

improvement after the initiation of HGT. HGT could lead to a slight curve correction and then causes a release of the apical tether on the spinal cord.

Some additional procedures were administrated in combination with traction to boost clinical and radiographic outcomes. Park [21] used an anterior release-HGT- posterior instrumentation protocol to correct severe pediatric spinal deformity getting 66.3% of major coronal curve correction and 62.7% of sagittal curve correction. Koptan [8] compared a three-staged correction by an anterior release, 2 weeks of halo-gravity traction then posterior instrumentation (TRN group) with a two-staged correction by anterior release then posterior instrumentation (SAP group), and found that the application of gradual traction over a limited period of 2 weeks in addition to anterior release led to better correction. Bao [22] reported a group of adult scoliosis patients with respiratory dysfunction undergoing HGT combined with assisted ventilation, and demonstrated that combined HGT and assisted ventilation would be beneficial to pulmonary function improvement in severe adult scoliosis cases. Halo-femoral traction was also popular in correcting severe scoliosis. Qiu [6] used an anterior release- halo femoral traction- posterior instrumentation to correct severe idiopathic and congenital scoliosis, and got a 57.5%. correction of major curve for idiopathic scoliosis and 45.2% for congenital scoliosis. Wang [23] used preoperative halo-femoral plus posterior vertebral column resection to correct extremely severe rigid spinal deformity with sharp angular curve > 150°, and achieved 69% correction of scoliosis and 66% correction of kyphosis. The present protocol was applied for the patients with good tolerance of heavy traction and without neurological compromise. If a patient had neurological compromise, we preferred a halo-gravity traction before correction surgery. The advantages of this protocol could be three folds: first, a long and difficult correction surgery for severe scoliosis was divided to two phases minimizing surgical complications and providing intermittent recovery period for patients;

second, posterior release had less complications and pulmonary compromise as compared to anterior release; third, heavy bi-directional traction by skull-femoral traction provided more traction forces and entailed less traction time as compared to HGT. In our cohort, correction rate of scoliosis reached 55% and kyphosis 58%. The contribution of traction to correction was 51% for scoliosis and 43% for kyphosis. As other forms of traction, skull-femoral traction after posterior release attained most of correction within 2 weeks, and after 3 weeks, the traction corrected deformity much slower than the first 2 weeks. 3 weeks of traction is enough for most patients.

Prevalence of traction-related complications ranged from 16 to 28% [24]. Pin-related complications ranked first, including pin loosening and superficial pin-site infection. In our study, pin-related complications occurred at 2 patients, both of which were infection. After debridement, infection was successfully controlled. The most concerning complication was neurological deficit caused by heavy weight traction [14, 25]. In our hospital, skull- femoral traction was always prescribed to adult patients, because they have better tolerance as compared to pediatric patients. However, there were still two cases of brachial plexus palsy and one case of femoral nerve palsy. After reducing traction weight, symptoms relived in all three patients. Deep vein thrombosis (DVT) may be a unique complication for skull-femoral traction, because the patients were immobilized during traction [26]. To avoid this complication, we recommended the use of anticoagulant therapy during traction [27]. Other complications included two cases of transient hematuria and one case of gastrointestinal symptoms, which were relieved by reducing traction weight. Generally, the incidence of complications of skull-femoral traction was not low, but transient and could be successfully managed.

Seventeen misplaced screws were observed at 12 patients at CT scans. At final surgery, we revised the positions of these screws. For some severe scoliosis, especially scoliosis associated with Marfan syndrome and neurofibromatosis-1, pedicles were extremely thin in concave side of apex region, and misplacement would be inevitable by free-hand technique. Staged correction protocol provides opportunity to revise misplaced screws that avoids neurological compromise and correction loss caused by misplaced screws. Only one case of incomplete neurological deficit occurred, and finally recovered. Traction may increase the tolerance of spinal cord to stretch trees and ischemia from correction of curve, diminishing risks of neurological complications.

The most significant limitation of this three-staged correction procedure was its inability to manage patients with pulmonary compromise because posterior release and screw placement should be performed prior to traction. A patient with pulmonary compromise may not tolerate fist stage surgery. In addition, bidirectional heavy weight traction was not suitable for pediatric patients in consideration of their poor tolerance. Finally, back pain and joint stiffness should also draw attention.

Another limitation of this study was unavailability of psychological status of patients receiving this complex treatment. Long time bed-bound heavy traction would pose significant mental stress on patients. Further study is needed to evaluate psychological status of these patients by using reliable questionnaires. In addition, heterogeneity of etiology was also a limitation. However, correlation analysis did not find correlation between etiology and surgical outcomes.

Conclusion

In conclusion, three- staged correction (one stage posterior release and screw placement, two stage skull-femoral traction and three stage posterior instrumentation) could effectively correct adult severe scoliosis. The incidence of complications of skull-femoral traction was not low, but transient and could be successfully managed.

Abbreviations
HGT: Halo-gravity traction; SFT: Skull-femoral traction

Acknowledgements
We would like to thank all participating patients, and MS Zhang Linlin for radiograph collecting.

Funding
This study was supported by the National Natural Science Foundation of China (81501932) and Science Foundation of Jiangsu Province (BK20150107) and China Postdoctoral Science Foundation (2015 M570440).

Authors' contributions
QJ, XLL, LZ and XL reviewed radiographs. QJ and SX performed statistical analysis and drafted the manuscript. ZZ, and QB gave administrative and intellectual support. ZZ and YQ conceived the study, finalized the manuscript and is responsible. All authors read and approved the final manuscript.

Competing interests
Zezhang Zhu is a member of the Editorial Board of BMC Musculoskeletal Disorder. The other authors declare that they have no competing interests.

Author details
[1]Department of Spine Surgery, the Affiliated Drum Tower Hospital of Nanjing University Medical School, 321 Zhongshan Road, Nanjing, China. [2]Intensive care unit, the Second Hospital of Nanjing, Southeast University, Nanjing, China.

References

1. Kandwal P, Goswami A, Vijayaraghavan G, Subhash KR, Jaryal A, Upendra BN, et al. Staged anterior release and posterior instrumentation in correction of severe rigid scoliosis (cobb angle >100 degrees). Spine Deform. 2016;4(4):296–303.
2. Chan CY, Lim CY, Shahnaz Hasan M, Kwan MK. The use of pre-operative halo traction to minimize risk for correction of severe scoliosis in a patient with Fontan circulation: a case report and review of literature. Eur Spine J. 2016;25(Suppl 1):245–50.
3. Aaro S, Ohlund C. Scoliosis and pulmonary function. Spine (Phila Pa 1976). 1984;9(2):220–2.
4. Danielsson AJ, Ekerljung L, Hallerman KL. Pulmonary function in middle-aged patients with idiopathic scoliosis with onset before the age of 10 years. Spine Deform. 2015;3(5):451–61.
5. Hamilton DK, Smith JS, Sansur CA, Glassman SD, Ames CP, Berven SH, et al. Rates of new neurological deficit associated with spine surgery based on 108,419 procedures: a report of the scoliosis research society morbidity and mortality committee. Spine (Phila Pa 1976). 2011;36(15):1218–28.
6. Qiu Y, Liu Z, Zhu F, Wang B, Yu Y, Zhu Z, et al. Comparison of effectiveness of halo-femoral traction after anterior spinal release in severe idiopathic and congenital scoliosis: a retrospective study. J Orthop Surg Res. 2007;2:23.
7. Rinella A, Lenke L, Whitaker C, Kim Y, Park SS, Peelle M, et al. Perioperative halo-gravity traction in the treatment of severe scoliosis and kyphosis. Spine (Phila Pa 1976). 2005;30(4):475–82.
8. Koptan W, ElMiligui Y. Three-staged correction of severe rigid idiopathic scoliosis using limited halo-gravity traction. Eur Spine J. 2012;21(6):1091–8.
9. Da Cunha RJ, Al Sayegh S, LaMothe JM, Letal M, Johal H, Parsons DL, et al. Intraoperative skull-femoral traction in posterior spinal arthrodesis for adolescent idiopathic scoliosis: the impact on perioperative outcomes and health resource utilization. Spine (Phila Pa 1976). 2015;40(3):E154–60.
10. Chen B, Yuan Z, Chang MS, Huang JH, Li H, Yang WZ, et al. Safety and efficacy of one-stage spinal osteotomy for severe and rigid congenital scoliosis associated with split spinal cord malformation. Spine (Phila Pa 1976). 2015;40(18):E1005–13.
11. Hedlund R. Pedicle subtraction osteotomy in degenerative scoliosis. Eur Spine J. 2012;21(3):566–8.
12. Suh SW, Modi HN, Yang J, Song HR, Jang KM. Posterior multilevel vertebral osteotomy for correction of severe and rigid neuromuscular scoliosis: a preliminary study. Spine (Phila Pa 1976). 2009;34(12):1315–20.
13. Koller H, Zenner J, Gajic V, Meier O, Ferraris L, Hitzl W. The impact of halo-gravity traction on curve rigidity and pulmonary function in the treatment of severe and rigid scoliosis and kyphoscoliosis: a clinical study and narrative review of the literature. Eur Spine J. 2012;21(3):514–29.
14. Lewis SJ, Gray R, Holmes LM, Strantzas S, Jhaveri S, Zaarour C, et al. Neurophysiological changes in deformity correction of adolescent idiopathic scoliosis with intraoperative skull-femoral traction. Spine (Phila Pa 1976). 2011;36(20):1627–38.
15. Zhang HQ, Gao QL, Ge L, Wu JH, Liu JY, Guo CF, et al. Strong halo-femoral traction with wide posterior spinal release and three dimensional spinal correction for the treatment of severe adolescent idiopathic scoliosis. Chin Med J. 2012;125(7):1297–302.
16. Watanabe K, Lenke LG, Bridwell KH, Kim YJ, Hensley M, Koester L. Efficacy of perioperative halo-gravity traction for treatment of severe scoliosis (>/=100 degrees). J Orthop Sci. 2010;15(6):720–30.
17. Kulkarni AG, Shah SP. Intraoperative skull-femoral (skeletal) traction in surgical correction of severe scoliosis (>80 degrees) in adult neglected scoliosis. Spine (Phila Pa 1976). 2013;38(8):659–64.
18. Sink EL, Karol LA, Sanders J, Birch JG, Johnston CE, Herring JA. Efficacy of perioperative halo-gravity traction in the treatment of severe scoliosis in children. J Pediatr Orthop. 2001;21(4):519–24.

19. Seller K, Haas S, Raab P, Krauspe R, Wild A. Preoperative halo-traction in severe paralytic scoliosis. Z Orthop Ihre Grenzgeb. 2005;143(5):539–43.

20. Sponseller PD, Takenaga RK, Newton P, Boachie O, Flynn J, Letko L, et al. The use of traction in the treatment of severe spinal deformity. Spine (Phila Pa 1976). 2008;33(21):2305–9.

21. Park DK, Braaksma B, Hammerberg KW, Sturm P. The efficacy of preoperative halo-gravity traction in pediatric spinal deformity the effect of traction duration. J Spinal Disord Tech. 2013;26(3):146–54.

22. Bao H, Yan P, Bao M, Qiu Y, Zhu Z, Liu Z, et al. Halo-gravity traction combined with assisted ventilation: an effective pre-operative management for severe adult scoliosis complicated with respiratory dysfunction. Eur Spine J. 2016;25(8):2416–22.

23. Wang Y, Xie J, Zhao Z, Li T, Zhang Y, Bi N, et al. Preoperative short-term traction prior to posterior vertebral column resection: procedure and role. Eur Spine J. 2016;25(3):687–97.

24. Yang C, Wang H, Zheng Z, Zhang Z, Wang J, Liu H, et al. Halo-gravity traction in the treatment of severe spinal deformity: a systematic review and meta-analysis. Eur Spine J. 2017;26(7):1810–6.

25. Bang-ping Q, Yong Q, Bin W, Yang Y, Ze-zhang Z. Brachial plexus palsy caused by halo traction before posterior correction in patients with severe scoliosis. Chin J Traumatol. 2007;10(5):294–8.

26. Mazzolai L, Aboyans V, Ageno W, Agnelli G, Alatri A, Bauersachs R, et al. Diagnosis and management of acute deep vein thrombosis: a joint consensus document from the European society of cardiology working groups of aorta and peripheral circulation and pulmonary circulation and right ventricular function. Eur Heart J. 2017. Feb 17.Epub.

27. Franco L, Giustozzi M, Agnelli G, Becattini C. Anticoagulation in patients with isolated distal deep vein thrombosis: a meta-analysis. J Thromb Haemost. 2017;15(6):1142–54.

Agreement among physiotherapists in assessing patient performance of exercises for low-back pain

Aurore Hermet[1*], Alexandra Roren[1,2,3], Marie-Martine Lefevre-Colau[1,2,3], Adrien Gautier[1], Jonathan Linieres[1], Serge Poiraudeau[1,2,3] and Clémence Palazzo[1,2,3]

Abstract

Background: There is no agreement for the performance assessment of patients who practice exercises.. (2 points to withdraw) This assessment is currently left to the physiotherapist's personal judgement. We studied the agreement among physiotherapists in rating patient performance during exercises recommended for chronic low-back pain (LBP).

Methods: A vignette-based method was used. We first identified ten exercises recommended for LBP in the literature. Then, 42 patients with chronic LBP participating in a rehabilitation program were videotaped during their performance of one of the ten exercises. A vignette was an exercise video preceded by clinical information. Ten physiotherapists from primary (4) and tertiary care (6) viewed the 42 vignettes twice, one month apart, and rated patient performance from zero (worse performance) to ten (excellent performance) by considering the position and duration of the contraction or stretching. Intra-class correlation coefficients (ICCs) and 95% confidence intervals (95% CIs) were computed to assess inter- and intra-rater reliability.

Results: The overall inter-rater agreement was fair (ICC 0.48 [95% CI 0.33–0.56]) but was better for stretching exercises (0.55 [0.35–0.64]) than strengthening exercises (0.42 [0.20–0.52]) and for tertiary-care physiotherapists (0.66 [0.54–0.76]) than primary-care physiotherapists (0.28 [0.09–0.37]). The intra-rater agreement was overall good (0.72 [0.57–0.81] to 0.88 [0.79–0.94]). It was better for stretching exercises (from 0.68 [0.46–0.81] to 0.96 [0.91–0.98]) than strengthening exercises (from 0.68 [0.38–0.84]) to 0.82 [0.56–0.92]).

Conclusion: The agreement in rating patient performance of exercises for LBP is good among physiotherapists trained in managing LBP but is low among non-trained physiotherapists.

Keywords: Physical therapists, LowBack pain, Rehabilitation, Exercise therapy, Agreement

Background

Exercise therapy decreases pain and improves function in musculoskeletal diseases [1–3]. Individually designed exercise programs are effective in healthcare settings [1, 4]. The exercise program is usually learned during supervised physical therapy sessions and is performed at home by the patient alone, so the patient must be able to self-actualize the exercises at the end of supervised sessions.

There is no standardised way to assess patient performance during exercises. In practice, the assessment is left to the physiotherapists' personal judgement. This judgement may result from an unconscious integration of various data such as their own beliefs and experience, patient characteristics (age, comorbidities), exercise characteristics, and the relationship with the patient [5]. Better assessment of patient performance could help to improve the teaching of exercises and determine how many physiotherapy sessions are required for one patient, to propose a more personalized treatment. Indeed, if the number of supervised sessions is not sufficient, the treatment can be ineffective and patients can stop home exercises because

* Correspondence: aurore.hermet@yahoo.fr
[1]Service de rééducation et réadaptation de l'appareil locomoteur et des pathologies du rachis, Hôpital Cochin AP-HP, Université Paris Descartes, PRES Sorbonne Paris Cité, Paris, France
Full list of author information is available at the end of the article

they do not feel able to practice alone. In contrast, if the number of supervised sessions is greater than needed, the exercises will be a waste of time both for the physiotherapist and the patient.. (2 points to withdraw) As well, we need to better understand why treatment fails for some patients and whether home exercises are correctly performed to better adapt the treatment strategy: if exercises are correctly performed, other treatments may be considered; otherwise, new learning sessions and advice may be necessary. Finally, patients may have doubts about their performance and should be advised promptly to avoid stopping the exercises. This advice could improve adherence to home exercises, which is a common problem in musculoskeletal-disease rehabilitation [6–8].

Low-back pain (LBP) is highly prevalent [9], disabling, and costly [10, 11] and represents the first cause for needing a physiotherapist in France [12, 13]. Numerous studies have shown the effectiveness of exercise therapy in reducing pain and improving function with this condition [1, 14, 15]. Therefore, LBP is an ideal condition to evaluate whether physiotherapists' judgement can be trusted and is reproducible.

The aim of this study was to assess the agreement among physiotherapists in rating patient performance during exercises recommended for LBP.

Methods

This is an intra- and inter-reliability study. Case-vignettes were used to study physiotherapists agreement [16] because these allow for different health providers to assess the same exercise performed by the same patient.

Development of vignettes

Identification of exercises to translate into vignettes

We identified the exercises recommended in LBP by a non-exhaustive literature review. One author (CP) searched MEDLINE and PEDRO databases for articles evaluating the effectiveness of exercises in LBP that were published in English from 1982 to 2012.

From the articles obtained, the steering committee of the study (including one physical medicine and rehabilitation physician, one rheumatologist and one physiotherapist expert in LBP) selected ten exercises: six strengthening exercises (two for back muscles, two abdominal muscles, one gluteus muscles and one trunk stabilizing exercise) with alternating contraction/rest periods of five seconds (five repetitions) and four stretching exercises (one for hamstrings, one gluteus muscles, one back muscles and one rectus femoris muscles) with a stretch of at least 20 s (Fig. 1).

Creation of vignettes

A vignette included brief clinical information for the patient (age, main co-morbidities that could affect the achievement of the exercise [e.g., knee osteoarthritis can affect the ability to kneel]), a short description of the exercise (e.g., used for strengthening back muscles), and a video of a patient performing the exercise.

After giving their consent, 42 patients with nonspecific chronic LBP participating in a supervised rehabilitation program in a tertiary-care hospital (Cochin hospital, Paris, France) were videotaped while they performed one

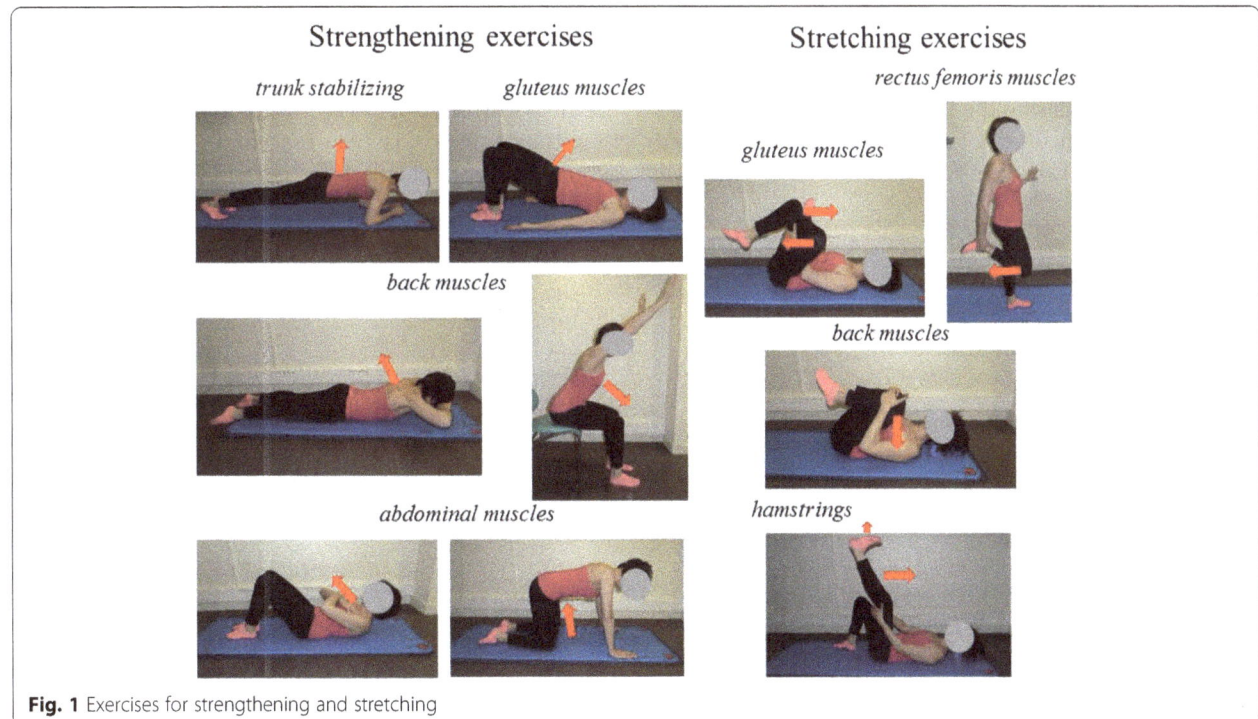

Fig. 1 Exercises for strengthening and stretching

of the specific exercises they had learned (at least four different patients performed the same exercise). An example of a vignette is shown in Additional file 1. The acquisition of videos was highly standardised to ensure reproducibility (Additional file 2).

Participants

All physiotherapists working in the rehabilitation department of the tertiary-care Cochin hospital were informed of the study and were asked to participate on a voluntary basis [15]. Six physiotherapists accepted to participate.

Six physiotherapists (staff personal contacts) working in primary care centres were informed of the study by e.mails. Four accepted to participate.

The experience was self-reported. They were asked: "Among your patients, what percentage of them have low back pain?" We considered physiotherapists to be experienced when more than 50% of their patients had low back pain and low experienced when less than 50% of their patients had low back pain.

Study design

The Fig. 2 shows the study design. Before scoring the vignettes, the physiotherapists provided the following information: age, gender, time working in the current job, experience in the management of LBP (proportion of patients with LBP they daily managed).

All rehabilitation center physiotherapists scored the 42 vignettes twice. The first scoring determined the inter-rater agreement and the second scoring (one month apart) determined the intra-rater agreement. For each vignette, they received the following instruction: "We ask you to assess the patient's ability to perform an exercise recommended for LBP. Taking into account the patient's position during the whole exercise, the duration of the contraction or the stretching, could you please note from zero (worse performance) to ten (excellent performance) the patient's ability to perform the following exercise?" The vignettes were saved on a personal computer and could be viewed individually by participants for one week. Participants were asked not to talk about the topic during the study period. The answers were anonymous. To assess intra-rater agreement, participants were asked one month later to rate the same vignettes in another random order and blind of their first answers.

The primary care physiotherapists received the same 42 vignettes by e-mail and rated them once. Because this process was time-consuming, a second scoring was not possible. Only inter-rater agreement could be assessed.

Finally, three other rehabilitation centre physiotherapists were asked to rate the performance of 16 patients doing exercises while they were being videotaped. Six months later, they rated the exercise videos of the same patients so we could compare the face-to-face assessment with the scoring of the exercise video.

Statistical analysis

We estimated the number of vignettes and participants needed for physiotherapists to assess agreement on the precision of the intra-class correlation coefficient (ICC), and on feasibility considerations (time needed to build a vignette, time needed for scoring, number of participants available). With 42 vignettes, each scored twice, and an expected inter-observer ICC of 0.60, the expected 95% confidence interval (95% CI) would be about 0.4 [17].

Data are described as median (range). As data had a near normal distribution, ICCs were used to assess intra- and inter-rater agreement. ICC estimates were calculated based on a single measurement, consistency, two-way mixed-effects model (ICC (3,1)). The bootstrap procedure (bias-corrected and accelerated bootstrap) was used to estimate 95% CIs. An ICC of 0 indicates chance agreement and 1 perfect agreement. We defined

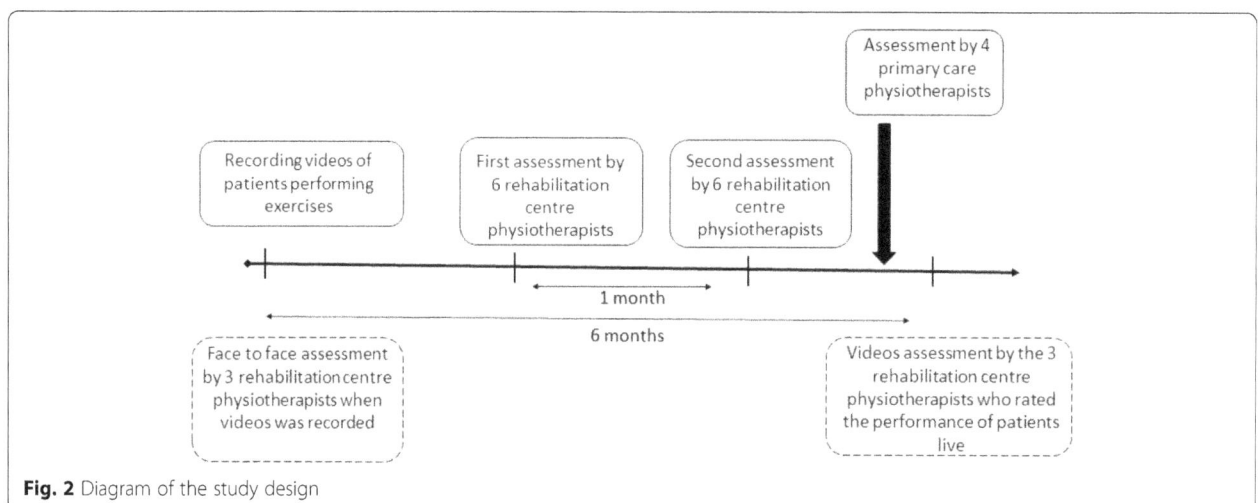

Fig. 2 Diagram of the study design

agreement as poor, ICC < 0.4; fair, 0.4 to 0.59; good, 0.6 to 0.74; and excellent, ≥0.75 [18]. Bland and Altman plotting was used to assess the quality of concordance among physiotherapists by the amplitude of the agreement intervals, with the upper and lower limits of agreement defined as the mean difference plus and minus 1.96 times the standard deviation of the differences.

Analyses involved use of R v3.1.2 (statistical software). Written consent was obtained for all participants. The study was approved by the local ethics committee (Comité d'évaluation éthique de l'INSERM (IRB00003888)).

Results

Ten physiotherapists participated in the study: six from the rehabilitation department of Cochin hospital and four from primary care. The median age was 26 years (range 23–42) and six were women. The physiotherapists from primary care were less experienced in managing LBP than those from tertiary care. Patients with LBP represented 80% of the patients managed in Cochin hospital, while in primary care patients with LBP were not always majority. Only one in four primary care physiotherapists had 60% of his patients with LBP. (Table 1).

Inter-rater agreement

Overall, the inter-rater agreement was fair for the ten physiotherapists (ICC 0.48 [95% CI 0.33–0.56]) (Table 2). The agreement was better for stretching exercises (0.55 [0.35–0.64]) than strengthening exercises (0.42 [0.20–0.52]), with an overlap of CI.

The agreement among physiotherapists from tertiary care was good (ICC 0.66 [0.54–0.76]) (Table 2). It was better for stretching exercises (0.73 [0.56–0.82]) than strengthening exercises (0.58 [0.32–0.71]) with an overlap of CI. During the second scoring of the vignettes (one month later), the agreement increased to 0.70 [0.58–0.77]); the agreement for strengthening exercises improved (0.65 [0.43–0.77]) but remained stable for stretching exercises (0.73 [0.57–0.82]) with an overlap of CI.

By contrast, the inter-rater agreement among primary care physiotherapists was poor (ICC 0.28 [0.09–0.37]) (Table 2). The agreement was better for strengthening

exercises (0.34 [0.07–0.48]) than stretching exercises (0.21 [− 0.01–0.28]) but remained low with an overlap of CI. One primary-care physiotherapist scored the vignettes differently from the others (higher or lower scores), especially for stretching exercises. Without this outlier, the global agreement was better (0.46 [0.23–0.51]) but still low; the agreement for strengthening exercises was low (0.29 [95% CI 0–0.46]) but was good for stretching exercises (0.70 [0.31–0.66]).

The amplitudes of the agreement intervals on a Bland– Altman plot (Fig. 3) indicated the quality of concordance among physiotherapists. The 5 and 95% CIs correspond to the limits of agreement. For the global preference, the graphs indicated that the mean of the differences among the raters was very close to zero, with plots having a double funnel shape. It shows a greater concordance for the highest scores (the most successful exercises) (*Bland and Altman plots for strengthening and stretching exercises in* Additional file 3).

Intra-rater agreement

The intra-rater agreement was very good for all physiotherapists (ICC 0.72 [95% CI 0.57–0.81] to 0.88 [0.79–0.94]) (Table 3). It was better for stretching exercises (from 0.68 [0.46–0.81] to 0.96 [0.91–0.98]) than strengthening exercises (from 0.68 [0.38–0.84] to 0.82 [0.56–0.92]).

Comparison between video and face-to-face assessment

The three physiotherapists who rated the performance of patients live and on video all work in the rehabilitation department of Cochin hospital. They did not participate in the rest of the study. They were older (median 31 years [range 29–45]) and more experienced (median time working in the current job seven years [range 6–20]) than the other physiotherapists.

The intra-rater agreement was excellent and very good for two physiotherapists (ICC 0.93 [95% CI 0.38–1.00] and 0.71 [0.1–0.9]), whereas the third one had low agreement (0.39 [− 0.34–0.72]) (Additional file 4).

Table 1 Physiotherapist (PT) characteristics

	All PTs n = 10	Rehabilitation centre PTs n = 6	Primary-care PTs n = 4
Age (years), median (range)	26 (23–42)	26 (23–42)	26 (25–29)
Female, n (%)	6 (60)	4 (67)	2 (50)
Time working in the current job (years), median (range)		6 (3–18)	4 (2–7)
Personal experience in LBP management: None Low (< 50%) High (> 50%)		high experience	low experience

Table 2 Inter-rater agreement for PTs rating patients' ability to perform exercises

Agreement	All PTs	Rehabilitation centre PTs		Primary-care PTs
		First assessment	Second assessment*	
Global	0.48 (0.32–0.56)	0.66 (0.54–0.76)	0.70 (0.58–0.77)	0.28 (0.09–0.37)
For strengthening exercises	0.42 (0.2–0.52)	0.58 (0.32–0.71)	0.65 (0.43–0.77)	0.34 (0.07–0.48)
For stretching exercises	0.55 (0.35–0.64)	0.73 (0.56–0.82)	0.73 (0.57–0.82)	0.21(– 0.01–0.28)

Data are intraclass correlation coefficients (ICCs) and 95% confidence intervals (95% CIs)
*1 month later

Discussion

This study shows a good agreement among tertiary care physiotherapists, experienced in the management of LBP, but a low agreement among primary care physiotherapists, who were less experienced in the management of LBP. The reliability was greater during the second assessment, suggesting that training physiotherapists can improve their agreement in assessing patient performance of exercises for low-back pain.

These discrepancies may arise from a recruitment bias, as the physiotherapits of the rehabilitation centre have the same background and are used to manage a very specific population of patients (ie those who are not improved after a primary care physiotherapy), whereas the primary care physiotherapists may have different background and expectations. As well, we found better agreement for stretching than strengthening exercises, which suggests that stretching exercises are easier to score than strengthening exercises, which may require more feedback.

Although the performance of patients during therapeutic exercises may be a strong predictor of the effectiveness of exercises, it has never been studied previously. When the patient is learning the personalised exercise program during supervised sessions, the ability to perform the exercises should be assessed regularly. Our study suggests that this assessment could be easily performed by physiotherapists experienced in LBP management or with specific training. The adequate number of

supervised sessions could be adapted to each patient, for more personalized care, which may be more effective. Moreover, regularly assessing patient performance when they practice therapeutic exercises at home could help determine when exercises are no longer performed adequately ("unlearning" curve) and when refreshing supervised sessions are required.

Adherence is a main issue for exercise therapy programs, especially home-based programs [19]. The World Health Organization has defined adherence as "the extent to which a person's behaviour taking medication, following a diet, and/or executing lifestyle changes, corresponds with agreed recommendations from a health care provider" [20]. By extension, exercise adherence is often considered the extent to which a patient acts in accordance with the advised interval, exercise dose, and exercise dosing [21]. This definition does not take into account the performance of the patient when performing the prescribed exercises, which may explain why adherence is almost never reported in studies assessing the effectiveness of home-based exercise programs. For example, in a systematic review of interventions to improve adherence to exercise for chronic musculoskeletal pain, only 4 of 42 studies used the accuracy of exercises performed to rate adherence. However, an accurate reporting of adherence seems essential to better address the treatment efficacy of home-based exercises programs in clinical studies [22]. Consequently, future studies evaluating the effectiveness of therapeutic exercises should include an assessment of patient performance. Patient performance could be assessed by physiotherapists on a numeric rating scale from zero to ten.

We also wondered if these results could be transposed to a face-to-face assessment, without a video. The intra-rater agreement was high for two physiotherapists but low for the third one, perhaps because he was a physiotherapist manager and therefore less involved in patient care and did not directly participate in teaching exercises to patients (Additional file 4). Thus, the judgment of the videos was close to live assessment. This finding has two major advantages: first, our results could be transposed to a face-to-face assessment and second, patient performance could be assessed

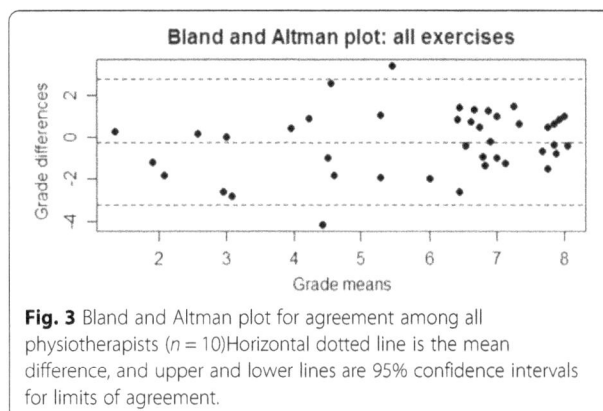

Fig. 3 Bland and Altman plot for agreement among all physiotherapists (*n* = 10)Horizontal dotted line is the mean difference, and upper and lower lines are 95% confidence intervals for limits of agreement.

Table 3 Intra-rater agreement for PTs rating patients' ability to perform exercises

PT number	Global	For strengthening exercises	For stretching exercises
1	0.74 (0.58–0.84)	0.68 (0.38–0.84)	0.78 (0.57–0.91)
2	0.72 (0.57–0.81)	0.71 (0.43–0.84)	0.68 (0.46–0.81)
3	0.86 (0.76–0.92)	0.79 (0.57–0.91)	0.92 (0.86–0.95)
4	0.82 (0.73–0.89)	0.81 (0.71–0.87)	0.84 (0.67–0.96)
5	0.86 (0.73–0.93)	0.82 (0.48–0.94)	0.88 (0.73–0.94)
6	0.88 (0.79–0.94)	0.82 (0.56–0.92)	0.96 (0.91–0.98)

Data are ICCs and 95% CIs

via "telemedicine", so that patients could be advised by a physiotherapist from their home.

This work has some limitations. A key limitation of this study as that COnsensus-based Standards for the selection of health (COSMIN) was not used to inform study design and decisions'. The number of physiotherapists was small, and there was a recruitment bias for the rehabilitation centre physiotherapists as they worked together. That is why we also wanted to include primary care physiotherapists. The confidence intervals could be wide because the numbers of physiotherapists were small. When the confidence intervals overlap, it was not possible to conclude that there is a definite difference But there was no overlap of confidence intervals when comparing the ICCs of the tertiary care physiotherapists with the ICCs of the primary care physiotherapists, suggesting a significative difference of reliability between them.. Finally, we focused on the exercises recommended for one particular condition, LBP, because this is a common problem with a significant socioeconomic impact. These results should be confirmed for other disorders, such as knee osteoarthritis or rotator cuff diseases.

Conclusion

The agreement among physiotherapists experienced in managing musculoskeletal disorder is good for using a ten-point scale to rate patient performance during exercises recommended for LBP. Training of less experienced physiotherapists is necessary. A ten-point scale could be used to assess patients performance in clinical studies evaluating the effectiveness of exercise therapy in LBP, but also in real life to determine the adequate number of physiotherapy sessions required and to help better understand the unlearning phenomenon of exercises.

This study is providing initial insights to determine the agreement among physiotherapists in assessing patient performance. Future studies will be needed to evaluate these findings in another population of physiotherapists and in other musculoskeletal disorders.

Abbreviations
95% CI: 95% confidence interval; ICC: Intra-class correlation coefficient; LBP: Low-back pain

Authors' contributions
AH collected the data, produced the statistics, and wrote the article. CP initiated the project, organized the study, produced the films and helped AH write the article. SP participated in the development and planning of the project. AR and MMLC participated in the organization of the study, helped for analysis and interpretation of the results. JL and AG participated in the design of the study, the creation of the vignettes and the interpretation of the results. All authors read and approved the final manuscript.

Competing interests
The authors declare that they have no competing interests.

Author details
[1]Service de rééducation et réadaptation de l'appareil locomoteur et des pathologies du rachis, Hôpital Cochin AP-HP, Université Paris Descartes, PRES Sorbonne Paris Cité, Paris, France. [2]CRESS, UMR 1153, INSERM, Paris, Institut fédératif de recherche handicap, INSERM/CNRS, Paris, France. [3]Institut Fédératif de Recherche Handicap, INSERM/CNRS, Paris, France.

References
1. Hayden JA, van Tulder MW, Malmivaara A, Koes BW. Exercise therapy for treatment of non-specific low back pain. Cochrane Database Syst Rev. 2005; 20(3):CD000335.
2. Thomas KS, Muir KR, Doherty M, Jones AC, O'Reilly SC, Bassey EJ. Home based exercise programme for knee pain and knee osteoarthritis: randomised controlled trial. BMJ. 2002;325(7367):752.
3. Deyle GD, Henderson NE, Matekel RL, Ryder MG, Garber MB, Allison SC. Effectiveness of Manual Physical Therapy and Exercise in Osteoarthritis of the Knee: A Randomized. Controlled Trial. Ann Intern Med. 2000;132(3):173.
4. Jonas S. Philips E. Boston: ACSM's Exercise in Medicine; 2009.
5. Edwards I, Jones M, Carr J, Braunack-Mayer A, Jensen GM. Clinical reasoning strategies in physical therapy. Phys Ther. 2004;84(4):312–30.
6. Friedrich M, Gittler G, Halberstadt Y, Cermak T, Heiller I. Combined exercise and motivation program: effect on the compliance and level of disability of patients with chronic low back pain: a randomized controlled trial. Arch Phys Med Rehabil. 1998;79(5):475–87.
7. Härkäpää K, Järvikoski A, Mellin G, Hurri H, Luoma J. Health locus of control beliefs and psychological distress as predictors for treatment outcome in low-back pain patients: results of a 3-month follow-up of a controlled intervention study. Pain. 1991;46(1):35–41.
8. Beinart NA, Goodchild CE, Weinman JA, Ayis S, Godfrey EL. Individual and intervention-related factors associated with adherence to home exercise in chronic low back pain: a systematic review. Spine J. 2013;13(12):1940–50.
9. van Oostrom SH, Monique Verschuren WM, de Vetl HC, Picavet HS. Ten year course of low back pain in an adult population-based cohort--the Doetinchem cohort study. Eur J pain Lond Engl. 2011;15(9):993-998.
10. Vos T, Flaxman AD, Naghavi M, Lozano R, Michaud C, Ezzati M, et al. Years lived with disability (YLDs) for 1160 sequelae of 289 diseases and injuries 1990-2010: a systematic analysis for the global burden of disease study 2010. Lancet. 2012;380(9859):2163–2196.

11. GBD 2013 DALYs and HALE Collaborators, CJL M, Barber RM, Foreman KJ, Abbasoglu Ozgoren A, Abd-Allah F, et al. Global, regional, and national disability-adjusted life years (DALYs) for 306 diseases and injuries and healthy life expectancy (HALE) for 188 countries, 1990–2013: quantifying the epidemiological. Transition Lancet. 2015;386(10009):2145–91.

12. Assurance-maladie, des soins de qualité pour tous. Lombalgies. La kinésithérapie et l'imagerie médicale souvent utilisées en excès. Faits marquants: 15 études P37–43. 2000.

13. HAS. Prise en charge massokinésithérapique dans la lombalgie commune: modalités de prescription. 2005.

14. Abenhaim L, Rossignol M, Valat JP, Nordin M, Avouac B, Blotman F, et al. The role of activity in the therapeutic management of back pain. Report of the international Paris task force on back pain. Spine. 2000;25(4 Suppl):1S–33S.

15. van Tulder M, Malmivaara A, Esmail R, Koes B. Exercise therapy for low back pain: a systematic review within the framework of the cochrane collaboration back review group. Spine. 2000;25(21):2784–96.

16. Bachmann LM, Mühleisen A, Bock A, ter Riet G, Held U, Kessels AGH. Vignette studies of medical choice and judgement to study caregivers' medical decision behaviour: systematic review. BMC. 2008;8:50.

17. Giraudeau B, Mary JY. Planning a reproducibility study: how many subjects and how many replicates per subject for an expected width of the 95 per cent confidence interval of the intraclass correlation coefficient. Stat Med. 2001;20(21):3205–14.

18. Shrout PE, Fleiss JL. Intraclass correlations: uses in assessing rater reliability. Psychol Bull. 1979;86(2):420–8.

19. Palazzo C, Klinger E, Dorner V, Kadri A, Thierry O, Boumenir Y, et al. Barriers to home-based exercise program adherence with chronic low back pain: patient expectations regarding new technologies. Ann Phys Rehabil Med. 2016;59(2):107–13.

20. Organization WH. Adherence to long-term therapies: evidence for action: World Health Organization; 2003. 230 p

21. Deka P, Pozehl B, Williams MA, Yates B. Adherence to recommended exercise guidelines in patients with heart failure. Heart Fail Rev. 2017;22(1):41–53.

22. Jordan JL, Holden MA, Mason EE, Foster NE. Interventions to improve adherence to exercise for chronic musculoskeletal pain in adults. Cochrane Database Syst Rev. 2010;1:CD005956.

12

General health factors may be a barrier to effective non-surgical multidisciplinary rehabilitation of common orthopaedic conditions in tertiary care settings

Shaun O'Leary[1,2]* [iD], Michelle Cottrell[1,3], Maree Raymer[2], David Smith[3] and Asaduzzaman Khan[1]

Abstract

Background: To explore patient characteristics predictive of a poor response to multidisciplinary non-surgical rehabilitation of three common orthopaedic conditions within a tertiary care service.

Methods: A retrospective audit of medical records of patients who had undergone multidisciplinary non-surgical management of their knee osteoarthritis (KOA, $n = 190$), shoulder impingement syndrome (SIS, $n = 199$), or low back pain (LBP, $n = 242$) within a multisite tertiary care service was undertaken. Standardised clinical measures recorded by the service at the initial consultation were examined using a base binary logistic regression model to determine their relationship with a poor response to management (ie. not achieving a minimal clinically important improvement in the condition disability measure pre-post management).

Results: Factors predictive of a poor response following non-surgical management included;; higher levels of anxiety (OR 1.11, $P < 0.02$) and lower functional score (OR 0.76, $P < 0.04$) for KOA, higher number of comorbidities (OR 1.16, $P < 0.03$) for SIS, and coexisting cervical or thorax pain (OR 2.1, $P = 0.04$) and lower pain self-efficacy (OR 0.98, $P = 0.02$) for LBP.

Conclusions: General health issues may present a barrier to achieving favourable outcomes in response to multidisciplinary non-surgical rehabilitation for the management of common orthopaedic conditions in a tertiary care setting. Clinicians may need to consider these broader patient issues when designing management strategies for patients with these conditions.

Keywords: Musculoskeletal, Shoulder impingement, Knee osteoarthritis, Low back pain, Predictors, Non-surgical management

Background

Chronic musculoskeletal conditions such as knee osteoarthritis (KOA), shoulder impingement syndrome (SIS) and low back pain (LBP) are one of the largest causes of disability in the community [1]. Often non-surgical management is the first line of care for these conditions. While non-surgical multidisciplinary management may benefit some patients with these conditions [2–4], modest outcomes from intervention trials indicate that many patients do not benefit. It would be clinically and economically advantageous to be able to identify characteristics of patients most likely to have a poor response to multidisciplinary non-surgical management. However, identifying patient characteristics of those at risk of not responding to this pathway of care is still a work in progress.

Studies identifying characteristics of patients potentially at risk of poor recovery from common musculoskeletal condition such as KOA, SIS, and LBP are emerging. However many studies only report factors associated with poorer outcome following surgery [5–13] or natural recovery [14]. Only a few studies have specifically investigated risk factors in the context of response to non-surgical rehabilitation [3, 15–19]. For example factors shown to be

* Correspondence: s.oleary@uq.edu.au
[1]School of Health and Rehabilitation Sciences, University of Queensland, Brisbane, Australia
[2]Physiotherapy Department, Royal Brisbane and Women's Hospital, Brisbane, Australia
Full list of author information is available at the end of the article

associated with poor response to physical interventions for KOA include patellofemoral pain, anterior cruciate ligament laxity, and greater height [15]. Similarly, symptom severity, poorer patient expectations, low self-efficacy, compensable claims history, and co-morbidities have been reported as some of the potential risk factors for a poor response to non-surgical rehabilitation in shoulder conditions [3, 16–18]. Pain severity and psychological factors such as catastrophizing or depressed mood have also been identified as predictive of a poor response to non-surgical management of LBP [19].

There are also some methodological limitations in this field of research investigating risk factors for a poor response to non-surgical rehabilitation. For example studies may only focus on a particular domain such as clinical severity [17], physical findings [20], psychosocial factors [21], or adherence to recommended management strategies [22–25]. Furthermore some studies limit their investigation to the response to unimodal interventions (eg. manipulation) only [26, 27] or in response to treatment from a single professional discipline (eg. physiotherapy) [16, 19]. A final, but particularly relevant limitation is that studies may be confined to a primary care setting [14, 19]. This may have implications when findings are extrapolated to those patients managed in secondary or tertiary care settings where both the patient demographic and the specifics of the non-surgical service and interventions may be very different. Clearly it is challenging for any single predictive study to account for all potential risk factors, patient populations, intervention types, or variations in service settings.

The aim of this study is to further explore potential predictors of a poor response to the non-surgical management of KOA, SIS, and LBP, but is focused to a multidisciplinary intervention conducted within a tertiary care setting. It describes a retrospective audit of medical records from a representative sample of patients with known standardised service relevant clinical outcome measures and assessment items, taken over a course of non-surgical multidisciplinary rehabilitation for their orthopaedic condition within a multisite tertiary healthcare service.

Methods
Study design
A retrospective medical record audit was undertaken at seven public hospitals in Queensland, Australia. All cases included in the audit were patients of a standardised statewide physiotherapy-led orthopaedic tertiary service within Queensland Health Hospital facilities between July 2008 and June 2010. These patients had been selected from specialist orthopaedic outpatient waiting lists following a triage process to undergo a course of non-surgical multidisciplinary (physiotherapy, occupational therapy, dietetics, and/or psychology) management for their KOA, SIS, or LBP. Each patient's management (duration of management period,

disciplines consulted) had been pragmatically based on the initial examination findings of the triaging service team leader (who was a physiotherapist) and the clinical discretion of the involved discipline-specific treatment providers.

This project received multisite ethical approval from the Institutional Medical Research Ethics Committee (HREC/10/QRBW/455). Public Health Act approval was obtained from each of the public hospitals permitting access to medical records without the need for informed consent.

Sample size estimation
Based on multiple regression modelling, it had been calculated that at least 192 patient cases for each condition were required to achieve a power of 80% with 5% level of significance (effect size 0.10), accounting for the number of potential predictor variables included for each condition (27 KOA, 27 SIS, 29 LBP). This calculation also accounted for approximately 10% missing data.

Criteria for a poor response to outcome (dependent variable)
A poor response to management for each patient case was determined by evaluating if they had achieved a minimal clinically important difference (MCID) based on the change scores of the region-specific disability questionnaires between the initial consultation and discharge. The MCID scores were used as the intent of the study was to specifically identify prognostic factors relevant to patients who have a poor response (ie. did not achieve MCID) from the studied intervention as they are the patients of the highest priority to identify clinically.

These region-specific disability questionnaires are routinely recorded pre (initial consultation) and post-intervention (at discharge from the service) and included the -.

1. Western Ontario and McMaster Universities Osteoarthritis Index (WOMAC) for the KOA group: This measure is used to evaluate the condition of patients with osteoarthritis of the knee and hip, and includes factors such as pain, stiffness, and physical functioning [28, 29]. In this study the WOMAC was scored using the relevant items from the Knee Injury and Osteoarthritis Outcome Score [30, 31] that is routinely measured for patients with KOA in the service, but could not be used due to the lack of published MCID. The MCID of the WOMAC has been reported as a reduction in score of 10 points or greater [32].
2. Shoulder Pain and Disability Index (SPADI) for the SIS group: This measure contains items for the domains of shoulder pain and disability (eg, self-care,

lifting) and has a reported MCID of a 20 point reduction or greater [33].

3. Oswestry Disability Index (ODI) for the LBP group: This index is used to quantify disability for low back pain and contains items concerning pain intensity and function (eg. lifting, self-care) and has a MCID of a 10 point reduction or greater [34].

Change scores between the initial consultation and discharge from the service for each patient case were dichotomized (binary outcome) as either not achieving (reference outcome of a poor response) or achieving, the MCID for the relevant outcome measure.

Potential predictor variables (independent variables)

Potential predictor variables were comprised of routine clinical information recorded at the patient's initial consultation with the service team leader. This information included questionnaires and recorded information from the patient interview. These assessment items have progressively been selected over the development of the service by the team leaders to be clinically informative for the patient population. It was decided a priori that physical examination measures would not be collected for the purpose of this audit due to the known lack of standardisation for recording these items across the different sites and between team leaders. The included potential predictor variables (including units of measurement) are described below and in Table 1:

1. Demographic and general health information including age (years), gender (female/male), Body Mass Index (kilogram/meters^2), comorbidities (number), and medications (number).

2. The Assessment of Quality of Life questionnaire (4 Dimension - utility measure score/1) which is a measure of health-related quality of life incorporating four domains (Independent Living, Mental Health, Relationships, Senses) [35].

3. Psychological questionnaires including the Depression, Anxiety and Stress Scale (DASS-21) that measures dimensions of depression (score/42), anxiety (score/42), and stress (score/42) [36], and the Pain Self-Efficacy Questionnaire (score/60). This assesses the confidence of people with ongoing pain in performing activities (eg. household chores, socialising, work) while in pain and is related to measures of pain-related disability, coping strategies, concordance to management programs, and functional outcomes [37].

4. Patient reported symptom characteristics including symptom severity (Pain Visual Analogue Scale Score/100 mm) [38], symptom distribution (extracted from medical record body chart that

matched predetermined potential symptom regions as listed for each condition in Table 1), symptom duration (months), and mechanisms of onset (traumatic onset/not traumatic) of the condition.

5. Functional deficits as evaluated by the Patient Specific Functional Scale (score/10) that has been shown to be valid and responsive measure of function in patients with musculoskeletal disorders [39].

6. Prior management pathway for the condition including any previous consultations with orthopaedic medical specialists (yes/no), or previous surgery (yes/no) for the same condition.

7. Any documented radiological findings specifically investigating the patient's condition matching predetermined potential radiological findings, as listed for each condition in Table 1.

Audit and data extraction

Auditing was undertaken by a single investigator (M.C) and the process is depicted in Fig. 1. Potential cases were initially identified from the service database according to body region managed ($n = 1252$; 510 knees, 284 lumbar, 458 shoulders) and their medical records reviewed. Only cases that included both pre- and post-intervention region-specific questionnaire scores were included ($n = 887$; 284 knees, 328 shoulders, 275 lumbar). Further cases were then excluded if they did not meet the eligibility criteria for the three orthopaedic conditions resulting in a total of 631 eligible cases (KOA, $n = 190$; SIS, $n = 199$; LBP, $n = 242$).

The inclusion criteria for the conditions included; 1/ persistent knee pain in addition to radiologically identified knee osteoarthritis for the KOA group, 2/ reported pain in the lumbar/buttock region with or without leg symptoms for the LBP group, and 3/patients in the SIS group had to have been diagnosed with sub-acromial impingement syndrome and/or rotator cuff disease, with no indication of adhesive capsulitis, acromioclavicular joint injury, or recent or recurrent glenohumeral joint dislocation/subluxation/fracture. For all three conditions, cases had been naturally excluded by the standard service screening process, which excluded those presenting with potentially serious medical conditions requiring urgent referral to the medical specialist, or those not consenting to undertake non-surgical rehabilitation.

Statistical analysis

All statistical analysis was performed using SPSS (version 20). The analysis was conducted separately for each of the musculoskeletal conditions (KOA, SIS, LBP) but followed an identical approach. Firstly the potential predictor variables (ie. patient demographics, quality of life and psychological measures, symptom characteristics, functional measure, prior management, radiological findings)

Table 1 Group means (± standard deviation) for the variables tested for their relationship with not achieving a minimal clinically important difference (MCID) in outcome in response to the non-surgical multidisciplinary management of KOA, SIS, and LBP

Variables	Knee Osteoarthritis (n = 190)	Shoulder Impingement Syndrome (n = 199)	Low Back Pain (n = 242)
Age (years)	59.61 ± 10.48	60.75 ± 12.95	51.52 ± 15.02
Gender (% male)	39%*	45%*	44%
Body Mass Index (kilogram/meters²)	33.23 ± 7.29	30.51 ± 7.41	30.87 ± 7.73
Comorbidities (number)	3.26 ± 2.17	3.03 ± 2.24*	2.53 ± 2.17
Medications (number)	4.86 ± 3.6	5.22 ± 4.59	4.54 ± 4.41
Quality of Life (utility score/1)	0.5 ± 0.26*	0.53 ± 0.26	0.44 ± 0.26
Depression, Anxiety and Stress Scale			
Depression (score/42)	8.35 ± 10.21*	7.68 ± 9.92	10.45 ± 10.19
Anxiety Score (score/42)	6.23 ± 7.42*	5.74 ± 7.65	9.01 ± 8.76
Stress Score (score/42)	9.92 ± 9.53*	10.1 ± 10.15	13.83 ± 10.47
Pain Self-Efficacy (score/60)	34.89 ± 14.88*	37.04 ± 16.01	31.29 ± 14.87*
Pain Severity (score/100 mm)	56.36 ± 21.94	57.67 ± 23.5	58.03 ± 20.99
Function (score/10)	3.81 ± 1.71*	3.41 ± 1.96	3.85 ± 1.52
Symptom Duration (months)	61.09 ± 82.25	24.89 ± 57.4	93.19 ± 112.61*
Traumatic Onset (% traumatic, (n))	17% (32)	29% (57)	12% (30)
Previous Consultation (% yes, (n))	13% (24)	4% (8)	12% (28)*
Previous Surgery (% yes, (n))	13% (24)	0.5% (1)	5% (12)

Symptom Distribution (% cases, n) as recorded in the medical record body chart:
   Knee Osteoarthritis – Pain reported; lower back/pelvic/hip region (40.53%, 77), lower leg (12%, 23), bilateral knee (40%, 76)*. *Shoulder Impingement Syndrome* – Pain reported; cervical (27%, 53), acromioclavicular (16%, 32), forearm (29%, 58), bilateral shoulder (16%, 31). *Low Back Pain* - Pain reported; bilateral lower back 74% (178), one leg 47% (114)*, both legs 21% (51), thoracic and/or cervical region 16% (39)*. Paraesthesia and/or anaesthesia reported in the legs 41% (99).

Radiological Findings (% cases, n) as reported in medical records:
   Knee Osteoarthritis – Medial (89%, 169), lateral (45%, 86) or patella (64% (122) compartment osteoarthritis, or tri-compartmental osteoarthritis (30%, 56). Osteoarthritis rated as severe (42%, 80)*. Reported meniscus pathology (25%, 47), valgus (9%, 18) or varus (18% 35) alignment. *Shoulder Impingement Syndrome* – Glenohumeral (19%, 37) or acromioclavicular (51%, 101) joint osteoarthritis, subacromial bursa distension (53%, 106), supraspinatus (67%, 134), infraspinatus (5%, 10)*, or subscapularis (15%, 30) muscle tendon tears. Multiple rotator cuff tendon tears; 1 (53%, 105), 2 (14%, 28), 3 (3%, 5). *Low Back Pain* – Lumbar degenerative changes (71%, 171), disc pathology (63%, 153), vertebral body pathology (18%, 44), zygopophyseal joint pathology (29%, 70), neural compression (43%, 103)*, spondylolisthesis (18%, 44), canal stenosis (31%, 75), foraminal stenosis (24%, 59).

*denotes variables with a univariate relationship ($p \leq 0.1$) with a non-MCID in outcome. Further details regarding some variables are provided in the footnote

were tested for a univariate relationship with the clinical management outcome of interest (ie. non- MCID of either the WOMAC, SPADI, or ODI) using independent-samples t-tests for continuous variables, and chi-square tests for categorical variables. Variables with a univariate relationship with the clinical outcome of a significance level of $p \leq 0.1$ were retained as potential prediction variables [40]. Potential predictor variables were entered into a base binary logistic regression model which commenced with a full model, sequentially removing the most insignificant variables until all remaining were significant. This process was repeated for all three conditions separately to determine the most accurate set of variables for the prediction of a non-MCID outcome. Odds Ratios (OR) and 95% confidence intervals for significant variables were calculated. Standardised residuals of the fitted models were examined for outliers and no outliers were identified in each of the three models.

Results

At baseline the region-specific disability questionnaire scores (± standard deviation) were 51.94% (18.24%) for the WOMAC (KOA group), 59.29% (21.8%) for the SPADI (SIS group), and 40.24% (15.31%) for the ODI (LBP group). Overall 98/190 (51.58%) of patients with KOA, 93/199 (46.73%) of patients with SIS, and 120/242 (49.59%) of patients with LBP, fit the criteria as a non-responder (ie. not achieving a MCID). The patient characteristics showing a univariate relationship with a non-MCID outcome in response to non-surgical management of KOA, SIS, and LBP are shown in Table 1.

Following logistic regression analysis, factors predictive of a non-MCID outcome included higher levels of anxiety (OR 1.11, 95% CI 1.03–1.21, $p < 0.02$) and lower functional score (OR 0.76, 95% CI 0.59–0.97, $p < 0.03$) for KOA, higher number of comorbidities (OR 1.16, 95% CI 1.02–1.32, $p < 0.03$) for SIS, and coexisting cervical or thorax

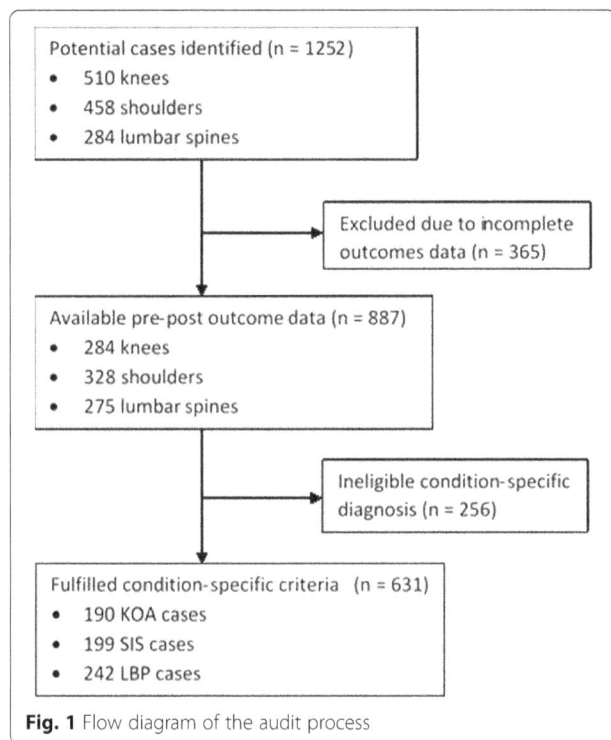

Fig. 1 Flow diagram of the audit process

pain (OR 2.1, 95% CI 1.02–4.4, p = 0.04) and lower pain self-efficacy (OR 0.98, 95% CI 0.96–1, p = 0.02) for LBP (Table 2). A Hosmer and Lemeshow goodness of fit test was conducted for all estimated models, and their insignificance (p > 0.28) suggest that the estimated models were a good fit to the sample data.

Discussion

The findings of this study indicate that general health factors potentially present some barrier to effective non-surgical multidisciplinary rehabilitation of common orthopaedic conditions managed in the tertiary care setting. The findings share both similarities and discrepancies with previous literature, albeit many of the previous studies performed in primary care settings. For example the psychological factors observed to be predictive of a poor response in KOA (higher levels of anxiety) and LBP (lower pain self-efficacy) are consistent with those previously reported for LBP (catastrophizing, depressed mood) [19] and shoulder disorders (patient expectations, self-efficacy) [16]. Similarly higher comorbidity has been observed as a risk factor for poorer outcome in shoulder disorders in this current study and in previous studies [16, 18]. In general findings are also consistent with factors identified in a systematic review to be generic prognostic indicators of poor recovery such as widespread pain, higher disability, and comorbid psychological factors [14].

Interestingly only one variable specific to the condition (low functional capacity in KOA) in this study was predictive of a poor response. No other condition-specific measures including those relating to symptoms (severity, duration), mechanisms of onset, previous management, or radiological findings were found to be related to a poor response to rehabilitation. This is in contrast to previous studies that have shown condition-specific factors to be associated with poor response to rehabilitation for KOA (pain severity, ligament laxity, pain during physical examination) [15] and shoulder conditions (pain severity and duration [18, 41], subacromial injection response [3], acromion morphology [17]). It should be acknowledged however, that this discrepancy may reflect the limited condition-specific factors that were measured in this study, including the lack of physical assessment measures. Irrespective, the findings of this study have an important message for clinicians managing these disorders to consider the total patient presentation when considering prognostic indicators of recovery and not just factors directly related to the condition.

Table 2 Patient characteristics demonstrating a relationship with not achieving a minimal clinically important difference (MCID) following the non-surgical management of KOA, SIS, and LBP

Condition	No MCID Mean ± Standard Deviation or % (n)	MCID (Reference) Mean ± Standard Deviation or % (n)	Adjusted OR (95% Confidence Intervals)
Low Back Pain			
Cervical and/or thoracic pain			
Present	66.7% (26)	33.3% (13)	2.1 (1.02–4.4)[A]
Absent	46.3% (94)	53.7% (109)	
Pain Self Efficacy Score	28.82 ± 13.81 (120)	33.72 ± 15.51 (122)	0.98 (0.96–1)[A]
Shoulder Impingement Syndrome			
Comorbidities	3.55 ± 2.31 (133)	2.77 ± 2.28 (124)	1.16 (1.02–1.32)[A]
Knee Osteoarthritis			
Psychological Anxiety	7.89 ± 8.91 (91)	4.54 ± 5.02 (89)	1.11 (1.03–1.21)[A]
Patient Specific Functional Scale	3.37 ± 1.38 (53)	4.19 ± 1.88 (62)	0.76 (0.59–0.97)[A]

Significant at [A]P < 0.05

It should be noted that the strength of the relationship between some of the predictive variables and not achieving a MCID in outcome was relatively modest (OR range 0.76–2.1). For example the anxiety level of the KOA group not achieving a MCID (7.89 points) is at the lower end of the mild anxiety category (8–9 points) [36]. Irrespective, these patient characteristics observed prior to management suggests the presence of a more severe or complex condition (widespread pain, low functional capacity, comorbidity, low pain self-efficacy, higher anxiety) that may potentially affect the individual's capacity to achieve a satisfactory benefit from non-surgical multidisciplinary management. Certainly the findings of this exploratory study warrants further investigation of these and other patient characteristics in their capacity to identify at risk patients. This is especially the case as predictive characteristics may be different between musculoskeletal conditions and between different health settings (primary versus tertiary).

Limitations

There are limitations of this study due its retrospective methodology. These include unrecorded, missing, or illegible information within the medical records. Additionally other potentially useful variables such as physical examination findings were not included as they had not been recorded in a standardised manner across participating sites. Therefore, there may be other informative clinical variables not evaluated in this retrospective study which justifies further prospective investigation, with the aim of eventually developing effective screening tools to identify at risk patients. It should also be noted that there are limitations associated with dichotomising clinical outcomes (ie. not achieving/achieving a MCID). While MCID scores were purposefully used in this study to specifically identify prognostic factors relevant to patients who report a poor response, potentially regression modelling based on the original score may give better power in predictor selection and effect estimations. Despite these limitations, the use of measures collected in the clinical environment in this study, combined with the collection of data at seven tertiary hospital sites, strengthens the potential clinical meaningfulness of the findings.

Conclusions

General health issues (eg. coexisting conditions, psychological factors) are potential barriers to effective non-surgical multidisciplinary rehabilitation of common orthopaedic conditions in tertiary care. Specifically the findings suggest that factors other than just the biological severity of the orthopaedic condition may impact the patient's response to rehabilitation. From a clinical perspective, the early identification of prognostic indicators of a poor response in an individual patient should be considered within the context of management planning for that patient.

Abbreviations
KOA: Knee Osteoarthritis; LBP: Low Back Pain; MCID: Minimal Clinically Important Difference; ODI: Oswestry Disability Index; OR: Odds Ratio; SIS: Shoulder Impingement Syndrome; SPADI: Shoulder Pain and Disability Index; WOMAC: Western Ontario and McMaster Universities Osteoarthritis Index

Acknowledgements
SOL was supported by a Health Practitioner Research Fellowship (Queensland Health and University of Queensland (NHMRC CCRE Spinal Pain, Injury and Health)). The investigators would like to thank the Orthopaedic Physiotherapy Screening Clinic and Multidisciplinary Services Clinical Leaders as well as Medical Records staff at the participating hospital sites; Royal Brisbane and Women's Hospital, Ipswich Hospital, Princess Alexandra Hospital, Logan Hospital, Gold Coast Hospital, Townsville Hospital, and Redcliffe Hospital.

Funding
This study was funded by a Royal Brisbane and Women's Hospital Research Project Grant. This funding body had no role in the design of the study and collection, analysis, and interpretation of data and in writing the manuscript.

Authors' contributions
SOL contributed to the study design and preparation, data collection process, data analysis and interpretation, and manuscript preparation. MC contributed to the data collection process, data analysis and interpretation, and manuscript preparation. MR contributed to the study design and preparation, data collection process, data analysis and interpretation, and manuscript preparation. DS contributed to the study design and preparation, data collection process, and manuscript preparation. AK contributed to the study design and preparation, data analysis and interpretation, and manuscript preparation. All authors read and approved the final manuscript.

Competing interests
The authors declare that they have no competing interests.

Author details
[1]School of Health and Rehabilitation Sciences, University of Queensland, Brisbane, Australia. [2]Physiotherapy Department, Royal Brisbane and Women's Hospital, Brisbane, Australia. [3]Physiotherapy Department, Ipswich Hospital, Ipswich, Australia.

References
1. Vos T, Flaxman AD, Naghavi M, Lozano R, Michaud C, Ezzati M, et al. Years lived with disability (YLDs) for 1160 sequelae of 289 diseases and injuries 1990-2010: a systematic analysis for the global burden of disease study 2010. Lancet. 2012;380:2163–96 Epub 2012/12/19.
2. Bennell KL, Hunter DJ, Hinman RS. Management of osteoarthritis of the knee. Br Med J. 2012;345:e4934.
3. Cummins CA, Sasso LM, Nicholson D. Impingement syndrome: temporal outcomes of nonoperative treatment. J Shoulder Elb Surg. 2009;18:172–7.
4. Airaksinen O, Brox JI, Cedraschi C, Hildebrandt J, Klaber-Moffett J, Kovacs F, et al. Chapter 4. European guidelines for the management of chronic nonspecific low back pain. Eur Spine J. 2006;15(Suppl 2):S192–300.
5. Franklin PD, Li W, Ayers DC. The Chitranjan Ranawat award: functional outcome after total knee replacement varies with patient attributes. Clin Orthop Relat Res. 2008;466:2597–604.
6. Lingard EA, Katz JN, Wright EA, Sledge CB. Predicting the outcome of total knee arthroplasty. J Bone Joint Surg Am. 2004;86-A:2179–86.
7. Nunez M, Nunez E, del Val JL, Ortega R, Segur JM, Hernandez MV, et al. Health-related quality of life in patients with osteoarthritis after total knee replacement: factors influencing outcomes at 36 months of follow-up. Osteoarthr Cartil. 2007;15:1001–7 Epub 2007/04/13.
8. Judge A, Arden NK, Cooper C, Kassim Javaid M, Carr AJ, Field RE, et al. Predictors of outcomes of total knee replacement surgery. Rheumatology. 2012;51:1804–13 Epub 2012/04/26.
9. Henn RF 3rd, Kang L, Tashjian RZ, Green A. Patients' preoperative expectations predict the outcome of rotator cuff repair. J Bone Joint Surg Am. 2007;89:1913–9.

10. Oh JH, Kim SH, Ji HM, Jo KH, Bin SW, Gong HS. Prognostic factors affecting anatomic outcome of rotator cuff repair and correlation with functional outcome. Arthroscopy. 2009;25:30–9.

11. Oh JH, Kim SH, Kang JY, Oh CH, Gong HS. Effect of age on functional and structural outcome after rotator cuff repair. Am J Sports Med. 2010;38:672–8.

12. Tashjian RZ, Henn RF, Kang L, Green A. Effect of medical comorbidity on self-assessed pain, function, and general health status after rotator cuff repair. J Bone Joint Surg Am. 2006;88:536–40.

13. Sinikallio S, Aalto T, Airaksinen O, Herno A, Kroger H, Savolainen S, et al. Lumbar spinal stenosis patients are satisfied with short-term results of surgery - younger age, symptom severity, disability and depression decrease satisfaction. Disabil Rehabil. 2007;29:537–44.

14. Mallen CD, Peat G, Thomas E, Dunn KM, Croft PR. Prognostic factors for musculoskeletal pain in primary care: a systematic review. Br J Gen Pract. 2007;57:655–61.

15. Deyle GD, Gill NW, Allison SC, Hando BR, Rochino DA. Knee OA: which patients are unlikely to benefit from manual PT and exercise? J Fam Pract. 2012;61:E1–8 Epub 2012/01/06.

16. Chester R, Jerosch-Herold C, Lewis J, Shepstone L. Psychological factors are associated with the outcome of physiotherapy for people with shoulder pain: a multicentre longitudinal cohort study. Br J Sports Med. 2018;52:269–75.

17. Taheriazam A, Sadatsafavi M, Moayyeri A. Outcome predictors in nonoperative management of newly diagnosed subacromial impingement syndrome: a longitudinal study. MedGenMed. 2005;7:63.

18. Rodeghero JR, Cleland JA, Mintken PE, Cook CE. Risk stratification of patients with shoulder pain seen in physical therapy practice. J Eval Clin Pract. 2017; 23:257–63.

19. Bergbom S, Boersma K, Overmeer T, Linton SJ. Relationship among pain catastrophizing, depressed mood, and outcomes across physical therapy treatments. Phys Ther. 2011;91:754–64.

20. Wang JC, Horner G, Brown ED, Shapiro MS. The relationship between acromial morphology and conservative treatment of patients with impingement syndrome. Orthopedics. 2000;23:557–9 Epub 2000/06/30.

21. Daubs MD, Norvell DC, McGuire R, Molinari R, Hermsmeyer JT, Fourney DR, et al. Fusion versus nonoperative care for chronic low back pain: do psychological factors affect outcomes? Spine (Phila Pa 1976). 2011;36:S96–109 Epub 2011/10/05.

22. Carr AJ. Barriers to the effectiveness of any intervention in OA. Best Pract Res Clin Rheumatol. 2001;15:645–56.

23. Butterworth SW. Influencing patinet adherance to treatment guidelines. J Manag Care Pharm. 2008;14:S21–S5.

24. La Montagna G, Tirri G, Cacace E. Quality of life assessment during six months of NSAID treatment [Gonarthritis and quality of life (GOAL) study]. Clin Exp Rheumatol. 1998;16:49–54.

25. O'Reilly S, Muir K, Doherty M. Effectiveness of home exercise on pain and disability from osteoarthritis of the knee: a randomised controlled trial. Ann Rheum Dis. 1999;58:15–9.

26. Childs JD, Fritz JM, Flynn TW, Irrgang JJ, Johnson KK, Majkowski GR, et al. A clinical prediction rule to identify patients with low back pain most likely to benefit from spinal manipulation: a validation study. Ann Intern Med. 2004;141:920–8.

27. Flynn T, Fritz J, Whitman J, Wainner R, Magel J, Rendeiro D, et al. A clinical prediction rule for classifying patients with low back pain who demonstrate short-term improvement with spinal manipulation. Spine (Phila Pa 1976). 2002;27:2835–43 Epub 2002/12/18.

28. Bellamy N, Buchanan WW, Goldsmith CH, Campbell J, Stitt LW. Validation study of WOMAC: a health status instrument for measuring clinically important patient relevant outcomes to antirheumatic drug therapy in patients with osteoarthritis of the hip or knee. J Rheumatol. 1988;15:1833–40.

29. Roos EM, Klassbo M, Lohmander LS. WOMAC osteoarthritis index. Reliability, validity, and responsiveness in patients with arthroscopically assessed osteoarthritis. Western Ontario and MacMaster Universities. Scand J Rheumatol. 1999;28:210–5.

30. Roos EM, Roos HP, Lohmander LS, Ekdahl C, Beynnon BD. Knee injury and osteoarthritis outcome score (KOOS)--development of a self-administered outcome measure. J Orthop Sports Phys Ther. 1998;28:88–96.

31. Roos EM, Lohmander LS. The knee injury and osteoarthritis outcome score (KOOS): from joint injury to osteoarthritis. Health Qual Life Outcomes. 2003;1:64.

32. Angst F, Aeschlimann A, Michel BA, Stucki G. Minimal clinically important rehabilitation effects in patients with osteoarthritis of the lower extremities. J Rheumatol. 2002;29:131–8.

33. Ekeberg OM, Bautz-Holter E, Keller A, Tveita EK, Juel NG, Brox JI. A questionnaire found disease-specific WORC index is not more responsive than SPADI and OSS in rotator cuff disease. J Clin Epidemiol. 2010;63:575–84 Epub 2009/10/20.

34. Lauridsen HH, Hartvigsen J, Manniche C, Korsholm L, Grunnet-Nilsson N. Responsiveness and minimal clinically important difference for pain and disability instruments in low back pain patients. BMC Musculoskelet Disord. 2006;7:82 Epub 2006/10/27.

35. Richardson J, Hawthorne G. The Australian quality of life (AQoL) instrument: psychometric properties of the descriptive system and inital validation. Australian Studies of Health Service Administration. 1998;85:315–42.

36. Henry JD, Crawford JR. The short-form version of the depression anxiety stress scales (DASS-21): construct validity and normative data in a large non-clinical sample. Br J Clin Psychol. 2005;44:227–39.

37. Nicholas M. The pain self-efficacy questionnaire: taking pain into account. Eur J Pain. 2007;11:153–63.

38. Fries J, Spitzer P, Kranes G, Holman H. Measurement of patient outcome in arthritis. Arthritis Rheum. 1980;23:137–45.

39. Stratford P, Gill C, Westaway M, Binkley J. Assessing disability and change on individual patients: a report of a patient specific measure. Physiother Can. 1995;47:258–63.

40. Freedman DA. A note on screening regression equations. Am Stat. 1983;37: 152–5.

41. Kuijpers T, van der Windt DA, Boeke AJ, Twisk JW, Vergouwe Y, Bouter LM, et al. Clinical prediction rules for the prognosis of shoulder pain in general practice. Pain. 2006;120:276–85.

13

Cohort identification of axial spondyloarthritis in a large healthcare dataset: current and future methods

Jessica A. Walsh[1]*[iD], Shaobo Pei[2], Gopi K. Penmetsa[1], Jianwei Leng[2], Grant W. Cannon[2], Daniel O. Clegg[1] and Brian C. Sauer[2]

Abstract

Background: Big data research is important for studying uncommon diseases in real-world settings. Most big data studies in axial spondyloarthritis (axSpA) have been limited to populations identified with billing codes for ankylosing spondylitis (AS). axSpA is a more inclusive concept, and reliance on AS codes does not produce a comprehensive axSpA study population. The first objective was to describe our process for establishing an appropriate sample of patients with and without axSpA for developing accurate axSpA identification methods. The second objective was to determine the classification performance of AS billing codes against the chart-reviewed axSpA reference standard.

Methods: Veteran Health Affairs clinical and administrative data, between January 2005 and June 2015, were used to randomly select patients with clinical phenotypes that represented high, moderate, and low likelihoods of an axSpA diagnosis. With chart review, the sampled patients were classified as Yes axSpA, No axSpA or Uncertain axSpA, and these classification assignments were used as the reference standard for determining the positive predictive value (PPV) and sensitivity of AS ICD-9 codes for axSpA.

Results: Six hundred patients were classified as Yes axSpA (26.8%), No axSpA (68.3%), or Uncertain axSpA (4.8%). The PPV and sensitivity of an AS ICD-9 code for axSpA were 83.3% and 57.3%, respectively.

Conclusions: Standard methods of identifying axSpA patients in a large dataset lacked sensitivity. An appropriate sample of patients with and without axSpA was established and characterized for developing novel axSpA identification methods that are anticipated to enable previously impractical big data research.

Keywords: Spondyloarthropathy, Ankylosing spondylitis, Databases, Health services research

Background

Big data research is necessary for studying uncommon diseases and outcomes in real-world settings [1]. Big data research is particularly important for spondyloarthritis (SpA), since concepts of SpA have broadened in recent years [2]. The axial SpA (axSpA) concept was introduced in 2009 [3], when it became apparent from advances in imaging and treatment that nearly one-half of patients with an axial inflammatory arthritis phenotype were excluded from traditional axSpA definitions (i.e. ankylosing spondylitis [AS]) [4]. Despite the growing recognition of more inclusive axSpA concepts, big data axSpA studies continue to be limited to the AS subtype [5–9], since there are no billing codes for non-AS subtypes. In more broadly defined axSpA populations, little is known about real-life outcomes, such as comorbidities, mortality, diagnostic and treatment patterns, health care utilization , and costs [10]. New methods of identifying axSpA patients are needed for a wide range of big data research in axSpA.

In order to develop and evaluate new axSpA identification methods, an appropriate sample of patients with and without axSpA is needed [11]. The ideal approach is to screen patients from the general population and classify them as having or not having axSpA. This approach is impractical for uncommon diseases, like axSpA, since

* Correspondence: jessica.walsh@hsc.utah.edu
[1]Division of Rheumatology School of Medicine, 30 North 1900 East, Salt Lake City, UT 84132, USA
Full list of author information is available at the end of the article

tens of thousands of patients would need to be screened to identify a sufficient number of axSpA patients for research.

For feasibility purposes, patient populations are frequently enriched with patients at high risk of having the outcome of interest [12, 13]. For example, in an axSpA radiographic progression study, the population may consist of patients at elevated risk for structural disease progression (elevated C-Reactive Protein or baseline syndesmophytes) [14]. A disadvantage of this high-risk sampling approach is that the generalizability of the study results is limited by excluding lower risk patients (i.e. the results of the radiographic progression studies cannot be applied to axSpA patients without an elevated CRP or baseline syndesmophytes).

An alternative approach is to include both patients with high and low risk of disease. The sampled population is enriched for the disease of interest by including a greater percentage of patients at high risk than occurs in the general population. To improve generalizability, people at low risk are also required to be included in the sampled population. Compared to the distribution of high and low risk people in the general population, people at high risk for the disease are over-sampled and people at low risk are under-sampled [15]. This risk stratification sampling approach balances the advantages of feasibility with enrichment of high risk patients vs. generalizability with inclusion of low risk patients.

The first objective of this study was to describe our sampling strategy and chart-review process for establishing an appropriate sample of patients with and without axSpA for the future development of accurate axSpA identification methods for big data research. The second objective was to determine the classification performance of the International Classification of Diseases-Ninth Revision (ICD-9) code for AS against the chart-reviewed axSpA reference standard.

Methods

Design, setting, and data sources

This retrospective study used data from Veterans enrolled in the Veterans Health Administration (VHA). The data source was the Corporate Data Warehouse, a national repository of data from the VHA medical record system (VistA) and other VHA clinical and administrative systems [16]. The patient Integration Control Number was used to link patients across VHA stations. Data were housed and analyzed within the Veterans Affairs Informatics and Computing Infrastructure (VINCI) [17].

Patient sampling strategy

The sampled population consisted of 600 randomly selected Veterans with conditions representing high (n = 200), moderate (n = 200), and low (n = 200) risk

for axSpA, between January 1, 2005 to June 30, 2015. Structured Query Language (SQL) server newid function was used for randomization [18]. Veterans were considered by clinical experts to be at high risk for having axSpA if they had ≥1 AS ICD-9 code or a clinically available positive HLA-B27 result. Veterans with ICD-9 codes for sacroiliitis or a non-AS SpA subtypes (psoriatic arthritis, undifferentiated spondyloarthritis, reactive arthritis, and enteropathic arthritis) were categorized as moderate axSpA risk. The low risk category included patients with chronic back pain or other diseases that may mimic SpA [rheumatoid arthritis, diffuse idiopathic skeletal hyperostosis (DISH), crystal arthritis (gout and pseudogout), and other types of inflammatory arthritis (connective tissue disease, vasculitis, polymyalgia rheumatic, sarcoidosis, Paget's disease)].

AxSpA classification by chart review

Methods for classifying patients as having or not having axSpA occurred in multiple steps. First, clinical experts determined concepts that were expected to be useful for classification assignments. The concept categories included diagnostic language, disease features, laboratory results, and medications. Diagnostic language included statements affirming or negating the presence of SpA or an alternative diagnosis (i.e. "Mr. X has ank spond...", "there is no evidence of spondyloarthritis", or "her back pain is due to a herniated disk". Disease features included language affirming or negating sacroiliitis, uveitis, enthesitis, inflammatory arthritis, dactylitis, psoriasis, inflammatory bowel disease, and syndesmophytes. Disease modifying anti-rheumatic drugs (DMARDs) included apremilast, leflunomide, methotrexate, sulfasalazine, adalimumab, certolizumab, etanercept, golimumab, infliximab, rituximab, and ustekinumab. Laboratory results included HLA-B27 positivity, elevated erythrocyte sedimentation rate, elevated C-reactive protein, rheumatoid factor, and anti-cyclic citrullinated protein.

Second, data were extracted for the 600 sampled patients. Four types of data were included: provider notes, imaging reports, laboratory results, and medications. For provider notes, all Text Integration Utility notes from primary care, rheumatology, orthopedics, gastroenterology, dermatology, ophthalmology, physical medicine and rehabilitation, pain clinics, geriatrics, emergency medicine, urgent care, and podiatry were extracted. Imaging reports were extracted with note titles indicating inclusion of a joint (neck, shoulder, elbow, wrist, hand, finger, pelvis, sacroiliac joint, hip, spine, knee, ankle, feet, and toe). The laboratory results were extracted by their Logical Observation Identifiers Names and Codes (LOINC) [19]. Quality review and revisions were used to ensure correct mapping and to standardize laboratory values. DMARD exposure data were extracted for all DMARDs dispensed during the study period.

Third, annotation software (eHOST [20]) was adapted and applied to the 600 sampled patients. A customized user interface was built for eHOST that enabled reviewers to efficiently view the extracted provider notes, imaging, laboratory results, and medications on a single screen, for the purpose of making patient-level classifications. Data were extracted and displayed in a manner that maintained the sequential nature and prioritization of the relevant documents. Annotation functions were designed for the reviewers to highlight and annotate the sections of text that were used to make classification decisions. Classification categories for axSpA status included Yes axSpA, No axSpA, and Uncertain axSpA. The uncertain category was assigned to patients with conflicting information or an axSpA diagnosis without additional information to support an axSpA diagnosis.

Two rheumatologists (JAW and GKP) independently annotated and classified the sampled patients. Classification guidelines were developed and revised. The protocol required reviewers, at a minimum, to assess specific types of documents (rheumatology consults and most recent rheumatology note, all articular imaging reports, dermatology notes, etc.). Additionally, the eHOST software was programmed to pre-annotate (highlight) every mention of terms relevant to axSpA (ankylosing spondylitis, spondyloarthr*, iritis, uveitis, dactylitis, enthesitis, erosion, *B27, etc.) in each document. After completing the initial annotation of the required documents (without pre-annotation), the reviewers annotated the pre-annotated terms that were not captured with the chart reviewers' previous annotation, to minimize the risk of overlooking data relevant to classification assignments. Both reviewers completed chart review classifications in batches of 20 until inter-rater agreement exceeded 85%. Discrepancies were adjudicated. After the 85% inter-rater agreement goal was achieved, the remainder of the sampled population was classified by a single reviewer.

Characterizing the chart-reviewed population and evaluating AS ICD-9 codes

The demographics and health care utilization of the sampled patients were described in three groups: Yes axSpA, No axSpA, and Uncertain axSpA. Health care utilization was measured with duration of active VA system use during the study period (time between initial and most recent encounter with a provider or medication dispensation) and mean number of provider visits per year. The PPV of an AS ICD-9 code for axSpA was calculated in all patients with ≥1 ICD-9 code for AS [21]. The sensitivity of an AS ICD-9 code for axSpA was calculated in the subset who were *not* specifically selected to the sampled population because of an AS ICD-9 code. For PPV and sensitivity calculations, patients with sufficient evidence of axSpA (Yes axSpA)

were compared to patients with insufficient evidence of axSpA (No axSpA and Uncertain axSpA). For confidence intervals, exact binomial confidence intervals were used for categorical variables and normal approximation was used for continuous variables.

Results
Patient population

During the study period, 9,803,429 Veterans participated in the VHA system. Patients eligible for selection into the sampled population included Veterans with ICD-9 codes for specific diseases or a laboratory result that placed them at high, moderate and low risk for axSpA (Table 1). Six hundred Veterans were randomly selected, including 0.83% of Veterans from the high risk stratum ($n = 200$), 0.25% from the moderate risk stratum ($n = 200$), and 0.01% from the low risk stratum ($n = 200$). Among the 600 sampled Veterans, 162 (27.0%) were classified as Yes axSpA, 409 (68.2%) were classified as No axSpA, and 29 (4.8%) were classified as Uncertain axSpA (Table 2). Within the group selected from the high risk stratum, 87% with an AS ICD-9 code were classified as Yes axSpA, while 38% of patients with a clinically available positive HLA-B27 result were classified as Yes axSpA. In the moderate risk groups, 27% with an ICD-9 code for a non-AS SpA subtype were classified as Yes axSpA and 7% with a sacroiliitis ICD-9 code were classified as Yes axSpA. In the low risk category, 2% of patients with an ICD-9 code for a SpA mimic were classified as Yes axSpA, and 1% of patients with ICD-9 codes chronic back pain were classified as Yes axSpA. The demographics and health care utilization patterns of the sampled population were similar between the Yes axSpA group and the No axSpA group, with the exception of younger age (56.2 vs. 59.9) and higher percentage of males (95.7% vs. 88.8%) in the Yes axSpA group (Table 3).

Performance of AS diagnosis codes for classifying axSpA

Among the 156 axSpA patients with an AS ICD-9 code, the PPV of the AS ICD-9 code for axSpA was 83.3% (Fig. 1). Within the 75 axSpA patients who were *not* specifically selected to into the sampled population because of an AS ICD-9 code, the sensitivity of an AS ICD-9 code for axSpA was 57.3%.

Discussion

We established and characterized an appropriate sample of patients with and without axSpA for developing novel axSpA identification methods and for evaluating AS billing codes in axSpA patients. This population is enriched with axSpA patients and is representative of more generalizable disease states (i.e. chronic back pain). Additionally, patients were included with diseases that may mimic axSpA (DISH, peripheral psoriatic arthritis,

Table 1 Selection of patients sampled for the chart review population

Subgroups	Subgroup Criteria (ICD-9 or laboratory data)	No. of Veterans	No. of Veterans selected to chart review population	% from each risk stratum selected to the chart review population (95% CI)
High risk for axSpA				
Ankylosing spondylitis	720.0	15,862	100	0.83 (0.72–0.96)
HLA-B27 positivity	positive B27 test result	8168	100	
Moderate risk for axSpA				
Sacroiliitis	720.2	50,603	100	0.25 (0.21–0.28)
SpA subtype other than AS			100[a]	
Spondyloarthritis NOS	720.8x and/or 720.9x	6319		
Reactive arthritis	711.x and/or 99.3	1072		
Psoriatic arthritis	696.0	22,625		
Enteropathic arthritis	713.1 AND either 555.x OR 556.x	521		
Low risk of axSpA				
Chronic back pain	(≥2 ICD-9 codes for back pain ≥3 months apart [724.1, 724.2, 724.5])	2,069,644	100	0.01 (0.01–0.01)
Non-SpA rheumatologic disease			100[a]	
DISH	721.6	2963		
Crystal arthritis	274.x and/or 712.x	675,799		
Rheumatoid arthritis	714.x	143,620		
Other inflammatory arthritis	CTD (710.x), vasculitis (273.2, 446.0, 446.4, 446.5, 446.7), PMR (725), Paget's (731.0), sarcoidosis (135)	135,608		

[a]25 patients from each subcategory of spondyloarthritis NOS, reactive arthritis, psoriatic arthritis, enteropathic arthritis, DISH, crystal arthritis, rheumatoid arthritis, and other inflammatory arthritis

crystal arthritis, etc.) to maximize the ability of axSpA identification methods to differentiate between axSpA and axSpA mimics. These sampled patients will be used to identify and prioritize data that differentiate between patients with and without axSpA, for the development of novel axSpA classification algorithms.

The evaluation of the AS ICD-9 code demonstrated a reasonably high PPV for axSpA (83.3%). This is similar to the PPV of ≥1 AS ICD-9 code for AS reported in a Veteran population attending rheumatology clinics

(83%) [22]. However, the PPV estimates in both of these studies are likely overestimated compared to the PPV in the general population, since these population were enriched with AS patients, and PPV estimates increase when the prevalence of the underlying condition increases.

The sensitivity of the AS ICD-9 code for axSpA was low (57%). Not all patients with axSpA have AS, since axSpA also includes non-AS subtypes. However, it is likely that providers used the AS ICD-9 code as a proxy for non-AS axSpA subtypes, since there are no billing

Table 2 AxSpA classification by chart review

	All	High risk for axSpA		Moderate risk for axSpA		Low risk for axSpA	
	No. [%] (95% CI) n = 600	AS No. (95% CI) n = 100	HLA-B27+ No. (95% CI) n = 100	Non-AS SpA subtype No. (95% CI) n = 100	Sacroiliitis No. (95% CI) n = 100	SpA mimics No. (95% CI) n = 100	Chronic back pain No. (95% CI) n = 100
Yes AxSpA	162 [27.0] (23.5–30.7)	87 (78.8–92.9)	38 (28.5–48.3)	27 (18.6–36.8)	7 (2.9–13.9)	2 (0.2–7.0)	1 (0.0–5.5)
No AxSpA	409 [68.2] (64.3–71.9)	4 (1.1–9.9)	57 (46.7–66.9)	63 (52.8–72.4)	89 (81.2–94.4)	97 (91.5–99.4)	99 (94.6–100.0)
Uncertain AxSpA	29 [4.8] (3.3–6.9)	9 (4.2–16.4)	5 (1.6–11.3)	10 (4.9–17.6)	4 (1.1–9.9)	1 (0.0–5.5)	0 (0.0–3.6)

No. number, CI confidence interval

Table 3 Patient characteristics and health care utilization in chart review population

	Yes axSpA (n = 162)			No axSpA (n = 409)			Uncertain axSpA (n = 29)		
	No./Mean	SD/%	95% CI	No./Mean	SD/%	95% CI	No./Mean	SD/%	95% CI
Age	56.2	13.5	54.1, 58.3	60.0	13.2	58.7, 61.2	58.1	14.3	52.9, 63.3
Gender (Male)	155	95.7	91.3, 98.3	363	88.8	85.3, 91.7	28	96.6	82.2, 99.9
Race									
White	128	79.0	71.9, 85.0	305	74.6	70.1, 78.7	22	75.9	56.5, 89.7
Black	18	11.1	6.7, 17.0	63	15.4	12.0, 19.3	4	13.8	3.9, 31.7
Other	2	1.2	0.2, 4.4	6	1.5	0.5, 3.2	0	0.0	0.0, 11.9
Unknown	14	8.6	4.8, 14.1	35	8.6	6.0, 11.7	3	10.3	2.2, 27.4
Ethnicity									
Non-Hispanic	144	88.9	83.0, 93.3	367	89.7	86.4, 92.5	27	93.1	77.2, 99.2
Hispanic	7	4.3	1.8, 8.7	19	4.6	2.8, 7.2	2	6.9	0.9, 22.8
Unknown	11	6.8	3.4, 11.8	23	5.6	3.6, 8.3	0	0.0	0.0, 11.9
Geographic region									
Southeast	57	35.2	27.9, 43.1	153	37.4	32.7, 42.3	14	48.3	29.5, 67.5
North Atlantic	35	21.6	15.5, 28.7	84	20.5	16.7, 24.8	7	24.1	10.3, 43.5
Midwest	30	18.5	12.9, 25.4	68	16.6	13.2, 20.6	2	6.9	0.9, 22.8
Continental	22	13.6	8.7, 19.8	58	14.2	11.0, 17.9	4	13.8	3.9, 31.7
Pacific	18	11.1	6.7, 17.0	46	11.2	8.4, 14.7	2	6.9	0.9, 22.8
Duration of active VA system use during study period (years)	9.3	2.0	9.0, 9.6	8.9	2.4	8.7, 9.2	9.0	2.2	8.2, 9.8
#Provider visits/ year during active system use period	43.6	39.3	37.5, 49.6	45.9	42.6	41.7, 50.0	25.5	27.3	15.6, 35.5

No. number, *VA* Veteran Affairs, *CI* confidence interval

codes for non-AS axSpA subtypes. While precise usage patterns of AS billing codes remain unknown, the lack of an AS ICD-9 code in 43% of axSpA patients over the 10.5 year study period, demonstrated that nearly one-half of axSpA patients were not identifiable with the only ICD-9 billing code that indicates that presence of inflammatory axial arthritis.

Strengths of this study include the large sample size and access to a medical record system that enabled consistent data capture across VHA sites throughout the United States. Furthermore, the chart review process was feasible for comprehensive review of multiple types of data for several hundred patients over a period exceeding 10 years. Another strength was the clinical expertise of the chart reviewers. As rheumatologists specializing in SpA within the VA system, both reviewers are experienced with the intricacies of axSpA patient care and documentation within the VA system.

This study was limited by the inability of chart reviewers to directly interact with patients or access digital

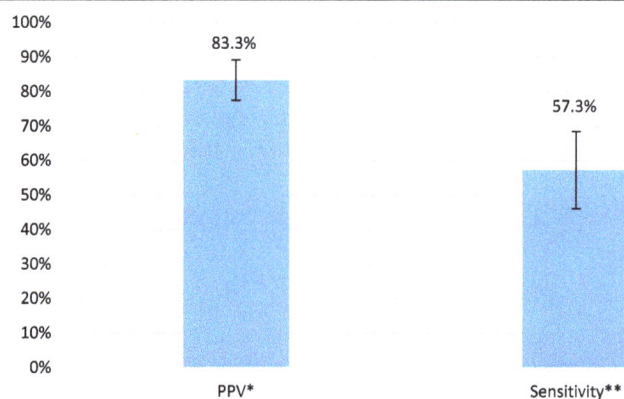

Fig. 1 Positive predictive value and sensitivity of ankylosing spondylitis ICD-9 code for AxSpA. PPV = positive predictive value. *n = 156 Veterans with an AS ICD-9 code. **n = 75 Veterans with AxSpA who were *not* selected to the chart review sample specifically for an AS ICD-9 code

radiologic images (radiology reports were reviewed). Thus, classification decisions had to be made with incomplete and otherwise imperfect data. These data limitations inevitably led to classification errors, particularly in patients with sparse data. Since patients with early or mild axSpA are expected to have fewer encounters than established and severe axSpA patients, the classification process was likely more accurate with established and more severe axSpA than early and milder axSpA [23]. Another limitation is that ICD-10 codes for axSpA were not evaluated, since the study period preceded the implementation of ICD-10 codes. It is anticipated that ICD-10 codes will be similarly limited with axSpA cohort identification, since ICD-10 codes do not include non-AS axSpA subtypes.

Conclusion

There is an unmet need for accurate methods of identifying axSpA patients in large datasets. We established and characterized an appropriate sample of patients for developing axSpA identification methods that are anticipated to enable a wide array of previously impractical big data studies in axSpA.

Abbreviations

AS: Ankylosing spondylitis; axSpA: Axial spondyloarthritis; DISH: Diffuse idiopathic skeletal hyperostosis; ICD: International Classification of Diseases; PPV: Positive predictive value; SpA: Spondyloarthritis; VHA: Veterans Health Administration

Funding

Funding for this project was provided by the Marriott Daughters Foundation and the Rheumatology Research Foundation Scientist Development Award. The funding Foundations were uninvolved in study design, data collection, analyses, and manuscript preparation. Support for Dr. Cannon was provided in part by Specialty Care Center of Innovation, Veterans Health Administration and Department of Veterans Affairs, Health Services Research and Development.

Authors' contributions

JAW contributed to study design, chart review, data analyses, data interpretation, and manuscript preparation. SP analyzed and interpreted patient data. GKP classified and characterized patients with chart review. JL customized software for chart review and prepared data for chart review. GWC contributed to study design and data interpretation. DOC contributed to study design and data interpretation. BCS contributed to study design and data interpretation. All authors read and approved the final manuscript.

Competing interests

The authors declare that they have no competing interests.

Author details

[1]Division of Rheumatology School of Medicine, 30 North 1900 East, Salt Lake City, UT 84132, USA. [2]George E. Wahlen Veteran Affairs Medical Center, 500 Foothill Boulevard, Salt Lake City, UT 84148, USA.

References

1. Lee CH, Yoon H-J. Medical big data: promise and challenges. Kidney Res Clin Pract. 2017;36:3–11.
2. Garg N, van den Bosch F, Deodhar A. The concept of spondyloarthritis: where are we now? Best Pract Res Clin Rheumatol. 2014;28:663–72.
3. Rudwaleit M, van der Heijde D, Landewé R, Listing J, Akkoc N, Brandt J, et al. The development of assessment of SpondyloArthritis international society classification criteria for axial spondyloarthritis (part II): validation and final selection. Ann Rheum Dis. 2009;68:777–83.
4. Poddubnyy D, Sieper J. Similarities and differences between nonradiographic and radiographic axial spondyloarthritis: a clinical, epidemiological and therapeutic assessment. Curr Opin Rheumatol. 2014;26: 377–83.
5. Walsh JA, Adejoro O, Chastek B, Park Y. Treatment patterns of biologics in US patients with ankylosing spondylitis: descriptive analyses from a claims database. J Comp Eff Res. 2018;7:369–80.
6. Deodhar A, Mittal M, Reilly P, Bao Y, Manthena S, Anderson J, et al. Ankylosing spondylitis diagnosis in US patients with back pain: identifying providers involved and factors associated with rheumatology referral delay. Clin Rheumatol. 2016;35:1769–76.
7. Walsh JA, Song X, Kim G, Park Y. Evaluation of the comorbidity burden in patients with ankylosing spondylitis treated with tumor necrosis factor inhibitors using a large administrative claims data set. J Pharm Health Serv Res. 2018;9:115–21.
8. Lu MC, Koo M, Lai NS. Incident spine surgery in patients with ankylosing spondylitis: a secondary cohort analysis of a nationwide, population-based health claims database. Arthritis Care Res (Hoboken). 2017; https://doi.org/10.1002/acr.23478.
9. Wysham KD, Murray SG, Hills N, Yelin E, Gensler LS. Cervical Spinal Fracture and Other Diagnoses Associated With Mortality in Hospitalized Ankylosing Spondylitis Patients. Arthritis Care Res (Hoboken). 2017;69:271–7.
10. Wang R, Ward MM. Epidemiology of axial spondyloarthritis: an update. Curr Opin Rheumatol. 2018;30:137–43.
11. Sarmiento RF, Dernoncourt F. Improving patient cohort identification using natural language processing. In: Secondary analysis of electronic health records. Cham: Springer; 2016. p. 405–17.
12. Macklin EA, Blacker D, Hyman BT, Betensky RA. Improved design of prodromal Alzheimer's disease trials through cohort enrichment and surrogate endpoints. J Alzheimers Dis. 2013;36(3):475–86.
13. Cohen G, Hilario M, Sax H, Hugonnet S, Geissbuhler A. Learning from imbalanced data in surveillance of nosocomial infection. Artif Intell Med. 2006;37:7–18.
14. Baraliakos X, Listing J, Rudwaleit M, Haibel H, Brandt J, Sieper J, et al. Progression of radiographic damage in patients with ankylosing spondylitis: defining the central role of syndesmophytes. Ann Rheum Dis. 2007;66:910–5.
15. Wang X, Zhou J, Wang T, George SL. On Enrichment Strategies for Biomarker Stratified Clinical Trials. J Biopharm Stat. 2017;21:1–17.
16. Fihn S, Francis J, Clancy C, Neilson C, Nelson K, Rumsfeld J, et al. Insights from advanced analytics at the veteran health administration. Health Aff. 2014;33:1203–11.
17. US Department of Veterans Affairs "VINCI Central. VA Informatics and Computing Infrastructure (VINCI). 2017. http://www.hsrd.research.va.gov/for_researchers/vinci/ . Accessed 6 Feb 2018.
18. Marcelo De Barros M, Gidewall K. Selecting Rows Randomly from a Large Table. 2008. https://msdn.microsoft.com/en-us/library/cc441928.aspx. Accessed 3 July 2018.
19. Loinc: The universal standard for identifying health measurements, observations, and documents. https://loinc.org/. Accessed 29 June 2018.
20. Chris Jianwei Leng CJ, South B, Shuying S. eHOST: The Extensible Human Oracle Suite of Tools. 2012. https://orbit.nlm.nih.gov/browse-repository/software/nlp-information-extraction/62-ehost-the-extensible-human-oracle-suite-of-tools. Accessed 6 Feb 2018.
21. Parikh R, Mathai A, Parikh S, Chandra Sekhar G, Thomas R. Understanding and using sensitivity, specificity and predictive values. Indian J Ophthalmol. 2008;56:45–50.
22. Singh JA, Holmgren AR, Krug H, Noorbaloochi S. Accuracy of the diagnoses of spondylarthritides in veterans affairs medical center databases. Arthritis Rheum. 2007;57:648–55.
23. Walsh JA, Pei S, Burningham Z, Penmetsa G, Cannon GW, Clegg DO, et al. Use of Disease-modifying Antirheumatic Drugs for Inflammatory Arthritis in US Veterans: Effect of Specialty Care and Geographic Distance. J Rheumatol. 2018;45:430–6.

14

Biomechanical comparison of screw-based zoning of PHILOS and Fx proximal humerus plates

Ali Jabran[1], Chris Peach[1,2], Zhenmin Zou[1] and Lei Ren[1*]

Abstract

Background: Treatment of proximal humerus fractures with locking plates is associated with complications. We aimed to compare the biomechanical effects of removing screws and blade of a fixed angle locking plate and hybrid blade plate, on a two-part fracture model.

Methods: Forty-five synthetic humeri were divided into nine groups where four were implanted with a hybrid blade plate and the remaining with locking plate, to treat a two-part surgical neck fracture. Plates' head screws and blades were divided into zones based on their distance from fracture site. Two groups acted as a control for each plate and the remaining seven had either a vacant zone or blade swapped with screws. For elastic cantilever bending, humeral head was fixed and the shaft was displaced 5 mm in extension, flexion, valgus and varus direction. Specimens were further loaded in varus direction to investigate their plastic behaviour.

Results: In both plates, removal of inferomedial screws or blade led to a significantly larger drop in varus construct stiffness than other zones. In blade plate, insertion of screws in place of blade significantly increased the mean extension, flexion valgus and varus bending stiffness (24.458%/16.623%/19.493%/14.137%). In locking plate, removal of screw zones proximal to the inferomedial screws reduced extension and flexion bending stiffness by 26–33%.

Conclusions: Although medial support improved varus stability, two inferomedial screws were more effective than blade. Proximal screws are important for extension and flexion. Mechanical consequences of screw removal should be considered when deciding the number and choice of screws and blade in clinic.

Keywords: Proximal humerus fractures, Biomechanical testing, Locking plate, Blade plate

Background

Proximal humerus fractures are relatively common injuries, accounting for 5–8% of all fractures [1, 2]. They are more prevalent in the over-60 female population group [3]. Incidence of these fractures, especially in the elderly patients after low energy falls, is increasing due to the growing elderly population with osteoporosis [4]. Younger patients, however, generally sustain them by high energy traumas [5].

Approximately 80% of proximal humerus fractures are stable with low displacement of fracture fragments, so their conservative management has proven to be

successful with high patient satisfaction [6]. The remaining 15–20% fracture cases are characterised by instability and significant displacements so surgical intervention is required to restore stability, improve chances of bone healing and allow early rehabilitation. Although there are many implants available for treatment of these fractures, the optimum method of fracture fixation is unclear [7].

Since the development of locking technology several decades ago, biomechanical studies have shown advantages of locking plates over conventional non-locking and blade plates [8–10]. Clinical studies, on the other hand, reveal high complication rates with their use, often necessitating revision surgery [11–13]. Common complications include varus deformity, screw cut-out and screw penetration through the humeral head and into the

---

* Correspondence: lei.ren@manchester.ac.uk
[1]School of Mechanical, Aerospace and Civil Engineering, University of Manchester, Sackville Street, Manchester M13 9PL, UK
Full list of author information is available at the end of the article

glenohumeral joint [14–16]. In light of this, Gardner et al. suggested the importance of medial support for maintaining fracture reduction [17].

Although positive outcomes have been achieved with the medial insertion of autologous bone grafts, fibular allograft, calcium phosphate bone cement and inferomedial screws in plates, there is no golden standard for the medial support reconstruction [13, 18–21]. Despite this, inferomedial screws have become a common feature of recent locking plate design. One such plate is the PHILOS (Proximal Humerus Internal Locked System) plate (Synthes, Paoli, Pennsylvania, USA) that allows fixed angle insertion of two locking inferomedial screws. With a similar design philosophy, the Equinoxe Fx plate (Exactech, Gainsville, FL) is a hybrid fixed angle blade plate that provides the option of implanting inferomedial locking screws or a blade. The rationale for a hybrid system that allows both blade and screws in a single plate is to reap the most from the mechanical benefits of locking screw technology and the fracture buttressing provided by the increased surface area of a blade. There is a scarcity of literature on the mechanical contribution of the blade- or screw-based inferomedial support as compared to screws of other parts of the proximal humerus plate.

The aim of this study was two-fold. Firstly, we aimed to determine the effect of lack of medial support, both in form of inferomedial locking screws and blade, on the extension, flexion, valgus and varus bending stiffness of humeri treated with either PHILOS or Fx plate. Secondly, we aimed to investigate the effect of removal of other humeral head screws on the extension, flexion, valgus and varus bending stiffness of humeri treated with either PHILOS or Fx plate.

Methods

Forty-five left synthetic humeri (model 1028; Pacific Research Laboratories, Vashon, WA, USA) were obtained and divided into nine groups, each containing five specimens. Five groups were implanted with 90 mm stainless steel PHILOS locking plate and the remaining four groups were implanted with 80 mm stainless steel Fx fixed-angle locking blade plate.

Screws and blades of both PHILOS and Fx plate were numbered and then categorised into several zones based on their positions on the plates (Fig. 1). Of the five groups implanted with PHILOS plate, four had either zone 1, 2, 3 or 4 screws missing (P1-P4) while the fifth group (P0) acted as the control configuration group as it

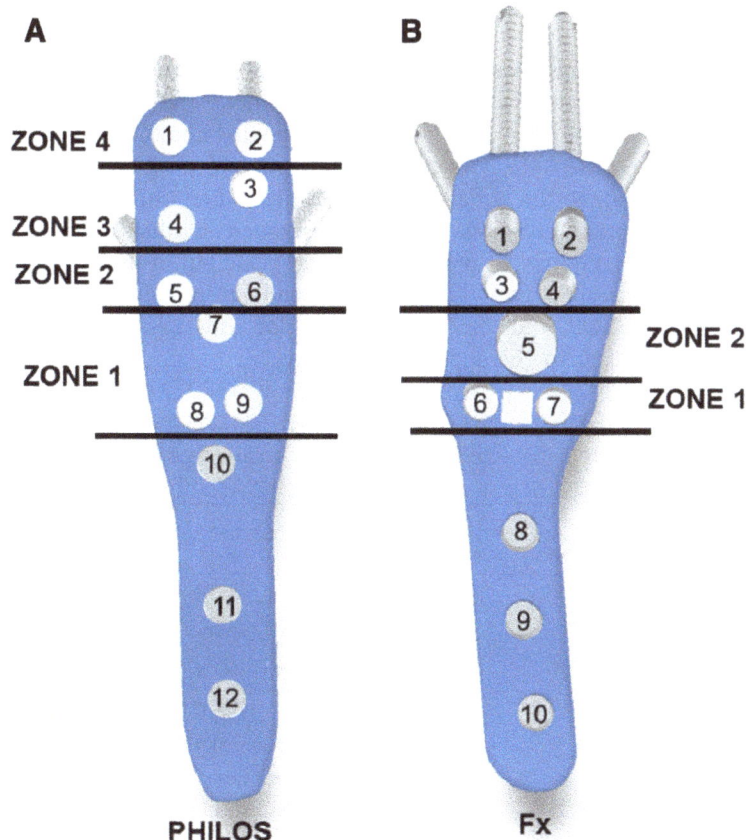

Fig. 1 Numbering and zoning of screws and blade holes on PHILOS plate (a) and Fx plate (b) based on their proximity to fracture gap]

had all the zones filled. Similarly, two of the four groups implanted with Fx plate had either zone 1 (F1) or zone 2 (F2) missing while the specimens from the third group had the blade swapped with two inferomedial locking screws (F3). The fourth Fx group had all the zones filled and acted as a control configuration group (F0). Details of the screw and blade choice for each plate configuration are tabulated in Table 1. Length of screws and blades were selected so that their tips abutted the subchondral bone, with the aim of achieving maximum screw purchase. This was determined in trial studies using the depth gauges provided by the manufacturers.

All specimens were potted in cement blocks to allow easy clamping of the humeral heads to the testing machine during the biomechanical tests (Fig. 2). The blocks were cubic so that by setting each of their four faces parallel to either the sagittal or frontal planes, loads could be applied along the anatomically accurate directions. With the shaft clamped vertically, humeral head was placed into a 100 cm^3 cubic mould. A cement mixture, consisting of standard, general purpose (Portland limestone) cement, rapid mix cement and water, was prepared by a ratio of 4:1:2.5 by volume. For homogeneity, the three were mixed using an electric mixer and then poured into the mould. The resulting mixture submerged the humeral head and was left for 48 h in the mould to dry.

Once removed from the mould, specimens were sawed at shaft to a length of 210 mm from humeral head apex. A 10 mm half-cut was created at the surgical neck. To simplify the process of fixating the plate onto humerus, plates were attached to the bone prior to the removal of the fracture piece. A half-cut was carried out to ease the removal of the fracture piece later and also to prevent damage caused to the plate.

The superior ends of the PHILOS and Fx plate were positioned 30 and 12 mm distal to the superior greater tuberosity. Once the plates were snug to the bone, screws holes were drilled and screws were implanted, starting from the shaft screws. All specimens were implanted according to the manufacturers' guidelines. The plates had similar procedures for specimen preparation, with small differences because of design features such as the blade insertion required in Fx plate. For the Fx plate, blades were inserted using a blade osteotome and held in position by shoulders grub screws. After implantation, the removal of the 10-mm block of bone was achieved by cutting through the other side of the bone to meet the previous two cuts and simulate a two-part fracture (corresponding to Neer classification). The block of bone was gently knocked out to prevent damage to the plate or any of the screws.

All forty-five specimens were subjected to both elastic (varus, valgus, extension and flexion bending five times) and plastic testing (varus bending once). For elastic testing, specimens were placed in an Instron 4500 universal materials testing machine (Instron, Canton, MA, USA) such that the humeral shaft was in a horizontal orientation. The specimens were then clamped rigidly at their proximal end by a custom fixture. The testing machine was installed with a semi-circular prismatic shaft holder. This way, crosshead was in contact with the humeral shaft at a distance of 30 mm from the specimen's distal end (Fig. 3). Five-millimetre displacement was applied at 1 mm/s along the frontal plane to achieve varus cantilever bending and the crosshead was then retracted back to its original position. This displacement was applied five times, after which the specimen was offloaded and repositioned so that it could be displaced along the frontal plane but in the opposite direction to induce valgus bending. In a similar manner, displacement was applied along the sagittal plane for extension and flexion bending.

Table 1 Length (mm) and descriptions of the screws and blades for the PHILOS plates and Fx plate configuration groups. Emboldened cells correspond to where combination differs from the control. Types of screws, cancellous, cortical locking and cortical compression, are denoted by CA, CO-L and CO-C, respectively

Configuration Group	Screw Number											
	1	2	3	4	5	6	7	8	9	10	11	12
P0 (Control)	40	40	45	50	42	42	None	50	50	32	30	30
P1 (No Zone 1)	40	40	45	50	42	42	None	None	None	32	30	30
P2 (No Zone 2)	40	40	45	50	None	None	None	50	50	32	30	30
P3 (No Zone 3)	40	40	None	None	42	42	None	50	50	32	30	30
P4 (No Zone 4)	None	None	45	50	42	42	None	50	50	32	30	30
F0 (Control)	29, CA	29, CA	44, CA	44, CA	50	45, Blade		26, CO-L	32, CO-C	26, CO-L	N/A	N/A
F1 (No Zone 1)	29, CA	29, CA	44, CA	44, CA	50	None		26, CO-L	32, CO-C	26, CO-L	N/A	N/A
F2 (No Zone 2)	29, CA	29, CA	44, CA	44, CA	None	45, Blade		26, CO-L	32, CO-C	26, CO-L	N/A	N/A
F3 (Swap Blade with Screws)	29, CA	29, CA	44, CA	44, CA	50	44, CA	44, CA	26, CO-L	32, CO-C	26, CO-L	N/A	N/A

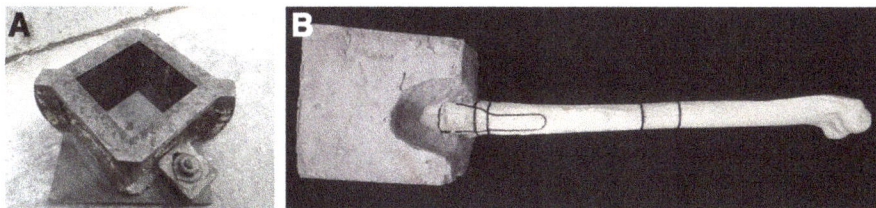

Fig. 2 Specimen preparation: Cubic mould (**a**) was filled with cement mix and humerus. After the block dried, humerus (**b**) was marked with positions of plate and cuts

Based on the load and displacement data recorded from the testing machine, peak load at 5 mm (F_5) and elastic stiffness (K) were determined for each direction.

Subsequently, plastic testing was conducted on all specimens to investigate their varus stability under large displacements. For this, the position of the constructs was similar to that for the varus elastic tests. Specimens were displaced at a rate of 0.05 mm/s until a 15-mm displacement was achieved. After an eight-minute intermission, the displacement was resumed at the same rate until a 30-mm displacement was obtained. Based on the trial studies, 30 mm was found to be large enough to ensure that all the specimens were in the plastic region of their load-displacement curve. For these tests, load at 30 mm (F_{30}) and those before and after the 15-mm intermission (F_{15a} and F_{15b}) were determined using the load-displacement data.

The statistical analyses of the experimental data were conducted using the SPSS 22.0 software (IBM, NY, USA). The effects on specimen groups' stiffness and load values were analysed by using a linear mixed model approach by taking intra- and inter-subject variability into account.

The fixed effect in the analysis was the configuration group while the specimens and their trials were set as the random effects. Dependent variables in the elastic test data were K and F_5 but in plastic test data, they

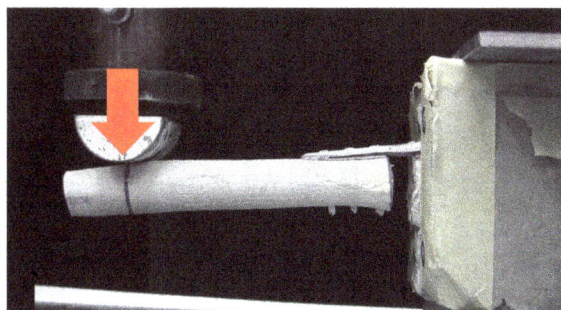

Fig. 3 Mechanical testing set-up used to apply varus cantilever displacement (red arrow) and determine bending loads and stiffness. Load was applied to the humeral shaft in a cantilever fashion while humeral head was potted inside the cement block

were F_{15a}, F_{15b} and F_{30}. The pair-wise difference was tested using Fisher's least significant difference (LSD) multiple comparison based on the least-squared means.

Results

Elastic testing results

For both plates, the trends in the mean peak loads among configuration groups were similar to those obtained for their mean stiffness (Figs. 4 & 5). No implant failure or screw pull-out was observed for any specimen during all tests. Out of all zones tested for PHILOS plate, removal of zone 1 screws in P1 had the greatest effect on valgus and varus stability, leading to 23 and 28% drop in mean stiffness (mean stiffness: 4.671/4.726 N/mm) when compared to the control group P0 (Table 2). In the order of decreasing effect on varus stiffness with their removal, zone 1 screws were followed by screws of zone 2 (5.867 N/mm), zone 3 (6.059 N/mm) and zone 4 (6.268 N/mm). This not only highlighted the importance of inferomedial screws for varus stability but also the likely link between the screws' position and varus stiffness. Removal of zone 1 screws had least impact on mean stiffness values in extension and flexion (7.956/6.349 N/mm). For loading along these two directions, removal of zone 2 led to the largest drop (33 and 31%) in mean stiffness (6.349/6.887), followed by the removal of screws of zone 3 (6.644/7.045 N/mm), zone 4 (6.871/7.377 N/mm) and zone 1 (7.956/8.284 N/mm).

In extension, flexion, valgus and varus testing of Fx plate, mean stiffness with the swapping of the blade with inferomedial screws in F3 (10.915/11.127/8.245/8.663 N/mm) was higher than the control group F0 (Table 3), followed by the removal of 6.5 mm screws in F2 (8.122/8.990/6.623/7.094 N/mm) and blade in F1 (7.734/8.248/6.332/5.619 N/mm). Like the removal of zone 1 screws in PHILOS plate, removing blade in Fx plate (F1) led to a larger decrease in valgus and varus stiffness (8 and 26%) than the removal of 6.5 mm screw (F2) when compared to control group F0. However, unlike the PHILOS plate configuration groups where zone 2 screws had a greater effect on extension and flexion than screws from zone 1, 6.5 mm screw in the Fx plate had less impact on extension and flexion stiffness than the removal of the

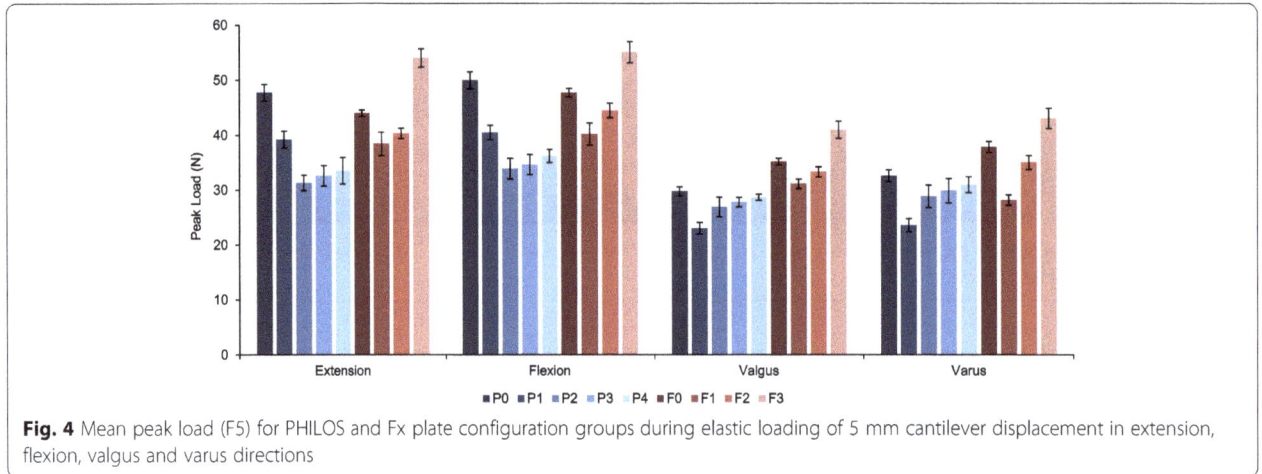

Fig. 4 Mean peak load (F5) for PHILOS and Fx plate configuration groups during elastic loading of 5 mm cantilever displacement in extension, flexion, valgus and varus directions

blade (8.1218/8.990 vs 7.734/8.248 N/mm). Swapping the blade with screws led to a statistically significant increase in extension, flexion, valgus and varus stiffness than the control group (10.915/11.127/8.245/8.663 vs 8.770/9.541/6.900/7.590 N/mm).

Results from the statistical analysis of the PHILOS configuration groups showed that there were statistically significant differences (P values less than 0.05) between stiffness and load values of all configuration group pairs, except two cases (Additional file 1 and Additional file 2). These were P3 and P4 in extension, and P2 and P3 in flexion. As for the pairwise comparison of the Fx plate configuration groups, there were statistically significant differences between peak loads and stiffness values of all configuration pairs (Additional file 3).

Plastic testing results

For both plates, the load trends recorded for the plastic tests among the configuration groups were similar to those recorded for elastic varus tests (Fig. 6). This showed that the conclusions drawn from varus elastic

test tests remained relevant even when specimens were subjected to larger displacements. There were statistically significant differences for all configuration group pairs (Additional file 4 and Additional file 5) with only one exception, which were the F_{15b} values for the F0 and F2 configuration group pair.

Discussion

The decision of how many and which screws to implant or leave out is a crucial one that is frequently made by clinicians. We believe that this decision is based on many factors including the screw's location, orientation and geometry. There is very little information in the literature on the optimal number of screws for a given fracture, with two studies recommending the insertion of at least five screws in the humeral head including at least one inferomedial screw [22, 23].

Although biomechanical models do exist for guidance on optimal selection of these factors, they are often based on simple fracture types and loadings. Thus, conclusions drawn from them are not fully applicable and

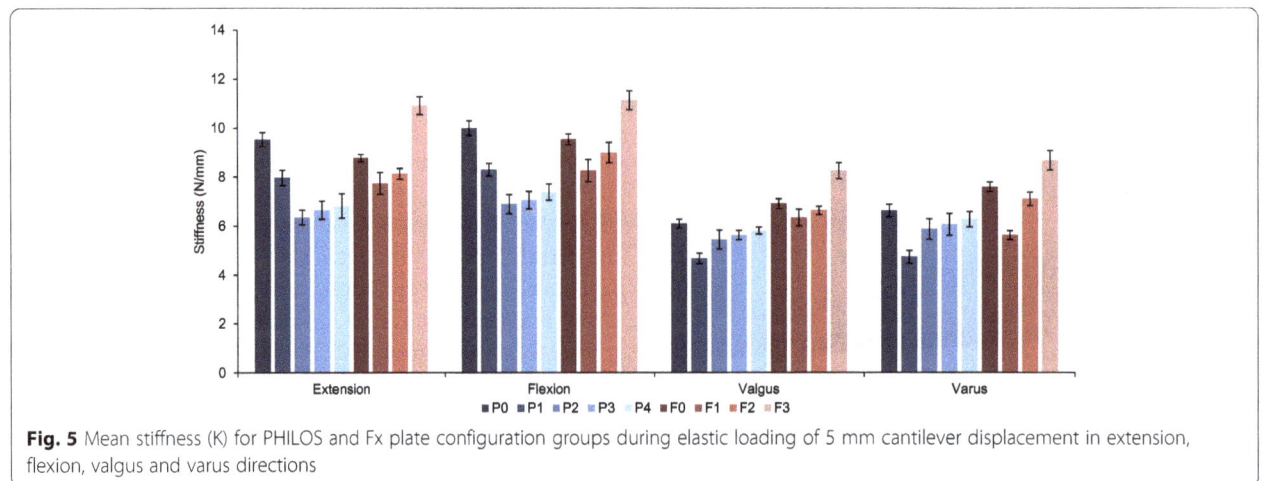

Fig. 5 Mean stiffness (K) for PHILOS and Fx plate configuration groups during elastic loading of 5 mm cantilever displacement in extension, flexion, valgus and varus directions

Table 2 Mean stiffness (K) and load values (F) for all PHILOS plate configuration groups, along extension, flexion, valgus and varus, with their respective standard deviations (S.D.). K and F5 denote stiffness and peak load values obtained during elastic tests while F15a and F15b are loads at 15 mm before and after eight-minute intermission and F30 is the load at 30 mm during plastic tests

	P0 (SD)	P1 (SD)	P2 (SD)	P3 (SD)	P4 (SD)
Extension					
K (N/mm)	9.533 (0.286)	7.956 (0.314)	6.349 (0.299)	6.644 (0.365)	6.819 (0.495)
F_5 (N)	47.749 (1.510)	39.191 (1.580)	31.295 (1.425)	32.597 (1.842)	33.501 (2.415)
Flexion					
K (N/mm)	9.997 (0.298)	8.284 (0.257)	6.887 (0.391)	7.045 (0.357)	7.377 (0.331)
F_5 (N)	49.981 (1.569)	40.475 (1.336)	33.846 (1.876)	34.601 (1.850)	36.152 (1.196)
Valgus					
K (N/mm)	6.091 (0.181)	4.671 (0.2150)	5.439 (0.386)	5.623 (0.189)	5.804 (0.140)
F_5 (N)	29.746 (0.815)	23.041 (1.065)	26.907 (1.769)	27.765 (0.852)	28.659 (0.537)
Varus					
K (N/mm)	6.609 (0.256)	4.726 (0.259)	5.867 (0.417)	6.059 (0.443)	6.268 (0.317)
F_5 (N)	32.561 (1.075)	23.601 (1.183)	28.826 (2.041)	29.862 (2.205)	30.951 (1.436)
F_{15a} (N)	75.590 (3.049)	46.636 (1.843)	53.759 (1.513)	62.235 (1.941)	65.012 (2.632)
F_{15b} (N)	71.558 (3.303)	42.376 (2.141)	50.199 (2.118)	58.432 (1.878)	62.693 (3.592)
F_{30} (N)	115.531 (6.336)	70.077 (3.446)	81.238 (3.127)	95.103 (2.901)	103.216 (5.422)

ought to be taken with caution especially with regards to treatment of complex fractures like proximal humerus fractures. Nevertheless, they are beneficial for understanding the results obtained in this study.

Effects of screw location

A commonly studied analytical model in the literature is that of the bending behaviour of two-part fracture in a cylindrical bone specimen treated with a plate [24–26]. Regarding this, Smith et al. defined the plate working length as the distance between the closest two screws on either side of the fracture gap [25]. We kept the number of shaft screws constant so the plate working length could only be changed by the filling or emptying of zones neighbouring the fracture gap.

Table 3 Mean stiffness (K) and load values (F) for all Fx plate configuration groups, along extension, flexion, valgus and varus, with their respective standard deviations (S.D.). K and F5 denote stiffness and peak load values obtained during elastic tests while F15a and F15b are loads at 15 mm before and after eight-minute intermission and F30 is the load at 30 mm during plastic tests

	F0 (SD)	F1 (SD)	F2 (SD)	F3 (SD)
Extension				
K (N/mm)	8.770 (0.156)	7.734 (0.445)	8.122 (0.220)	10.915 (0.362)
F_5 (N)	43.979 (0.596)	38.394 (2.151)	40.357 (0.927)	54.071 (1.651)
Flexion				
K (N/mm)	9.541 (0.221)	8.248 (0.454)	8.990 (0.424)	11.127 (0.385)
F_5 (N)	47.711 (0.775)	40.160 (2.033)	44.479 (1.321)	55.095 (1.922)
Valgus				
K (N/mm)	6.900 (0.200)	6.332 (0.339)	6.623 (0.170)	8.245 (0.324)
F_5 (N)	35.131 (0.617)	31.096 (0.855)	33.260 (0.919)	40.946 (1.600)
Varus				
K (N/mm)	7.590 (0.196)	5.619 (0.180)	7.094 (0.280)	8.663 (0.391)
F_5 (N)	37.792 (0.990)	28.151 (0.946)	35.001 (1.277)	43.059 (1.833)
F_{15a} (N)	84.470 (1.547)	81.472 (2.665)	73.545 (1.303)	90.735 (2.439)
F_{15b} (N)	79.304 (2.507)	78.650 (2.327)	70.296 (1.547)	87.577 (2.294)
F_{30} (N)	134.391 (3.574)	128.636 (2.339)	123.032 (6.161)	141.294 (3.487)

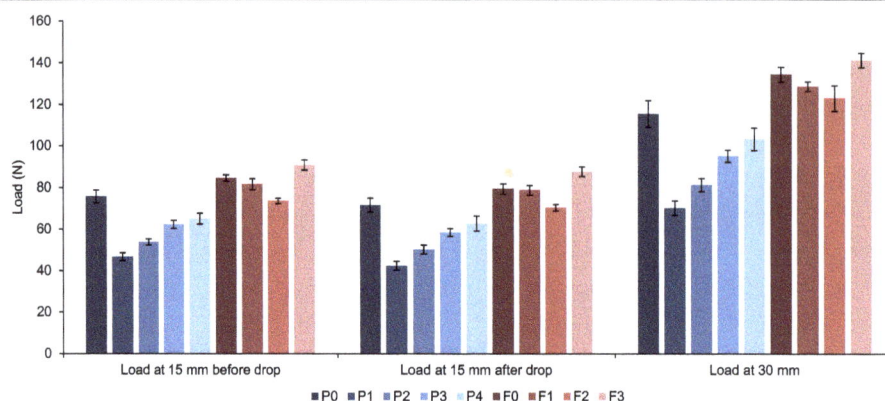

Fig. 6 Mean peak loads (F) for PHILOS and Fx plate configuration groups during plastic loading at 15 mm displacement before (F_{15a}) and after (F_{15b}) eight-minute intermission and at 30 mm displacement (F_{30})

If this length is kept too short, the overall construct stiffness is increased but so is the risk of high-stress concentration, straining and eventual failure of the plate at the section around the fracture gap [27]. These negative effects are more profound in the osteopenic bone where the bone-metal interface is weak, leading to screws cut-out, the second fracture at plate end and reduction in the micromotion needed for postoperative callus formation [28–30].

In response to this, the concept of 'semi-rigid' plates arose, where some flexibility and movement is permissible at the fracture site in order to absorb the load energy and reduce the strain at the bone-metal interface [31, 32]. However, care must be taken during fracture healing to prevent excessive movements keep the fracture fragments undisturbed and intact enough to avoid early failure [28].

This flexibility could be achieved by keeping the screws holes near fracture site empty to increase the working length and keep stress and strain low and well distributed. This comes at the expense of a reduction in overall construct stiffness and stability. For example, removing zone 1 screws in PHILOS plate increased the moment arm which reduced the cantilever load required to produce the same moment, leading to reduced stiffness. Mechanically, this is similar to the case of a cantilever beam with a concentrated load at the free end where maximum deflection of the beam has a cubic relationship with its arm length.

In our study, P2, P3 and P4 configuration groups had zone 1 screws in place, so the working length was fixed. This would imply that for a given load direction, the bending stiffness of these configurations would be same. Instead, the effect of screw removal on overall construct stiffness decreased from zone 2 to 3 and eventually zone 4. This decline at each proximal progression is possibly because leaving out zone 2 screws created a gap in the plate. Further, this omission of screws near the fracture

site affected the plate stability and construct stiffness. For P3 constructs, zone 1 and 2 screws were already present between zone 1 and the fracture gap. So, theoretically, they would exhibit higher stiffness than constructs with P2 configuration. Similarly, P4 constructs had zone 1, 2 and 3 screws in place and were stiffer than P3 constructs. Therefore, as the gap in the plate was made more proximal from the fracture gap, its influence over fracture gap stability and the construct stiffness diminished.

Based on these principles acquired from the simple analytical model, one could argue that it is the proximity of a zone to the fracture gap that dictates its importance in construct stability, as demonstrated by Stoffel et al. [27]. In varus and valgus bending, this was indeed true as the zones could be listed in the following order of reducing the effect on construct stiffness: zone 1, 2, 3 and 4.

Effects of screw orientation

In extension and flexion bending, zone 2 screws had the largest effect on construct stiffness, followed by screws of zone 3, 4 and 1. This implies that for these two directions, construct stability is controlled by other factors in addition to screw placement. The inadequacy of the aforementioned model to predict this behaviour is possibly because it does not account for complex humerus geometry and the fact that PHILOS plate allows implantation of several, multidirectional screws in each zone.

The angle between the zone's screw pairs and the plate midline seems to affect the extension and flexion bending stiffness. The near-parallel screw pairs had a lower impact on construct stability than diverging and converging screws. Zone 2 screws of PHILOS plate diverged by a relatively large angle while zone 3 screws had convergent trajectories. Zone 4 and 1 screws, on the other hand, were almost parallel to each other.

We believe that there are two main motives behind a screw orientation choice. The first is purely mechanical: to achieve enhanced stability along the load direction of interest. We observed this for extension and flexion where orienting the screws in these directions yielded higher stiffness. The second motive is biological: to connect regions of the humeral head with low bone quality to those of high bone quality such as the medial region [33, 34].

Medial support in plates, both in form of screws and blade, targets the inferomedial region. Importance of these screws for minimising humeral head collapse in varus bending is well known, but less so on that of the blade [22, 35, 36]. In a similar fashion to PHILOS plate's zone 1 screws, the importance of the blade for varus stability in the Fx plate was manifested when it was removed, causing a 26% drop in varus mean stiffness, more than any of the other three directions. However, since the bone specimen we used was made out polyurethane foam with relatively uniform density, the superior performance of medial support was not attributable to the better bone mineral density. Instead, we believe that the main factor was the proximity of the screws and blade to the fracture site. The use of synthetic bone was both an advantage and disadvantage of our study. It was an advantage in the sense that it highlighted that medial support is vital for varus stability, irrespective of local variations in bone mineral density. At the same time, it was a simplification of the in vivo scenario and thus demands future testing on cadaveric specimens.

Effects of screw geometry

Despite the significant importance of medial support over other zones, particularly in varus, a large difference was found between the medial support provided by zone 1 screws than that by the blade. Fx plate control group (F0) had superior varus and valgus stiffness values than PHILOS plate control group (P0) suggesting the advantage of using a blade. Swapping the Fx plate's blade with locking screws increased construct stiffness even further, not only in varus but also in the other three directions. This could be an issue of geometry and consequently the indirect locking mechanism of the blade. Unlike most conventional blade plates, Fx plate and its blade exist as two separate parts. In order to connect the two, the blade is placed into its slot on the plate and two grub screws are inserted on the plate, just above its blade's shoulders. This way, it is held in its place by the interference between its shoulders and the grub screws connected to the plate. There is also a geometrical mismatch between the rectangular cross-section of blade's shoulders and the circular screw holes. Loosening of the grub screws would allow the blade to toggle and slide out. On the contrary, the two inferomedial screws

do not rely on any grub screws and directly lock to the plate. In this way, they have longer effective working length and thus less toggling when subjected to bending. This issue of getting the blade, which has non-locking shoulders, to fix more rigidly to the plate should be addressed in future plate design.

The Fx plate's large central hole in zone 2 permits the insertion of a 6.5 mm locking screw. Our results showed that when compared to the blade and the inferomedial screws, this screw had less impact on construct stiffness in all four bending directions. In light of our understanding of the effect of screw's proximity to fracture gap in PHILOS plate, this is understandable since the 6.5 mm screw is more distant from the fracture than zone 1. We hypothesise that if two small screws both offset from plate midline were used instead of one large 6.5 mm screw, the bending stiffness, particularly in extension and flexion cantilever bending would be improved since the offset would increase the second moment of area. One advantage of the current large central hole is that it allows deployment of bone-void filler. Biomechanical benefits of cement augmentation have been demonstrated in several studies [37–42]. It may be useful, in future studies, to take the most stable configuration group from this study (F3), use bone cement in place of the 6.5 mm screw and investigate whether its augmentation further improves stability.

One way to modify the geometry of a screw or a blade is by changing its length. We idealised the screw purchase by keeping the screws long enough to achieve subchondral bone abutment. Due to the irregular geometry of the humeral head, screws were of varying lengths. Their possible influence on the mechanical performance of different zones can, therefore, not be ignored. Glenohumeral perforation of the screws is one of the leading complications associated with angle stable plates [14, 15, 43]. Using screws of shorter length may prevent screw perforation but can also lead to poor bone anchorage since the density of the cancellous bone in the subchondral region is relatively high [44]. As a consequence of this, the construct can lose its stability and collapse in varus.

Conclusions

Addition of medial support, both in form of screws and blade, improved mean varus bending stiffness of PHILOS and Fx plate specimens and we attribute this to their proximity to fracture gap. However, further studies on cadaveric specimens are needed to account for the effects of bone density on screw anchorage. Results showed that the type of medial support matters. In the Fx plate, the medial support provided by inferomedial screws exhibited significantly superior extension, flexion, valgus and varus bending than that by the blade.

Screw pairs placed proximal to the fracture gap played a significant role on extension and flexion bending stiffness, possibly owing to their non-parallel orientation. Hence, in appreciation of the complexity of in vivo loading of the humerus, we conclude that for general stability all four zones are critical as they have a synergistic relationship and clinical decisions ought to be made depending on the nature of the fracture being treated. The relatively low effect of the use of large 6.5 mm screw in Fx plate as compared to that of zone 2 screws on PHILOS plate demands a further mechanical investigation.

It is hoped that findings of the present study will provide valuable information to the clinicians with the decision making involved in selecting the optimal number and configuration for a given fracture case. It is also hoped that the design choices discussed in this study, especially with regards to the location, orientation and geometry of the screws and the locking mechanism of blades, will assist the design of future proximal humerus plates with enhanced mechanical and clinical performance.

Additional files

Additional file 1: Raw experimental data for calculation of mean stiffness and peak loads and for performing statistical analysis. (XLSX 73 kb)

Additional file 2: P values for elastic stiffness and peak load values of PHILOS plate configuration groups, obtained from their pairwise comparison statistical analysis (DOCX 17 kb)

Additional file 3: P values for elastic stiffness and peak load values of Fx plate configuration groups, obtained from their pairwise comparison statistical analysis. (DOCX 16 kb)

Additional file 4: Results of pairwise comparison statistical analysis: P values for plastic load at 15 mm displacement before (F_{15a}) and after (F_{15b}) eight-minute intermission and at 30 mm displacement (F_{30}), for PHILOS plate configuration groups. (DOCX 15 kb)

Additional file 5: Results of pairwise comparison statistical analysis: P values for plastic load at 15 mm displacement before (F_{15a}) and after (F_{15b}) eight-minute intermission and at 30 mm displacement (F_{30}), for Fx plate configuration groups. (DOCX 15 kb)

Funding

This research was partly supported by the projects of UK Engineering Physical Science Research Council (EP/K019759/1 and EP/I033602/1). DePuy Synthes (West Chester, PA, USA) granted funding for the purchase of the PHILOS plates used in the biomechanical tests. DePuy Synthes (West Chester, PA, USA) was not involved in the design of the study and collection, analysis, and interpretation of data and in writing the manuscript.

Authors' contributions

AJ conducted tests, performed data analysis and literature study and prepared manuscript. CP was involved in manuscript editing and discussion on the clinical aspects of the study. ZZ contributed to the design of mechanical tests. LR was the supervisor of study including mechanical testing design was involved in manuscript editing. All authors read and approved the final manuscript.

Competing interests

Dr. Chris Peach has a consultancy agreement with Exactech Inc. in relation to educational activity and not in relation to products in this article. All authors of this manuscript have no other affiliations with or involvement in any organization or entity with any financial interest (such as honoraria; educational grants; participation in speakers' bureaus; membership, employment, consultancies, stock ownership, or other equity interest; and expert testimony or patent-licensing arrangements), or non-financial interest (such as personal or professional relationships, affiliations, knowledge or beliefs) in the subject matter or materials discussed in this manuscript.

Author details

[1]School of Mechanical, Aerospace and Civil Engineering, University of Manchester, Sackville Street, Manchester M13 9PL, UK. [2]Department of Shoulder and Elbow Surgery, University Hospital of South Manchester, Southmoor Road, Wythenshawe, Manchester M23 9LT, UK.

References

1. Nayak NK, Schickendantz MS, Regan WD, Hawkins RJ. Operative Treatment of Nonunion of Surgical Neck Fractures of the Humerus. Clin Orthop Relat Res. 1995;:200–5.
2. Volgas D a, Stannard JP, Alonso JE. Nonunions of the humerus. Clin Orthop Relat Res. 2004;:46–50.
3. Lind T, Kroner K, Jensen J. The epidemiology of fractures of the proximal Humerus. Arch Orthop Trauma Surg. 1989;108:285–7.
4. Bengner U, Johnell O, Redlund-Johnell I. Changes in the incidence of fracture of the upper end of the humerus during a 30-year period. A study of 2125 fractures. Clin Orthop Relat Res. 1988;:179–82.
5. Iannotti JP, Ramsey ML, Williams GR, Warner JJ. Nonprosthetic management of proximal humeral fractures. Instr Course Lect. 2004;53:403–16.
6. Clifford PC. Fractures of the neck of the humerus: a review of the late results. Injury. 1980;12:91–5.
7. Cofield RH. Comminuted fractures of the proximal humerus. Clin Orthop Relat Res. 1988;:49–57. http://www.ncbi.nlm.nih.gov/pubmed/3284683.
8. Weinstein DM, Bratton DR, Ciccone WJ, Elias JJ. Locking plates improve torsional resistance in the stabilization of three-part proximal humeral fractures. J Shoulder Elb Surg. 2006;15:239–43.
9. Siffri PC, Peindl RD, Coley ER, Norton J, Connor PM, Kellam JE. Biomechanical analysis of blade plate versus locking plate fixation for a proximal humerus fracture: comparison using cadaveric and synthetic humeri. J Orthop Trauma. 2006;20:547–54.
10. Seide K, Triebe J, Faschingbauer M, Schulz AP, Püschel K, Mehrtens G, et al. Locked vs. unlocked plate osteosynthesis of the proximal humerus - a biomechanical study. Clin Biomech. 2007;22:176–82.
11. Lee CW, Shin SJ. Prognostic factors for unstable proximal humeral fractures treated with locking-plate fixation. J Shoulder Elb Surg. 2009;18:83–8.
12. Owsley KC, Gorczyca JT. Fracture displacement and screw cutout after open reduction and locked plate fixation of proximal humeral fractures [corrected]. J Bone Joint Surg Am. 2008;90:233–40. https://doi.org/10.2106/JBJS.F.01351.
13. Hardeman F, Bollars P, Donnelly M, Bellemans J, Nijs S. Predictive factors for functional outcome and failure in angular stable osteosynthesis of the proximal humerus. Injury. 2012;43:153–8.
14. Egol KA, Ong CC, Walsh M, Jazrawi LM, Tejwani NC, Zuckerman JD. Early complications in proximal humerus fractures (OTA types 11) treated with locked plates. J Orthop Trauma. 2008;22:159–64. https://doi.org/10.1097/BOT.0b013e318169ef2a.
15. Brunner F, Sommer C, Bahrs C, Heuwinkel R, Hafner C, Rillmann P, et al. Open reduction and internal fixation of proximal humerus fractures using a proximal humeral locked plate: a prospective multicenter analysis. J Orthop Trauma. 2009;23:163–72.
16. Clavert P, Adam P, Bevort A, Bonnomet F, Kempf JF. Pitfalls and complications with locking plate for proximal humerus fracture. J Shoulder Elb Surg. 2010;19:489–94.
17. Gardner MJ, Weil Y, Barker JU, Kelly BT, Helfet DL, Lorich DG. The importance of medial support in locked plating of proximal humerus fractures. J Orthop Trauma. 2007;21:185–91.

18. Egol KA, Sugi MT, Ong CC, Montero N, Davidovitch R, Zuckerman JD. Fracture site augmentation with calcium phosphate cement reduces screw penetration after open reduction-internal fixation of proximal humeral fractures. J Shoulder Elb Surg. 2012;21:741–8.

19. Micic ID, Kim KC, Shin DJ, Shin SJ, Kim PT, Park IH, et al. Analysis of early failure of the locking compression plate in osteoporotic proximal humerus fractures. J Orthop Sci. 2009;14:596–601.

20. Hettrich CM, Neviaser A, Beamer BS, Paul O, Helfet DL, Lorich DG. Locked plating of the proximal Humerus using an Endosteal implant. J Orthop Trauma. 2012;26:212–5.

21. Zhang L, Zheng JY, Wang WL, Lin GM, Huang YJ, Zheng J, et al. The clinical benefit of medial support screws in locking plating of proximal humerus fractures: a prospective randomized study. Int Orthop. 2011;35:1655–61.

22. Erhardt JB, Stoffel K, Kampshoff J, Badur N, Yates P, Kuster MS. The position and number of screws influence screw perforation of the humeral head in modern locking plates: a cadaver study. J Orthop Trauma. 2012;26:E188–92.

23. Cohen M, Amaral MV, Monteiro M, Brandão BL, Motta Filho GR. Osteosynthesis of proximal humeral end fractures with fixed-angle plate and locking screws: technique and results. Rev Bras Ortop. 2009;44:106–11. https://doi.org/10.1016/S2255-4971(15)30056-2.

24. Gautier E. Biomechanics of Osteosynthesis by screwed plates. In: Poitout DG, editor. Biomechanics and biomaterials in orthopedics. London: Springer London; 2016. p. 341–72. https://doi.org/10.1007/978-1-84882-664-9_29.

25. Smith WR, Ziran BH, Anglen JO, Stahel PF. Locking plates: tips and tricks. J Bone Joint Surg Am. 2007;89:2298–307. https://doi.org/10.1097/00005131-200409000-00003.

26. Ellis T, Bourgeault CA, Kyle RF. Screw position affects dynamic compression plate strain in an in vitro fracture model. J Orthop Trauma. 2001;15:333–7.

27. Stoffel K, Dieter U, Stachowiak G, Gächter A, Kuster MS. Biomechanical testing of the LCP - How can stability in locked internal fixators be controlled? Injury. 2003;34 SUPPL. 2.

28. Brunner A, Resch H, Babst R, Kathrein S, Fierlbeck J, Niederberger A, et al. The Humerusblock NG: a new concept for stabilization of proximal humeral fractures and its biomechanical evaluation. Arch Orthop Trauma Surg. 2012; 132:985–92.

29. Gardner MJ, Nork SE, Huber P, Krieg JC. Less rigid stable fracture fixation in osteoporotic bone using locked plates with near cortical slots. Injury. 2010; 41:652–6.

30. Bottlang M, Doornink J, Byrd GD, Fitzpatrick DC, Madey SM. A nonlocking end screw can decrease fracture risk caused by locked plating in the osteoporotic diaphysis. J Bone Joint Surg Am. 2009;91:620–7. https://doi.org/10.2106/JBJS.H.00408.

31. Kralinger F, Gschwentner M, Wambacher M, Smekal V, Haid C. Proximal humeral fractures: what is semi-rigid? Biomechanical properties of semi-rigid implants, a biomechanical cadaver based evaluation. Arch Orthop Trauma Surg. 2008;28:205–10.

32. Sinha S, Kelly CP. Controversial topics in surgery. Ann R Coll Surg Engl. 2010; 92:631–4.

33. Hepp P, Lill H, Bail H, Korner J, Niederhagen M, Haas NP, et al. Where should implants be anchored in the humeral head? Clin Orthop Relat Res. 2003;: 139–47. doi:https://doi.org/10.1097/01.blo.0000092968.12414.a8.

34. Tingart MJ, Lehtinen J, Zurakowski D, Warner JJP, Apreleva M. Proximal humeral fractures: regional differences in bone mineral density of the humeral head affect the fixation strength of cancellous screws. J Shoulder Elb Surg. 2006;15:620–4.

35. Lescheid J, Zdero R, Shah S, Kuzyk PRT, Schemitsch EH. The biomechanics of locked plating for repairing proximal Humerus fractures with or without medial cortical support. J Trauma-Injury Infect Crit Care. 2010;69:1235–42.

36. Zhang W, Zeng LQ, Liu YJ, Pan Y, Zhang W, Zhang CQ, et al. The mechanical benefit of medial support screws in locking plating of proximal Humerus fractures. PLoS One. 2014;9

37. Gradl G, Knobe M, Stoffel M, Prescher A, Dirrichs T, Pape HC. Biomechanical evaluation of locking plate fixation of proximal humeral fractures augmented with calcium phosphate cement. J Orthop Trauma. 2013;27: 399–404.

38. Kwon BK, Goertzen DJ, O'Brien PJ, Broekhuyse HM, Oxland TR. Biomechanical evaluation of proximal humeral fracture fixation supplemented with calcium phosphate cement. J Bone Joint Surg Am. 2002;84A:951–61.

39. Kathrein S, Kralinger F, Blauth M, Schmoelz W. Biomechanical comparison of an angular stable plate with augmented and non-augmented screws in a newly developed shoulder test bench. Clin Biomech. 2013;28:273–7.

40. Schliemann B, Seifert R, Rosslenbroich SB, Theisen C, Wahnert D, Raschke MJ, et al. Screw augmentation reduces motion at the bone-implant interface: a biomechanical study of locking plate fixation of proximal humeral fractures. J Shoulder Elb Surg. 2015;24:1968–73.

41. Unger S, Erhart S, Kralinger F, Blauth M, Schmoelz W. The effect of in situ augmentation on implant anchorage in proximal humeral head fractures. Inj J Care Inj. 2012;43:1759–63.

42. Roderer G, Scola A, Schmolz W, Gebhard F, Windolf M, Hofmann-Fliri L. Biomechanical in vitro assessment of screw augmentation in locked plating of proximal humerus fractures. Inj J Care Inj. 2013;44:1327–32.

43. Olerud P, Ahrengart L, Ponzer S, Saving J, Tidermark J. Internal fixation versus nonoperative treatment of displaced 3-part proximal humeral fractures in elderly patients: a randomized controlled trial. J Shoulder Elb Surg. 2011;20:747–55. https://doi.org/10.1016/j.jse.2010.12.018.

44. Frich LH, Jensen NC. Bone properties of the humeral head and resistance to screw cutout. Int J Shoulder Surg. 2014;8:21–6. https://doi.org/10.4103/0973-6042.131851.

15

The impact of capsular repair on the risk for dislocation after revision total hip arthroplasty – a retrospective cohort-study of 259 cases

Julia Jurkutat[1,3†], Dirk Zajonz[1,3†], Gerald Sommer[1,3], Stefan Schleifenbaum[1,3], Robert Möbius[3,5], Ronny Grunert[1,3,6], Niels Hammer[4] and Torsten Prietzel[2,3*] (iD)

Abstract

Background: Dislocation following total hip arthroplasty has to date not been resolved satisfactorily. Previous work has shown that using a less-invasive adaption of Bauer's lateral transgluteal approach with capsular repair significantly reduces dislocation rates in primary total hip arthroplasty. The aim of this retrospective cohort study was to assess whether this approach also helps to reduce the dislocation rate in revision total hip arthroplasty.

Methods: We analyzed revision total hip arthroplasty cases performed between 10/2005 and 12/2013 in our department, classifying capsular repair cases as study group and capsular resection cases as control group. The WOMAC score, the dislocations and the revisions were observed.

Results: A total of 259 cases were included, 100 in the study group and 159 in the control group. In the 12-month follow-up, dislocation rates were significantly lower in the study group (3%, $n = 3$) compared to the control group (21.4%, $n = 34$; $p = 0.001$). Overall follow-up periods were 49 and 79 months, revision frequencies were 10 and 29%, pain improvements were 5.5 compared to 4.4 and the WOMAC global scores averaged 2.0 ± 2.1 and 2.9 ± 2.6 for the study group and the control group, respectively.

Conclusion: The modified, less-invasive, lateral transgluteal approach with capsular repair was accompanied by an 86% reduction in dislocation rates when compared to the conventional technique with capsular resection via the anterolateral Watson-Jones-approach. Capsular repair is possible in about 60% of the revision total hip arthroplasty cases, may be considered as beneficial to avoid dislocation and can therefore be recommended.

Keywords: Capsular repair, Dislocation, Revision, THA

Background

Total hip arthroplasty (THA) is among the most frequently performed surgical procedures in the industrial world and was titled the operation of the twentieth century [1], providing a leap in patient satisfaction and quality of life in relation to hip-arthritis.

Nevertheless, THA dislocation remains a feared incident, representing the second leading complication and cause of revision surgery following aseptic THA loosening [2–5]. It even predominates in the early postoperative period – a devastating experience for both the affected patient and the responsible surgeon.

The risk of THA dislocation is usually reported to be between 7.5 and 14.4% after Revision THA (R-THA) - two to three times as high as after primary THA [6–9]. In reality, the dislocation rate is likely to be even higher, as not all dislocations can be recorded [10]. Thus, THA dislocation remains an ongoing problem that has yet to be solved.

* Correspondence: torsten.prietzel@helios-gesundheit.de
†Julia Jurkutat and Dirk Zajonz contributed equally to this work.
²Department of Orthopaedics and Trauma Surgery, HELIOS Clinic Blankenhain, Wirthstrasse 5, D-99444 Blankenhain, Germany
³ZESBO – Zentrum zur Erforschung der Stütz- und BewegungsOrgane, Semmelweisstrasse 14, D-04103, Leipzig, Germany
Full list of author information is available at the end of the article

Avoidance of capsular resection was already recommended in the early days of THA [11, 12]. Nevertheless, quite a few surgeons routinely excised it during R-THA. Current literature suggests that capsular repair [13, 14] and the use of larger prosthetic heads [15, 16] decrease the risk of THA dislocation.

To date, few studies exist on the benefits or disadvantages of capsular repair in R-THA [7, 17, 18] via the posterolateral approach.

Aiming at reduced dislocation rates, a less-invasive adaption of Bauer's lateral transgluteal approach was developed and deployed. In addition to the typical partial detachment and reconstruction of the ventral part of the iliotrochanteric muscles this procedure was focused on capsular repair, preserving the acetabular origin of the hip joint capsule. This modified technique has been shown to reduce dislocation rates by 88% in primary THA [13]. Since 10/2005 the technique has also been used in R-THA.

The aim of this study was to retrospectively analyze if this modified capsule-preserving technique could likewise reduce the dislocation rate after R-THA. We also wanted to determine whether this technique had adverse effects on the Western Ontario and McMaster Universities Osteoarthritis Index (WOMAC) score and pain scale change, clinical outcomes or subsequent revisions.

Methods

For decades, the conventional R-THA surgery with capsular resection has been successfully carried out in our department. In 2002, a modified, less invasive surgical technique with capsular repair was additionally introduced, based on the lateral transgluteal (Bauer) approach. Therefore, all R-THA cases treated in our Department in the timeframe between 10/2005 and 12/2013 were

identified via German Procedure Classification code 5–821 ('revision, exchange and removal of hip prosthesis', German modification of International Classification of Procedures in Medicine), included and retrospectively analyzed after approval of the study by the ethics committee of the University of Leipzig (044/14032016).

R-THA was defined as a surgical procedure involving an exchange of the acetabular component and/or liner, femoral stem and/or modular head, or any combination thereof.

Patients with dual-mobility cups, periprosthetic femur fracture, proximal femur replacement, periprosthetic joint infection, severe periarticular destruction, tumour disease or recent THA procedures (in the last 3 months) were excluded. The last exclusion criterion was used because of the assumption that the scarred regeneration of a neo-capsule takes at least 3 months [19]. Capsular repair cases were gathered in the study group (SG), capsular resection cases in the control group (CG) (see flow chart Fig. 1). One of the surgeons always aimed for a capsular repair, with the final decision taken during the operation, depending on whether it was feasible. The other surgeons involved routinely resected the capsule. Whether a capsular repair was sought or not was dependent on the scheduled surgeon and thus random. However, in terms of feasibility, selection bias is not completely excluded because the non-reparability of the capsule was most often caused by severe periarticular destruction.

Further patient-related data were taken from the anaesthesia records. A written consent declaration and a questionnaire were both sent to every patient. The latter was focused on the acquisition of the WOMAC score [20], the pre-operative and postoperative elevation of pain scale (retrospectively collected at the time of survey), the detection of dislocation incidents and further

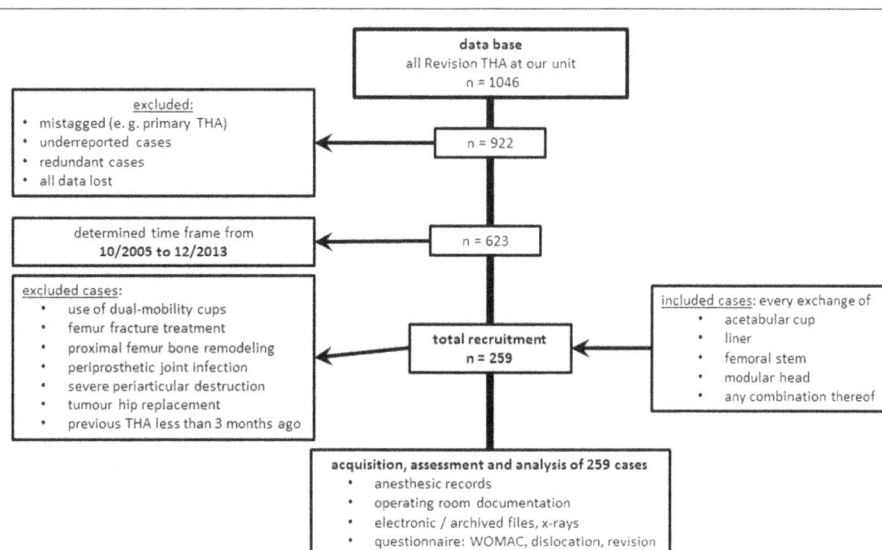

Fig. 1 Flow chart: Selection of cases

revision surgery. All non-responders were additionally contacted via telephone. In cases where the patients themselves were unable to give information (e.g. deceased patients), close relatives (spouse, partner, siblings, children) were asked to answer the key questions of dislocation and revision surgeries. Moreover, all available documentation and clinical imaging data were reviewed for potential dislocation incidents and revision surgery. A dislocation was considered if confirmed by X-ray or documented by a medical specialist. The date of the first dislocation was recorded to calculate dislocation rates in the 6-months and the 12-months follow-up. The appropriate medical case files were requested in cases where a closed reduction or revision surgery was performed elsewhere. The target variables were postoperative dislocation rates in the 12-months follow-up and total revision rates. If a revision occurred within 6 months after a dislocation of the same hip joint, it was rated as 're-revision due to dislocation'. Furthermore, the cutting-to-suture time, the postoperative hospital stay time as well as a pain scale and WOMAC indices were determined as secondary parameters.

In the timeframe between 10/2005 and 12/2013 623 R-THA-cases were treated in our department. Two hundred fifty-nine of this met the inclusion criteria and did not fulfil the exclusion criteria of this study. One hundred R-THA-cases were treated in the less-invasive capsule preserving technique via Bauer's lateral approach [21] and thus included in the SG. One hundred fifty-nine R-THA-cases were treated in the conventional technique with capsular resection via the anterolateral Watson-Jones-approach [22] and thus included in the CG.

Less-invasive surgical technique in R-THA including capsular repair

The modified technique was based on Bauer's lateral transgluteal approach [21], which is characterised by a lateral longitudinal skin incision and the detachment of the ventral part of the muscles, which attaches or originates ventrally to the greater trochanter. Connective tissues in

the plane of the hip joint capsule are incised in an inverted T-shape manner, preserving its acetabular origin completely [13]. In most cases the capsule was additionally incised cranially longitudinally, forming a U-flap of its ventrocranial section. In a few cases the removal of the internal layer of the capsule was necessary, while the outer layer was preserved. After the implantation and reduction of the prosthesis, both longitudinal capsular incisions (ventral and cranial) were closed by sutures (Fig. 2), while the transverse incision near the femoral neck base remained unclosed and served for insertion of a Redon drain [13]. After reconstruction of the muscles, the fascia and the subcutaneous layer the skin was routinely closed by a resorbable intracutaneous suture, so that no removal of suture material was necessary.

Conventional surgical technique in R-THA including capsular resection

The technique was based on the anterolateral approach (Watson-Jones-approach [22]).

The skin incision is slightly curved from distal-lateral to proximal-ventral. After the incision of the Tractus iliotibialis, the Musculus gluteus medius and minimus were incised near their attachment to the great trochanter and transverse to the direction of the muscle fibres. The connective tissues in the plane of the hip joint capsule were excised as completely as possible. Following the implantation and reduction of the prosthesis, a Redon drain was inserted and the muscles, the fascia and the subcutaneous layer were reconstructed. Finally, the skin was closed with clips that were removed after 10 days.

Statistics

Statistical analysis was carried out using EXCEL 2007 (Microsoft Corporation, Redmond, WA, USA) and SPSS STATISTICS version 23 (2015, IBM - International Business Machines Corporation, Armonk, NY, USA). The SG and the CG were compared with regards to epidemiological, implant-associated and surgery-specific data. Statistical evaluations were performed using

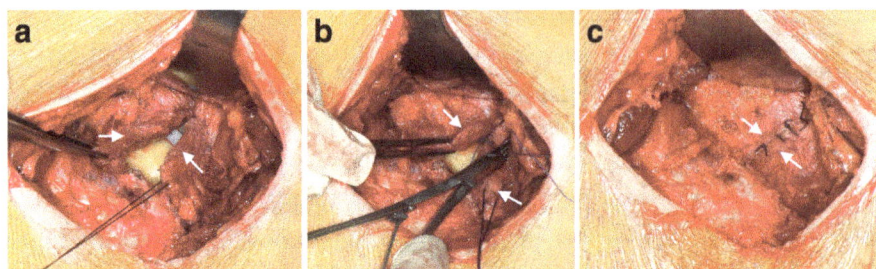

Fig. 2 Surgical technique of capsular repair (left hip joint): **a** Both capsular flaps (arrows) are neared by, **b** The ventral longitudinal incision is closed by suture, **c** Capsular repair is finished

independent Student's t-test, chi-square-test and Cox regression analysis. p-values of 0.05 or less were considered statistically significant, *p*-values of 0.01 or less were considered highly statistically significant.

Results

Patient cohort

Two hundred fifty-nine cases were included: 100 were identified retrospectively as belonging to the SG and 159 as belonging to the CG. The collected data and results comparing both groups are shown in Tables 1, 2, 3 and 4. One patient of CG (0.6%) died 11 months after surgery. A total of 45 patients (17%) passed away in the overall follow-up. The notes of the deceased were examined. In total 16 other patients were lost in the follow-up.

Thus, follow-up rate was 198 out of 259 (76%). The mean overall follow-up times were 49 months and 79 months ($p < 0.001$) for the SG and CG, respectively, with at least 12 months in all cases except one.

With respect to the epidemiological data there were no significant differences except for the co-existing morbidities classified according to the American Society of Anesthesiologists Physical Status Classification System (ASA) and the number of previous revisions (Table 1).

Both groups were similar and statistically non-different regarding the indication for surgery, which was limited to aseptic loosening, wear of liner and recurrent dislocation by the case selection criteria (see flow chart Fig. 1). The indications and surgical procedures were discussed and defined in our clinic-internal indication board. All treatments are based on the evaluated standard operating procedures (SOP) of our clinic.

Implant-related comparison

Differences in surgery- and implant-related data between the two groups were partly significant and are listed in Table 2. In the SG, the fixation technique used for most prostheses was cemented (35%), followed by hybrid (20%) and uncemented (19%). The larger part of the CG prostheses was implanted uncemented (48.5%), followed by cemented (15%).

The average number of the exchanged femoral stems was 14% in the SG and 24% in CG, whilst acetabular cups were exchanged at a rate of 25% in the SG and 12% in the CG. In summary, there were no significant differences between the two groups regarding the components exchanged during R-THA.

Mean femoral-head-size and acetabular-cup-size were similar in both groups (Table 2). The mean

Table 1 Epidemiologic Data

		Study group	Control group	p-value
Number of included cases		100	159	
Number of answered questionnaires		86 (86%)	112 (70%)	
Number of deceased patients		10 (10%)	35 (22%)	
Mean follow-up time		49 months min: 16 max: 90	79 months min: 23 max: 120	
Mean age at surgery		69.6 years min: 41 max: 87	68.5 years min: 23 max: 92	0.386
Mean body mass index (BMI)		28.3 min: 15.9 max: 42.5	28.6 min: 18.5 max: 63.8	0.726
ASA-classification	mean	2.4	2.5	0.011
	1	4%	Ø	
	2	56%	48%	
	3	40%	52%	
Gender male (♂) / female (♀)		♂ 41 (41%) ♀ 59 (59%)	♂ 57 (36%) ♀ 102 (64%)	
Side of procedure right (R) / left (L)		R 52 (52%) L 48 (48%)	R 84 (53%) L 75 (47%)	0.899
Number of previous revisions				0.015
none		93%	78%	
1		6%	17%	
≥ 2		1%	5%	

Table 2 Surgery- and Implant-Related Data

	Study group	Control group	p-value
Number of involved surgeons	1	7	
Mean experience of the surgeon in the field of orthopaedics at the time of surgery	17.2 ± 2.0 years	21.8 ± 7.7 years	
Mean acetabular cup size	56.6 mm min: 48 mm max: 68 mm	57.7 mm min: 48 mm max: 70 mm	0.085
Mean femoral head size	32.9 mm	32.7 mm	0.580
28 mm	14%	7%	
32 mm	50%	72%	
36 mm	36%	19%	
40 mm	Ø	Ø	
44 mm	Ø	1%	
48 mm	Ø	1%	
Mean femoral head size of dislocated cases	32.0 mm ($n = 3$)	33.0 mm ($n = 34$)	
Fixation:			0.001
Uncemented	19%	48.5%	
Hybrid (cemented stem)	20%	13%	
Inversed hybrid (cemented cup)	4%	2%	
Cemented	35%	15%	
No fixation (exchange of head or liner)	22%	21.5%	
Exchange of following components:			0.011
Femoral head and / or acetabular liner	22%	21%	
Acetabular cup	12%	25%	
Femoral stem	24%	14%	
Both cup and stem replacement	42%	40%	
Mean cutting-to-suture time	157 min min: 75 min max: 293 min	172 min min: 54 min max: 439 min	0.042
Mean period of post-operative hospitalization	9 d min: 5 d max: 19 d	17 d min: 6 d max: 83 d	0.001

head diameter of the dislocated cases was even 1 mm larger in the CG than in the SG (Table 2), which should actually result in a reduced dislocation risk in the CG. A higher dislocation tendency in the CG due to different head sizes is thereby excluded. The cutting-to-suture time was approximately 15 min longer in the CG ($p = 0.042$).

Comparison of postoperative parameters

The postoperative hospitalisation period was about 8 days longer in the CG than in the SG with 17 (range 6–83) vs. 9 (range 5–19) days, respectively ($p < 0.001$).

In the SG, the number of patients affected by dislocations was 3% (3/100) after 6 and 12 months compared to 19.5% (31/159) after 6 months and 21.5% (34/158)

Table 3 Results in the 12-months follow-up

	Study group	Control group	p-value
Dislocation after R-THA 12-months follow-up	**3% ($n = 3$)**	**21.5% ($n = 34$)**	0.001
Dislocation after R-THA 6 months follow-up	**3% ($n = 3$)**	**19.5% ($n = 31$)**	0.001
Number of dislocations 12 months follow-up			
1	2%	8%	
2	1%	5%	
≥ 3	Ø	8%	

Table 4 Results in the overall follow-up

	Study group	Control group	p-value
Mean overall follow-up time	49 months min: 16 max: 90	79 months min: 23 max: 120	
Cases with re-revision	10% ($n = 10$)	29% ($n = 46$)	
Revision due to dislocation	Ø ($n = 0$)	11% ($n = 17$)	
Time to re-revision			
Within 3 months	1%	16%	
Within 3 to 6 months	2%	2%	
More than 6 months	7%	11%	
Rate of revision surgeries			
1	9%	23%	
2	Ø	4%	
≥ 3	1%	2%	
Average pre-operative pain score	7.38	7.22	
Average post-operative pain score	1.91	2.83	
Difference of post–/pre-op. pain score	- 5.48	- 4.41	
Mean WOMAC			
Pain	1.47	2.32	
Stiffness	1.88	2.69	
Physical function	2.66	3.76	
Total score	2.00	2.92	

after 12 months in the CG, respectively ($p < 0.001$, Table 3). Because data evaluation for dislocation was restricted to the 12-months follow-up in this study, five late first-dislocation-cases (all from the CG, first dislocation occurred > 12 months after surgery) were considered "not dislocated" in order to keep the follow-up consistent for both groups. Thirty of totally 42 patients (71%) with one or more dislocations had their first dislocation incident within the first 3 months after R-THA surgery. After that period, the risk of dislocation was markedly reduced (see Fig. 3).

In the CG, 17 of 46 postoperative revisions (37%) were due to dislocation. Likewise, 17 of 39 dislocations in the CG (44%) caused surgical re-intervention within 6 months. Additionally, more than half of all patients (24/42; 57%) suffered multiple episodes of dislocations.

In terms of pain assessment, the average pain reduction postoperatively was lower in the CG with 4.41 in comparison to the SG with 5.48 (Table 4).

Moreover, all the WOMAC scores concerning pain, stiffness, physical function and global score, were better in the SG (Table 4).

Cox regression analysis

The results of Cox regression analysis, adjusted for the overall follow-up (Table 1), are given in Table 5. Taking into account the influencing factors capsular repair vs. resection, BMI, ASA, head size and fixation technique different hazard ratios could be determined. Taking capsular resection into account as an isolated factor, we have determined a hazard ratio of 4.1 compared to capsular repair (Table 5). When rating the Cox regression analysis, the small number of included dislocation events ($n = 32$) must be taken into account.

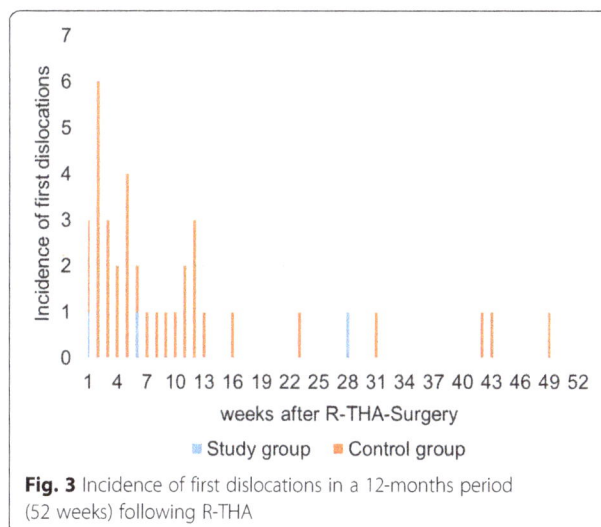

Fig. 3 Incidence of first dislocations in a 12-months period (52 weeks) following R-THA

Table 5 Cox regression analysis of major factors influencing dislocation and with isolated consideration of the factor capsular resection vs. repair (each adjusted for the follow-up, n = 32 events, 12.4% of the entire sample)

	Hazard Ratio	Confidence Interval	
		Lower	Upper
Major factors			
Capsular resection vs. repair	3.8	0.9	16.5
BMI	1.0	0.9	1.0
ASA	2.5	1.1	5.3
Head size	1.2	1.0	1.3
Fixation	1.1	1.0	1.5
Isolated factor capsular treatment			
Capsular resection vs. repair	4.1	0.9	17.8

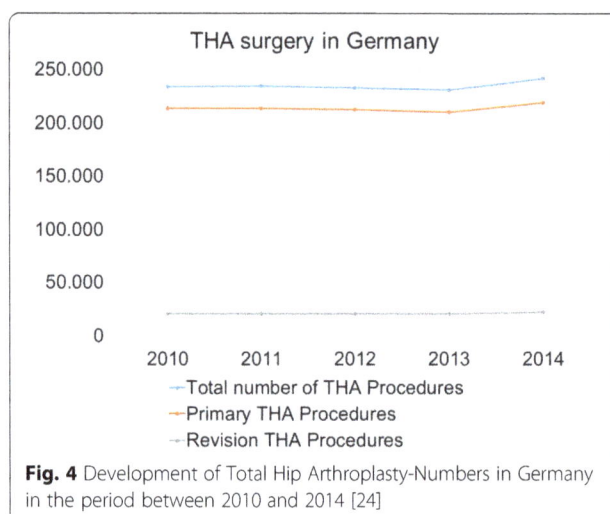

Fig. 4 Development of Total Hip Arthroplasty-Numbers in Germany in the period between 2010 and 2014 [24]

Discussion

Application of the less-invasive modification of Bauer's lateral transgluteal approach including capsular repair for R-THA lead to markedly reduced dislocation rates compared to the standard approach with capsular resection, indicated by 3% vs. 21% dislocation rates in a 12-months follow-up, respectively. Thus, according to these preliminary results, an estimated reduction of hip dislocations around 86% can be achieved if capsular repair is applied in combination with Bauer's lateral transgluteal approach in R-THA in contrast to the conventional technique with capsular resection via the anterolateral Watson-Jones-approach, similar to our findings in primary THA [13].

Dislocation is considered the second most common complication of THA and the second most common reason for R-THA [2–5] after aseptic loosening. In some studies, dislocation is even the leading cause for R-THA [23]. Dislocation rates ranging from 5 to 20% after R-THA [6, 7, 9]. A population-based study reported a dislocation rate of 14.4% in 12,956 cases of R-THA [8].

In Germany alone, the total number of annual THA procedures was larger than 240,000 in 2014 [24]. Surgeons are therefore faced with a considerable number of THA dislocations, accounting for thousands of cases despite relatively low dislocation rates. Growing numbers can be expected because of demographic change. The total number of THA procedures performed in Germany increased from 234,349 in 2010 to 241,673 in 2014 (increase of 3.1%) [24], whereas the number of R-THA increased from 20,652 in 2010 to 22,348 in 2014 and thus from an 8.8% (2010) to a 9.2% (2014) proportion of all THA procedures (Fig. 4). These data are in line with the Swedish register, showing a rise from 1426 R-THA performed in 2002 to 2283 in 2012, which means an increment of about 60% [2, 25]. It can be

assumed that the number of patients with osteoarthritis of the hip increases with higher life expectancy. This will lead to a rise in THA and R-THA procedures with their accompanying dislocation incidents. There are many patients suffering from recurrent instability and requiring further surgical intervention [26]. In addition to the medical importance of THA dislocation, the economic impact is similarly significant [27]. The combination of these factors indicates a need for the reduction of dislocation incidents.

Risk factors for THA dislocation

The causes of THA dislocation are variable and multi factorial, including patient-related factors (age, sex, indication, co-morbidities, lack of compliance), surgery-related factors (implant misalignment, surgical approach, soft tissue handling, experience of the surgeon), and implant-related factors (head diameter, design of the liner, head-neck-ratio) [28–30]. The most important factors listed here:

First, a correct cup position and orientation in the "safe zone" [31] or "landing zone" [32] is a prerequisite for avoiding impingement and dislocations.
Second, the posterolateral approach is associated with a significantly higher risk of dislocation [9].
Third, the use of larger (≥ 36 mm) or functionally larger head (bi- or tripolar hip endoprostheses) considerably decreases the dislocation rate after primary THA [15, 16, 33, 34] and R-THA [33, 34]. Forth, there is growing evidence that preserving and reconstructing the hip joint capsule may significantly lower the dislocation rates following primary THA [13, 14, 28, 35, 36] as well as R-THA [7, 17, 18].

A combination of capsular repair and using a larger head size may restore physical joint stability on a larger scale, provided by the permanent hip-stabilizing effects of atmospheric pressure, which continuously acts on the cross-sectional area of the prosthetic head, if the joint is hermetically sealed by either the hip capsule or connective tissues in the plane of the hip joint capsule [13, 35, 37–39].

Effects of capsular repair

The effects of capsular repair on dislocation rates after primary THA are reported in the literature. Some authors, analysing published reports on the effects of capsular repair on dislocation rates, found dislocation rates of 0% vs. 4% ($n = 790$) and 0.8% vs. 6.2% ($n = 284$) if capsular repair was performed instead of capsular resection [36]. Other studies reported about dislocation rates of 0.6% vs. 2.8% ($n = 1000$) [28] and of 0.7% vs. 4.8% ($n = 1515$) [40] if capsular repair was performed instead of capsular resection.

Other than these reports on capsular repair in primary THA, few studies can be found regarding capsular repair in combination with the posterolateral approach in R-THA. One of the aforementioned studies reported a dislocation rate of 2.5%, which was considerably lower than other reports in the literature [18]. One study including 47 R-THA cases with capsular reconstruction reported no dislocations [17]. Another group compared a capsular repair technique using 32-mm-heads ($n = 110$) with a capsular resection technique using 28-mm heads and found a reduced dislocation rate of 2.7% vs. 10.6% [7].

This study is the first to report on the decrease of dislocation rate following R-THA via Bauer's lateral transgluteal approach. The resulting 12-months dislocation rate of 3% in the study group is relatively low and comparable to a reported rate of 2.7% using a similar capsular repair technique via posterolateral approach [7]. The 12-months dislocation rate of 21.4% in our CG appears to be relatively high compared to dislocation rates of 5 to 20% reported in the literature [25, 26]. Equally, the 6-months dislocation rates of 19.5% in the CG appeared to be higher than the 14.4%, reported in another large population-based study [8]. In our series in total 14% of all R-THA patients suffered from dislocation, which is comparable to the aforementioned studies [8, 25, 26]. Most important is the 86% reduction in dislocations after R-THA in our SG relative to the CG. The follow-up of at least 16 months and response rates of 70% underline the power of our results, since the vast majority of dislocation incidents occur in the first 6 weeks and almost all dislocations in the first 12 months after surgery [13]. Furthermore, all other complications also occur predominantly in the first 6 months after surgery [26]. These early complications accounted for more than 70% of all complications in our study.

Postoperative hospital stay time was almost halved in the SG compared to the CG. In the study period, patients were only discharged after complete removal of suture material and with non-secreting dry wounds. Due to the routinely used resorbable intracutaneous suture in the SG, there was no suture removal required. Thus, SG patients could be discharged earlier and had a shorter postoperative hospital stay time. Furthermore, there were more revisions with cup exchange (isolated cup or complete THA-exchange) in the CG. This is probably responsible for the slightly longer operation time in the CG compared to the SG with more exchanges of head and liner or stem. The difference in the ASA classification was significant and less favorable for the CG. The huge discrepancies in the dislocation rates, however, could not be plausibly explained by this nonspecific factor. The small difference in BMI between the two groups has no practical relevance (Table 1). According to the WOMAC scores, the clinical outcomes of pain, stiffness, physical function and global outcome were worse in the CG. Furthermore, patients in the CG were faced with an increased risk of surgical re-intervention, considering revision rates of 29% within 79 months in the CG and 10% within 49 months in the SG. Epidemiological- and implant-related factors of this study cannot explain the resulting differences in dislocations between the SG and CG. The results of this study underline that capsular preservation and repair is of crucial importance to avoid early dislocations and subsequent revisions after R-THA-procedures.

Some authors supported this theory by pointing out that the highest risk for dislocation occurs immediately after surgery before any pseudo-capsule has reformed in patients with previous capsular resection [38]. Beyond that, another study demonstrated that a repaired posterior capsule remained intact in 90% of patients at 3-months follow-up [19]. This is in line with the higher rate of early dislocations in the CG-series of this study (Fig. 3) as well as in the capsular resection group of our previous study, analysing primary THA cases [13]. Both results can likely be explained by the absence of a hip capsule or scar tissue within the first 3 months following the R-THA or THA procedure in both capsular resection groups before a scarred capsule is formed.

Preservation and repair of the capsule, supported by the use of larger prosthetic heads if possible, helps to re-establish more of the pre-existing protection against dislocation, which is physiologically provided by the permanent hip stabilising effect of atmospheric pressure [38]. This mechanism seems to be one of the main factors, maybe even the leading factor, in the avoidance of THA dislocation [13, 35, 37–39]. This phenomenon has been described in detail by Prietzel et al. [35, 38]. A shorter postoperative hospitalization period demonstrates that the application of the modified, less-invasive, capsule preserving R-THA technique is accompanied by further medical and economic benefits.

Limitations

It was impossible to measure the acetabular inclination and anteversion angles in this study. However, a significant influence on the outcome is unlikely because senior surgeons with greater professional experience (Table 2) performed the R-THA-procedures in the CG.

The low number of patients included, the fact, that only one surgeon aimed at capsular repair (surgeons coincidentally assigned to the operation), the intraoperative decision-making about feasibility of capsular repair (possible selection bias), the differences in the overall follow-up periods, in the ASA classification and the number of previous revisions in both groups as well as a response rate of 70% were limitations of this study. Interpretability of Cox regression analysis was limited by the small number of dislocation events, especially in the study group with capsular repair ($n = 3$), in addition to the number of influencing factors investigated in the given study. As a further technical limitation, capsular reconstruction is impossible in about 40% of the R-THA-cases.

Conclusion

In this retrospective analysis of R-THA-procedures we found a significant reduction of cases affected by dislocations in the 12-months follow-up (minus 86%), when the modified less-invasive and capsule repairing technique via Bauer's lateral transgluteal approach was used instead of the conventional technique with capsular resection via the anterolateral approach. These results supplement and extend the existing literature's findings on capsular repair in R-THA using the posterolateral approach [7, 17, 18] and on capsular repair in primary THA [13, 14, 28, 36, 40].

With a lower re-revision rate and improved WOMAC scores, there was no evidence of the often postulated but to our knowledge not demonstrated disadvantages of capsular repair such as "capsular pain" or limited range of motion. As further advantages of the less invasive technique as a combination of capsular repair and resorbable intracutaneous suture, we found a significantly shorter postoperative hospitalisation period and even a shorter cutting-to-suture time. According to our experience, the less-invasive technique can be applied to approximately 60% of all R-THA cases.

Considering these medical and economic benefits, the modified, less-invasive capsular repairing approach in R-THA may be beneficial and can therefore be recommended.

Acknowledgements
The authors would like to thank Markus Seidel (Westsächsische Hochschule Zwickau, Fakultät Physikalische Technik/Informatik, PSF 201037, D-08012 Zwickau, Germany) for checking the statistics, Tamara Hildebrand for editing the questionnaires, Angela Steller for their help with the pictures and Aqeeda Singh for proofreading the paper as a native speaker.

Funding
This research study was not funded.

Authors' contributions
TP, RG and NH designed and supervised this study. JJ, GS, SS, RM, DZ and TP performed data collection and analysis. All authors have read and approved the manuscript. All authors agreed to authorship for this manuscript and gave their consent for publication. We confirm that all authors have the appropriate permissions and rights to the reported data.

Competing interests
The authors declare that they have no competing interests related to this study.

Author details
[1]Department of Orthopaedics, Trauma and Plastic Surgery, University Hospital Leipzig, Liebigstrasse 20, D-04103 Leipzig, Germany. [2]Department of Orthopaedics and Trauma Surgery, HELIOS Clinic Blankenhain, Wirthstrasse 5, D-99444 Blankenhain, Germany. [3]ZESBO – Zentrum zur Erforschung der Stütz- und BewegungsOrgane, Semmelweisstrasse 14, D-04103, Leipzig, Germany. [4]Department of Anatomy, University of Otago, Lindo Ferguson Building, 270 Great King St, Dunedin 9016, New Zealand. [5]Department of Anatomy, University of Leipzig, Semmelweisstraße 14, D-04103 Leipzig, Germany. [6]Fraunhofer Institute for Machine Tools and Forming Technology, 44, Nöthnitzer Straße, D-01187 Dresden, Germany.

References
1. Learmonth ID, Young C, Rorabeck C. The operation of the century: Total hip replacement. Lancet. 2007;370:1508–19. https://doi.org/10.1016/S0140-6736(07)60457-7.
2. Malchau H, Herberts P, Eisler T, Garellick G, Soderman P. The Swedish Total hip replacement register. J Bone Joint Surg Am. 2002;84-A(Suppl 2):2–20. https://doi.org/10.2106/00004623-200200002-00002.
3. Springer BD, Fehring TK, Griffin WL, Odum SM, Masonis JL. Why revision total hip arthroplasty fails. Clin Orthop Relat Res. 2009;467:166–73. https://doi.org/10.1007/s11999-008-0566-z.
4. Sadoghi P, Liebensteiner M, Agreiter M, Leithner A, Böhler N, Labek G. Revision surgery after total joint arthroplasty: a complication-based analysis using worldwide arthroplasty registers. J Arthroplast. 2013;28:1329–32. https://doi.org/10.1016/j.arth.2013.01.012.
5. Perka C, Haschke F, Tohtz S. Dislocation after Total Hip Arthroplasty. Z Orthop Unfall. 2012;150:e89–103, quiz e104–5. https://doi.org/10.1055/s-0031-1298419.
6. Werner BC. Instability after total hip arthroplasty. WJO. 2012;3:122. https://doi.org/10.5312/wjo.v3.i8.122.
7. Hummel MT, Malkani AL, Yakkanti MR, Baker DL. Decreased dislocation after revision total hip arthroplasty using larger femoral head size and posterior capsular repair. J Arthroplast. 2009;24:73–6. https://doi.org/10.1016/j.arth.2009.04.026.
8. Phillips CB, Barrett JA, Losina E, Mahomed NN, Lingard EA, Guadagnoli E, Baron JA, Harris WH, Poss R, Katz JN. Incidence rates of dislocation, pulmonary embolism, and deep infection during the first six months after elective Total hip replacement. J Bone Joint Surg Am. 2003;85-A(1):20–6.
9. Sanchez-Sotelo J, Berry DJ. Epidemiology of instability after total hip replacement. Orthop Clin North Am. 2001;32:543–52. vii
10. Devane PA, Wraighte PJ, Ong DCG, Horne JG. Do joint registries report true rates of hip dislocation? Clin Orthop Relat Res. 2012:3003–6.
11. Etienne A, Cupic Z, Charnley J. Postoperative dislocation after Charnley low-friction arthroplasty. Clin Orthop Relat Res. 1978;(132):19–23.
12. Charnley J. Low friction arthroplasty of the hip: theory and practice. Berlin: Springer Berlin Heidelberg; 1979.
13. Prietzel T, Hammer N, Schleifenbaum S, Adler D, Pretzsch M, Köhler L, et al. The impact of capsular repair on the dislocation rate after primary Total hip arthroplasty: a retrospective analysis of 1972 cases. Z Orthop Unfall. 2014; 152:130–43. https://doi.org/10.1055/s-0034-1368209.
14. Bottner F, Pellicci PM. Review: posterior soft tissue repair in primary total hip arthroplasty. HSS J. 2006;2:7–11. https://doi.org/10.1007/s11420-005-0134-y.

15. Howie DW, Holubowycz OT, Middleton R. Large femoral heads decrease the incidence of dislocation after total hip arthroplasty: a randomized controlled trial. J Bone Joint Surg Am. 2012;94:1095–102. https://doi.org/10.2106/JBJS.K.00570.

16. Bistolfi A, Crova M, Rosso F, Titolo P, Ventura S, Massazza G. Dislocation rate after hip arthroplasty within the first postoperative year: 36 mm versus 28 mm femoral heads. Hip Int. 2011;21:559–64. https://doi.org/10.5301/HIP.2011.8647.

17. Y-j L, L-c Z, Yang G-j, C-c Z, Wang W-l, Lin R-x, C-y C. Prevention of prothesis dislocation after the revision of total hip arthroplasty. Zhongguo Gu Shang. 2008;21:173–5.

18. Chivas DJ, Smith K, Tanzer M. Role of capsular repair on dislocation in revision total hip arthroplasty. Clin Orthop Relat Res. 2006;453:147–52. https://doi.org/10.1097/01.blo.0000238857.61862.34.

19. Pellicci PM, Potter HG, Foo LF, Boettner F. MRI shows biologic restoration of posterior soft tissue repairs after THA. Clin Orthop Relat Res. 2009;467:940–5. https://doi.org/10.1007/s11999-008-0503-1.

20. Stucki G, Meier D, Stucki S, Michel BA, Tyndall AG, Elke R, Theiler R. Evaluation of a German questionnaire version of the Lequesne cox- and gonarthrosis indices. Z Rheumatol. 1996;55:50–7.

21. Bauer R, Kerschbaumer F, Poisel S, Oberthaler W. The Transgluteal approach to the hip joint. Arch Orthop Traumat Surg. 1979;95:47–9. https://doi.org/10.1007/BF00379169.

22. Watson-Jones R.. Fractures of the neck of the femur. Br J Surg. 1936;XXIII(92): 787–808.

23. Dobzyniak M, Fehring TK, Odum S. Early failure in total hip arthroplasty. Clin Orthop Relat Res. 2006;447:76–8. https://doi.org/10.1097/01.blo.0000203484.90711.52.

24. Statistisches Bundesamt editor. Fallpauschalenbezogene Krankenhausstatistik (DRG-Statistik): Diagnosen, Prozeduren, Fallpauschalen und Case Mix der vollstationären Patientinnen und Patienten in Krankenhäusern. Wiesbaden: Statistisches Bundesamt; Fachserie 12 Reihe 6. 4–2015.

25. Garellick G, Kärrholm J, Lindahl H, Malchau H, Rogmark C, Rolfson O. Swedish National Hip Arthroplasty Register 2013. Annu Rep. 2013. ISBN 978-91-980507-5-2; ISSN 1654-5982.

26. Blom AW, Rogers M, Taylor AH, Pattison G, Whitehouse S, Bannister GC. Dislocation following total hip replacement: the Avon Orthopaedic Centre experience. Ann R Coll Surg Engl. 2008;90(8):658–62. https://doi.org/10.1308/003588408X318156.

27. Sanchez-Sotelo J, Haidukewych GJ, Boberg CJ. Hospital cost of dislocation after primary total hip arthroplasty. J Bone Joint Surg Am. 2006;88:290–4. https://doi.org/10.2106/JBJS.D.02799.

28. Goldstein WM, Gleason TF, Kopplin M, Branson JJ. Prevalence of Dislocation After Total Hip Arthroplasty Through a Posterolateral Approach with Partial Capsulotomy and Capsulorrhaphy. J Bone Joint Surg Am. 2001;83-A Suppl 2(Pt 1):2–7.

29. Meek RMD, Allan DB, McPhillips G, Kerr L, Howie CR. Epidemiology of dislocation after Total hip arthroplasty. Clin Orthop Relat Res. 2006;447:9–18. https://doi.org/10.1097/01.blo.0000218754.12311.4a.

30. Wetters NG, Murray TG, Moric M, Sporer SM, Paprosky WG, Della Valle CJ. Risk factors for dislocation after revision total hip arthroplasty. Clin Orthop Relat Res. 2013;471:410–6. https://doi.org/10.1007/s11999-012-2561-7.

31. Lewinnek GE, Lewis JL, Richard T, Compere CL, Zimmerman JR. Dislocations after total hip-replacement arthroplasties. J Bone Joint Surg Am. 1978;60(2): 217–20.

32. Elkins JM, Callaghan JJ, Brown TD. The 2014 frank Stinchfield award: the 'landing zone' for wear and stability in total hip arthroplasty is smaller than we thought: a computational analysis. Clin Orthop Relat Res. 2015;473:441–52. https://doi.org/10.1007/s11999-014-3818-0.

33. Zajonz D, Philipp H, Schleifenbaum S, Möbius R, Hammer N, Grunert R, Prietzel T. Larger heads compensate for an increased risk of THA dislocation in high-risk patients. Orthopade. 2015;44(5):381–91. https://doi.org/10.1007/s00132-015-3093-0.

34. Garbuz DS, Masri BA, Duncan CP, Greidanus NV, Bohm ER, Petrak MJ, et al. The frank Stinchfield award: dislocation in revision THA: do large heads (36 and 40 mm) result in reduced dislocation rates in a randomized clinical trial? Clin Orthop Relat Res. 2012;470:351–6. https://doi.org/10.1007/s11999-011-2146-x.

35. Prietzel T, Richter K-W, Pilz D, von Salis-Soglio G. The stabilizing effect of atmospheric pressure (AP) on hip joint subject to traction force – an experimental study. Z Orthop Unfall. 2007;145:468–75. https://doi.org/10.1055/s-2007-965255.

36. Pellicci PM, Bostrom M, Poss R. Posterior approach to Total hip replacement using enhanced posterior soft tissue repair. Clin Orthop Relat Res. 1998;355: 224–8. https://doi.org/10.1097/00003086-199810000-00023.

37. Grunert R, Schleifenbaum S, Möbius R, Sommer G, Zajonz D, Hammer N, Prietzel T. Are higher prices for larger fermoral heads in total hip arthroplasty justified from the perspective of health care economics? An analysis of costs and effects in Germany. Z Orthop Unfall. 2017;155(1):52–60. https://doi.org/10.1055/s-0042-113003.

38. Prietzel T, Hammer N, Schleifenbaum S, Kaßebaum E, Farag M, von Salis-Soglio G. On the permanent hip-stabilizing effect of atmospheric pressure. J Biomech. 2014;47:2660–5. https://doi.org/10.1016/j.jbiomech.2014.05.013.

39. Prietzel T, Drummer N, Farag M, Richter K-W, von Salis-Soglio G. The significance of the acetabular labrum for hip joint stability--an experimental study. Z Orthop Unfall. 2010;148:436–42. https://doi.org/10.1055/s-0029-1240586.

40. White RE, Forness TJ, Allman JK, Junick DW. Effect of posterior capsular repair on early dislocation in primary Total hip replacement. Clin Orthop Relat Res. 2001;393:163–7. https://doi.org/10.1097/00003086-200112000-00019.

16

Putative functional variants of lncRNA identified by RegulomeDB were associated with knee osteoarthritis susceptibility

Kejie Wang[1,2†], Minjie Chu[3†], Wenge Ding[2] and Qing Jiang[1,4*]

Abstract

Background: Knee osteoarthritis (KOA) is the most common form of chronic degenerative joint disease worldwide. Its incidence has increased in recent years. Aberrant expression profile of lncRNAs in damaged bone and cartilage of KOA patients has been reported recently, indicating its potential contributions in KOA development and a promising target for disease diagnosis and treatment. The aim of this study was to identify the association between genetic variation in lncRNA and KOA.

Methods: We retrieved relevant articles from the PubMed, Medline and Embase databases up to Jul 2017 investigating the association between lncRNA and the risk of osteoarthritis. There are 15 lncRNAs which show connection with osteoarthritis. We selected potential functional polymorphisms identified by RegulomeDB database in these lncRNAs. A case-control study was conducted which contained 278 KOA patients and 289 OA-free controls.

Results: Logistic regression analyses revealed that H19 rs2067051 T allele was significantly associated with decreased risk of KOA after adjusted for age, gender and BMI in recessive genetic model (OR = 0.63, P = 0.03) and additive genetic model (OR = 0.79, P = 0.03). MEG3 rs4378559 T allele was significantly associated with increased risk of KOA in additive genetic model (OR = 1.32, P = 0.04). Heterogeneity tests proved that H19 rs2067051, MEG3 rs4378559 and HOTTIP rs202384's risk effects on KOA were more remarkable for female, BMI ≥ 25 and younger age (age < 60), respectively.

Conclusion: The results indicate that potential functional genetic variation in lncRNA plays an important role in the pathogenesis of KOA.

Keywords: lncRNA, Osteoarthritis, Polymorphism, H19, MEG3, HOTTIP

Background

Knee osteoarthritis (KOA) is the most common joint disease worldwide, characterized by progressive degeneration of articular cartilage, synovitis, osteophyte formation, and subchondral bone sclerosis [1]. It can cause severe pain and physical disability thus substantially reduce elder people's quality of life [2, 3]. Although the incidence of osteoarthritis is still increasing, affecting approximately 10% of men and 18% of women over 60 years of age, its pathophysiology is still evolving and undetermined [4]. Twin-pair studies and family-based segregation analyses have showed clear evidence of a heritable component in the susceptibility of OA [5]. Researches have shown the evidence that genetic factors may play a vital role in the development of OA, although little of them have been identified so far.

Long noncoding RNAs (lncRNA) have been tentatively defined as a type of RNA molecule more than 200 nucleotides in length (while microRNAs are of 20–22 nucleotides in size) and are characterized by their complexity and diversity of sequences and mechanisms of action [6]. Several lncRNAs have been reported play an important role in the pathogenesis of osteoarthritis [7, 8]. Aberrant expression profile of lncRNAs in damaged bone and cartilage of OA patients has been reported recently,

* Correspondence: qingj@nju.edu.cn
†Kejie Wang and Minjie Chu contributed equally to this work.
[1]Department of Sports Medicine and Adult Reconstructive Surgery, Drum Tower Hospital Clinical College of Nanjing Medical University, Zhongshan Road 321, Nanjing 210008, Jiangsu, People's Republic of China
[4]The Center of Diagnosis and Treatment for Joint Disease, Drum Tower Hospital Affiliated to Medical School of Nanjing University, Nanjing 210008, Jiangsu, People's Republic of China
Full list of author information is available at the end of the article

indicating its potential contributions in OA development and a promising target for disease diagnosis and treatment [9]. However, the role of lncRNAs played in cartilage metabolism and their overall contributions to the degradation of chondrocyte extracellular matrix and the pathogenesis of OA are still not fully understood. Considering the important roles lncRNA played in cartilage anabolism and catabolism, we hypothesized that single nucleotide polymorphisms (SNPs) in lncRNA gene may individually or jointly contribute to the risk of osteoarthritis.

RegulomeDB, a database integrates a big collection of regulatory information from ENCODE and other data sources, is a powerful tool to choose functional SNPs in a specified chromosome region [10]. RegulomeDB presents a scoring system with categories ranging from 1 to 6 by the way of integrated annotations data on methylation, chromatin structure, protein motifs and binding. The lower RegulomeDB score indicates the stronger evidence for a variant to be located in a functional region.

Recently, many studies have used RegulomeDB to identify causal polymorphisms associated with human diseases such as cancer, polycystic ovary syndrome and so on [11, 12]. Thus in this case-control study, we explored KOA risk with lncRNA polymorphisms which are annotated in RegulomeDB.

Methods

Patients

In this study, Han Chinese KOA patients were recruited between June 2013 and August 2016 at the orthopaedics department, Changzhou No.1 people's hospital according to the American College of Rheumatology (ACR) diagnostic criteria for KOA [13]. Each patient had taken the affected knee's anteroposterior weight-bearing radiographs. Two orthopedics doctors provide a Kellgren–Lawrence (KL) score ranging from 0 to 4 assessed by the radiographic data [14]. Other knee joint diseases were excluded such as inflammatory arthritis (septic arthritis, rheumatoid, or autoimmune disease), posttraumatic arthritis, or knee joint developmental dysplasia. All healthy volunteer controls were frequency-matched to the case subjects by gender and age. The healthy control subjects reported no history of OA or other rheumatic diseases, which were included from the same hospital during the same period. Each participant was interviewed face-to-face to gather demographic data by two trained investigators. After signing informed consent at recruitment, peripheral blood of each participant was collected. All subjects were weighed with a calibrated beam balance to 0.1 kg, wearing the least possible clothes. Also their height was measured in centimeters using a stadiometer. The body mass index (BMI) was then calculated using the above data. This study was approved by the Human Research Ethics Committees of the Changzhou No.1 people's hospital.

LncRNAs and SNPs selection

We retrieved relevant articles from the PubMed, Medline and Embase databases up to Jul 2017 investigating the association between lncRNA and the risk of osteoarthritis. There are 15 lncRNAs reported related with osteoarthritis including UFC1, lncRNA-MSR (TMSB4XP6), PCGEM1, MEG3, HOTAIR, GAS5, PMS2L2 (uc011kep.2), RP11-445H22.4 (ENST00000427303), H19, CTD-2574D22.4 (ENST00000567795), lncRNA-CIR, HOTTIP, PACER, CILinc01 and CILinc02 [15–19].

Variant with lower RegulomeDB score indicates the variant is more strongly located in a functional region. Consequently, we selected SNPs with RegulomeDB scores ranging from 1 to 2b. Based on the data from UCSC database (GRCh37/hg19), regulomeDB database, the criteria of minor allele frequency (MAF) > 0.05 and linkage disequilibrium (LD) < 0.8 in Han Chinese, we found 10 potentially functional SNPs in these 15 lncRNAs.

DNA extraction and genotyping

Genomic DNA was extracted from leukocyte pellets by proteinase K digestion and phenol chloroform as described in previous study [20]. The genotype detecting was performed by Sequenom MassARRAY assay without knowing the status of case or control according to instructions of the manufacturer. Three SNPs genotyping were failure due to probe design. Finally, the left 7 SNPs successfully genotyped call rate were all above 95%. Over 10% specimens were randomly slected to be repeated with over 99% consistency and two blank (water) controls were tested in each 384-well plate for quality control.

Statistical analyses

The χ^2 test and Student's t-tests were used to analyze distribution differences of demographic characteristics and genotypes between cases and controls, for categorical variables and continuous variables respectively. Hardy–

Table 1 Distributions of select variables in OA cases and controls

Variables	Case	Control	P
	n = 278 (%)	n = 289 (%)	
Age, year (mean ± SD)	62.00 ± 10.55	61.13 ± 10.92	0.34
Gender			0.87
Male	82(29.5)	87(30.1)	
Female	196(70.5)	202(69.9)	
BMI	24.97 ± 3.26	23.84 ± 2.96	**< 0.01**
< 25	150(54.0)	189(66.5)	< 0.01
≥ 25	128(46.0)	95(33.5)	
KL classification			
1–2	135		
3–4	143		

Bold font presents P < 0.05

Weinberg equilibrium (HWE) was tested using a goodness-of-fit χ^2 test to compare the expected and observed genotype frequencies in controls for the distribution of each SNP. We use logistic regression to estimate odd ratios (ORs) and 95% confidence intervals (CIs) to evaluate the association with KOA susceptibility after adjusted for age, sex and BMI. We use the χ^2-based Q-test to measure the heterogeneity (ORs and 95% CIs) derived from corresponding subgroups to examine the differences between different subgroups. We also assessed the cumulative effects of the genotyped 6 SNPs using a risk score analysis with a linear of the SNP genotypes (coded as 0, 1, and 2) weighted by the regression coefficient. All of the statistical analyses were

Table 2 Logistic regression analysis of associations between selected polymorphisms and KOA risk

SNP	Genotype	Case	Control	OR (95%CI)	P	OR (95%CI)[a]	P[a]
H19 rs2067051	CC	162	142	1		1	
	TC	64	63	0.89(0.59–1.35)	0.58	0.87(0.57–1.35)	0.54
	TT	50	69	0.64(0.41–0.97)	**0.04**	0.61(0.39–0.95)	**0.03**
	TT + TC vs.CC			0.76(0.54–1.06)	0.11	0.73(0.52–1.04)	0.08
	TTvs.TC+ CC			0.66(0.44–0.99)	**0.05**	0.63(0.42–0.97)	**0.03**
	Additive			0.81(0.66–0.99)	**0.04**	0.79(0.64–0.98)	**0.03**
MEG3 rs4378559	CC	148	176	1		1	
	TC	108	98	1.31(0.92–1.86)	0.13	1.23(0.86–1.76)	0.26
	TT	21	14	1.78(0.88–3.63)	0.11	1.78(0.86–3.68)	0.12
	TT + TC vs.CC			1.37(0.98–1.91)	0.07	1.30(0.92–1.83)	0.13
	TT vs.TC+ CC			1.61(0.80–3.23)	0.18	1.65(0.81–3.35)	0.17
	Additive			1.32(1.01–1.74)	**0.04**	1.28(0.97–1.69)	0.08
MEG3 rs4906024	CC	88	80	1		1	
	TC	103	131	0.71(0.48–1.06)	0.10	0.72(0.48–1.09)	0.12
	TT	82	76	0.98(0.64–1.52)	0.93	1.04(0.67–1.62)	0.87
	TT + TC vs.CC			0.81(0.57–1.17)	0.26	0.84(0.58–1.21)	0.35
	TT vs.TC+ CC			1.19(0.82–1.72)	0.35	1.25(0.86–1.83)	0.24
	Additive			0.99(0.79–1.23)	0.90	1.02(0.81–1.27)	0.90
HOTTIP rs10233387	AA	62	80	1		1	
	GA	127	137	1.20(0.79–1.80)	0.39	1.22(0.80–1.85)	0.35
	GG	64	62	1.33(0.82–2.16)	0.24	1.49(0.91–2.45)	0.11
	GG + GA vs.AA			1.24(0.84–1.82)	0.28	1.30(0.88–1.93)	0.19
	GG vs.GA+ AA			1.19(0.79–1.77)	0.41	1.31(0.87–1.98)	0.20
	Additive			1.16(0.91–1.47)	0.24	1.22(0.95–1.57)	0.11
HOTTIP rs2023843	TT	92	108	1		1	
	CT	143	144	1.17(0.81–1.67)	0.41	1.23(0.85–1.78)	0.28
	CC	43	37	1.36(0.81–2.30)	0.24	1.52(0.89–2.58)	0.13
	CC + TC vs.TT			1.21(0.85–1.70)	0.29	1.29(0.90–1.83)	0.17
	CC vs.TC+ TT			1.25(0.78–2.00)	0.36	1.34(0.83–2.18)	0.24
	Additive			1.17(0.91–1.49)	0.22	1.23(0.96–1.58)	0.10
HOTAIR rs10783618	CC	157	159	1		1	
	TC	96	108	0.90(0.63–1.28)	0.56	0.90(0.63–1.29)	0.56
	TT	25	22	1.15(0.62–2.13)	0.65	1.18(0.63–2.20)	0.61
	TT + TC vs.CC			0.94(0.68–1.31)	0.73	0.94(0.67–1.33)	0.74
	TT vs.TC+ CC			1.20(0.66–2.18)	0.55	1.23(0.67–2.26)	0.51
	Additive			1.00(0.77–1.29)	0.99	1.00(0.77–1.30)	0.98

Bold font presents $P < 0.05$
[a]Adjusted for age, gender and BMI

performed with SPSS Statistics Version 17.0 or PLINK (http://www.cog-genomics.org/plink2/) software.

Results

The distribution of selected clinical variables between OA cases and controls was summarized in Table 1. In brief, the age and gender between two groups were comparable ($P > 0.05$).

Rs2067079 of GAS5 was excluded due to violation of Hardy–Weinberg equilibrium. The genotype distributions of the left 6 SNPs and their associations with KOA risk were presented in Table 2. The success rates of genotyping for all these SNPs were above 98%. Logistic regression analyses revealed that H19 rs2067051 T allele was significantly associated with decreased risk of KOA adjusted for age, gender and BMI in recessive genetic model (OR = 0.63, 95% CI: 0.42–0.97, $P = 0.03$) and additive genetic model (OR = 0.79, 95% CI: 0.64–0.98, $P = 0.03$). MEG3 rs4378559 T allele was significantly associated with the increased risk of KOA in additive genetic model without adjustment (OR = 1.32, 95% CI: 1.01–1.74, $P = 0.04$), but the association no longer existed after adjustment ($P = 0.08$). HOTTIP rs2023843 C allele showed boundary positive in additive genetic model after adjustment (OR = 1.23, 95% CI: 0.96–1.58, $P = 0.10$).

Further stratified analyses were conducted in four positive models as above mentioned (Table 3). Results showed that H19 rs2067051 T allele on KOA was more evidenced for female in recessive model (TT vs.TC+ CC) (P for heterogeneity was 0.01). MEG3 rs4378559 T allele on KOA risk was more obvious in BMI ≥ 25 in additive model (P for heterogeneity was 0.02). HOTTIP rs2023843

C allele on KOA was more distinct for younger age (age < 60) in additive model (P for heterogeneity was 0.03).

Cumulative effects of the 6 SNPs were conducted using a risk score analysis weighted by the regression coefficient (Table 4). The mean of cumulative risk score among KOA cases (0.38 ± 0.40) was higher than that among controls (0.29 ± 0.34) (P value for T test < 0.01). Logistic regression analyses revealed that risk score was significantly associated with increased risk of KOA adjusted for age, gender and BMI (OR = 2.21, 95% CI: 1.36–3.60, $P < 0.01$).

Discussion

In the current study, we conducted a case-control study to explore the association between genetic variants identified by RegulomeDB in candidate lncRNA genes and KOA. Our results confirm that putative functional variants H19 rs2067051 and MEG3 rs4378559 were associated with KOA susceptibility. Heterogeneity existed between different gender, BMI and age group for H19 rs2067051, MEG3 rs4378559 and HOTTIP rs202384 respectively, which means gene-environment interactions between genetic variants in lncRNA genes and these clinical data for KOA risk.

All RegulomeDB score of H19 rs2067051, MEG3 rs4378559 and HOTTIP rs2023843 were 2b. ChIP-seq data showed these polymorphisms binding to many proteins including EZH2, E2F6, REST and IKZF1 (http://regulome.stanford.edu/).

The development of osteoarthritis was ameliorated by inhibition of EZH2 through the Wnt/β-catenin pathway [21, 22]. E2F6 encodes a member of transcription factors which play an important role in the cell cycle controling [23]. A transcriptional repressor which represses neuronal genes in non-neuronal tissues was encoded by REST [24].

Table 3 Stratified analyses of rs2023843, rs2067051, and rs4378559 genotypes associated with patients of kOA by selected variables

	rs2067051 Additive			rs2067051 TTvs.TC+ CC			rs4378559 Additive			rs2023843 Additive		
	OR(95%CI)[a]	P^a	P_{het}^b	OR(95%CI)[a]	P^a	P_{het}^b	OR(95%CI)[a]	P^a	P_{het}^b	OR(95%CI)[a]	P^a	P_{het}^b
Age			0.12			0.18			0.17			**0.03**
age < 60	0.63(0.45–0.89)	0.01		0.41(0.21–0.84)	0.01		1.04(0.68–1.61)	0.86		1.64(1.11–2.44)	0.01	
age ≥ 60	0.90(0.68–1.19)	0.47		0.77(0.44–1.33)	0.34		1.56(1.07–2.27)	0.02		0.92(0.65–1.30)	0.63	
Gender			0.12			**0.01**			0.76			0.07
male	1.09(0.70–1.71)	0.69		1.92(0.75–4.91)	0.18		1.36(0.80–2.31)	0.25		1.78(1.09–2.90)	0.02	
female	0.73(0.57–0.93)	0.01		0.48(0.29–0.78)	0.00		1.24(0.89–1.72)	0.20		1.05(0.78–1.42)	0.75	
BMI			0.43			0.13			**0.02**			0.55
BMI < 25	0.76(0.57–1.00)	0.05		0.49(0.28–0.87)	0.01		1.02(0.72–1.43)	0.92		1.15(0.84–1.59)	0.38	
BMI ≥ 25	0.90(0.64–1.26)	0.54		0.96(0.50–1.86)	0.91		2.07(1.27–3.38)	0.00		1.35(0.90–2.04)	0.15	
KL			0.20			0.50			0.17			0.22
KL12	0.70(0.53–0.92)	0.01		0.56(0.32–0.98)	0.04		1.07(0.75–1.52)	0.72		1.41(1.03–1.93)	0.03	
KL34	0.89(0.69–1.16)	0.40		0.73(0.44–1.22)	0.23		1.51(1.07–2.11)	0.02		1.07(0.78–1.46)	0.68	

Bold font presents $P < 0.05$
[a]Adjusted for age, gender and BMI
[b]P value for heterogeneity test

Table 4 Cumulative risk scores of 6 SNPs on the risk of kOA

	Case	Control	P^a	OR(95%CI)^b	P^b
Risk score	0.38 ± 0.40	0.29 ± 0.34	**< 0.01**	2.21(1.36–3.60)	**< 0.01**

Bold font presents $P < 0.05$
[a] P for T test
[b] Adjust for age, gender, and BMI

IKZF1 encodes a transcription factor which belongs to the zinc-finger DNA-binding protein family, which correlates with chromatin remodeling [25]. IKZF1 participated in inflammation suggested that IKZF1 may contribute to osteoarthritis [26].

A 2.5 kb RNA Polymerase II dependent transcript was expressed from H19 and it is spliced, capped, polyadenylated, and finally exported into the cytoplasm [27]. MiR-675, which suppresses growth, is developmentally reversed in H19 [28]. It also participates in the development of OA through affecting the pathological processes including inflammatory response, extracellular matrix (ECM) disruption, angiogenesis and apoptosis. Research showed that H19 was up-regulated in OA compared with normal tissue and was a metabolic marker in damaged cartilage of OA patients or in cultured chondrocytes under hypoxic signaling condition [29, 30]. Rs2067051 of H19 has been verified connected with birth weight and coronary artery disease [31, 32]. Both high birth weight and coronary artery disease have relationship with higher BMI, which are crucial risk factors for KOA. In this study, we also found heterogeneity was existed for H19 rs2067051 in different gender group. It is already found that H19 represents a key factor which causes sex differences in the incidence of cholestatic liver injury in mice whose multidrug resistance 2 gene was knockout [33].

A maternally expressed lncRNA, which was named MEG3, was closely connected to inflammation-related diseases, for example knee osteoarthritis [34]. It revealed that MEG3 demonstrated low expression level in OA cartilage samples in rat model. It was also shown that MEG3 was down regulated and negatively correlated with VEGF expression levels in cartilage samples from knee osteoarthritis patients [34]. MEG3 knockdown could promoted chondrocytes proliferation and inhibited chondrocytes apoptosis induced by IL-1β possibly through miR-16/SMAD7 system [35].

HOTTIP, which participate in the process of osteoarthritis advance and endochondral ossification, showed higher expression level in OA cartilage in comparison to normal cartilage [36]. Through modulating intergrin-α1 either transcriptionally by HOXA13 or epigenetically by DNMT-3B, HOTTIP control cartilage destruction and development. Research data also indicated that HOTTIP could be potential diagnostic biomarker or therapeutic target for OA and other joint cartilage related disease.

Conclusions

In conclusion, our study suggested that potential functional genetic variation in lncRNA plays a crucial role in the pathogenesis of KOA. Further independent studies with different races and larger sample sizes are necessary to elucidate the molecular mechanisms underlying these findings.

Abbreviations
BMI: Body mass index; CIs: Confidence intervals; ECM: Extracellular matrix; HWE: Hardy–Weinberg equilibrium; KOA: Knee osteoarthritis; lncRNA: Long noncoding RNAs; ORs: Odd ratios; SNP: Single nucleotide polymorphisms

Funding
This study was supported by the guiding project of Health and Family Planning Commission of Changzhou (No.wz201514). This work was supported by National Natural Science Foundation of China (No. 81272017). This work was supported by the Projects of International Cooperation and Exchanges National Natural Science Foundation of China (No. 81420108021).

Authors' contributions
KJW and MJC drafted the first manuscript. KJW, MJC, WGD and QJ participated in study design, data acquisition, analysis and interpretation of data, critical review and final approval. KJW, WGD and QJ contributed with clinical expertise, conduct of patient visit procedures, data collection, data interpretation and final approval of the manuscript. KJW and MJC performed all statistical analyses. KJW, MJC and QJ contributed with data analysis and interpretation, critical review, and final approval of the manuscript.

Competing interests
Qing Jiang is a member of the editorial board (Section Editor) of BMC Musculoskeletal Disorders. The authors declare that they have no competing of interests.

Author details
[1]Department of Sports Medicine and Adult Reconstructive Surgery, Drum Tower Hospital Clinical College of Nanjing Medical University, Zhongshan Road 321, Nanjing 210008, Jiangsu, People's Republic of China. [2]Department of Orthopaedics, Changzhou No.1 People's Hospital, Changzhou 213003, Jiangsu, People's Republic of China. [3]Department of Epidemiology, School of Public Health, Nantong University, Nantong 226019, Jiangsu, People's Republic of China. [4]The Center of Diagnosis and Treatment for Joint Disease, Drum Tower Hospital Affiliated to Medical School of Nanjing University, Nanjing 210008, Jiangsu, People's Republic of China.

References
1. Zhuo Q, Yang W, Chen J, Wang Y. Metabolic syndrome meets osteoarthritis. Nat Rev Rheumatol. 2012;8:729–37.
2. Felson DT, Zhang Y. An update on the epidemiology of knee and hip osteoarthritis with a view to prevention. Arthritis Rheum. 1998;41:1343–55.
3. Felson DT. Developments in the clinical understanding of osteoarthritis. Arthritis research & therapy. 2009;11:203.
4. Glyn-Jones S, Palmer AJ, Agricola R, Price AJ, Vincent TL, Weinans H, et al. Osteoarthritis. Lancet. 2015;386:376–87.
5. Loughlin J. Genetic epidemiology of primary osteoarthritis. Curr Opin Rheumatol. 2001;13:111–6.
6. Perkel JM. Visiting "noncodarnia". BioTechniques. 2013;54(301):03–4.
7. Liu Q, Zhang X, Dai L, Hu X, Zhu J, Li L, et al. Long noncoding RNA related to cartilage injury promotes chondrocyte extracellular matrix degradation in osteoarthritis. Arthritis Rheumatol. 2014;66:969–78.
8. Liu Q, Hu X, Zhang X, Dai L, Duan X, Zhou C, et al. The TMSB4 pseudogene LncRNA functions as a competing endogenous RNA to promote cartilage degradation in human osteoarthritis. Molecular therapy : the journal of the American Society of Gene Therapy. 2016;24:1726–33.

9. Fu M, Huang G, Zhang Z, Liu J, Huang Z, Yu B, et al. Expression profile of long noncoding RNAs in cartilage from knee osteoarthritis patients. Osteoarthr Cartil. 2015;23:423–32.

10. ENCODE Project Consortium. An integrated encyclopedia of DNA elements in the human genome. Nature. 2012;489:57–74.

11. Khadzhieva MB, Kolobkov DS, Kamoeva SV, Ivanova AV, Abilev SK, Salnikova LE. Verification of the chromosome region 9q21 association with pelvic organ prolapse using RegulomeDB annotations. Biomed Res Int. 2015;2015:837904.

12. Hu L, Zhang Y, Chen L, Zhou W, Wang Y, Wen J. MAPK and ERK polymorphisms are associated with PCOS risk in Chinese women. Oncotarget. 2017;8:100261–8.

13. Altman R, Asch E, Bloch D, Bole G, Borenstein D, Brandt K, et al. Development of criteria for the classification and reporting of osteoarthritis. Classification of osteoarthritis of the knee. Diagnostic and therapeutic criteria Committee of the American Rheumatism Association. Arthritis Rheum. 1986;29:1039–49.

14. Kellgren JH, Lawrence JS. Radiological assessment of osteo-arthrosis. Ann Rheum Dis. 1957;16:494–502.

15. Chen WK, Yu XH, Yang W, Wang C, He WS, Yan YG, et al. lncRNAs: novel players in intervertebral disc degeneration and osteoarthritis. Cell proliferation. 2017;50:e12313.

16. Zhang L, Yang C, Chen S, Wang G, Shi B, Tao X, et al. Long noncoding RNA DANCR is a positive regulator of proliferation and Chondrogenic differentiation in human synovium-derived stem cells. DNA Cell Biol. 2017;36:136–42.

17. Zhang G, Wu Y, Xu D, Yan X. Long noncoding RNA UFC1 promotes proliferation of chondrocyte in osteoarthritis by acting as a sponge for miR-34a. DNA Cell Biol. 2016;35:691–5.

18. Pearson MJ, Philp AM, Heward JA, Roux BT, Walsh DA, Davis ET, et al. Long intergenic noncoding RNAs mediate the human chondrocyte inflammatory response and are differentially expressed in osteoarthritis cartilage. Arthritis Rheumatol. 2016;68:845–56.

19. Parasramka MA, Maji S, Matsuda A, Yan IK, Patel T. Long non-coding RNAs as novel targets for therapy in hepatocellular carcinoma. Pharmacol Ther. 2016;161:67–78.

20. Zhang CW, Zhang XL, Xia YJ, Cao YX, Wang WJ, Xu P, et al. Association between polymorphisms of the CYP11A1 gene and polycystic ovary syndrome in Chinese women. Mol Biol Rep. 2012;39:8379–85.

21. Chen L, Wu Y, Wang Y, Sun L, Li F. The inhibition of EZH2 ameliorates osteoarthritis development through the Wnt/beta-catenin pathway. Sci Rep. 2016;6:29176.

22. Trenkmann M, Brock M, Gay RE, Kolling C, Speich R, Michel BA, et al. Expression and function of EZH2 in synovial fibroblasts: epigenetic repression of the Wnt inhibitor SFRP1 in rheumatoid arthritis. Ann Rheum Dis. 2011;70:1482–8.

23. Ogawa H, Ishiguro K, Gaubatz S, Livingston DM, Nakatani Y. A complex with chromatin modifiers that occupies E2F- and Myc-responsive genes in G0 cells. Science. 2002;296:1132–6.

24. Bayram Y, White JJ, Elcioglu N, Cho MT, Zadeh N, Gedikbasi A, et al. REST final-exon-truncating mutations cause hereditary gingival fibromatosis. Am J Hum Genet. 2017;101:149–56.

25. Ueta M, Hamuro J, Nishigaki H, Nakamura N, Shinomiya K, Mizushima K, et al. Mucocutaneous inflammation in the Ikaros family zinc finger 1-keratin 5-specific transgenic mice. Allergy. 2017;73(2):395–404.

26. Chrousos GP, Kino T. Ikaros transcription factors: flying between stress and inflammation. J Clin Invest. 2005;115:844–8.

27. Seidl CI, Stricker SH, Barlow DP. The imprinted air ncRNA is an atypical RNAPII transcript that evades splicing and escapes nuclear export. EMBO J. 2006;25:3565–75.

28. Keniry A, Oxley D, Monnier P, Kyba M, Dandolo L, Smits G, et al. The H19 lincRNA is a developmental reservoir of miR-675 that suppresses growth and Igf1r. Nat Cell Biol. 2012;14:659–65.

29. Xing D, Liang JQ, Li Y, Lu J, Jia HB, Xu LY, et al. Identification of long noncoding RNA associated with osteoarthritis in humans. Orthop Surg. 2014;6:288–93.

30. Steck E, Boeuf S, Gabler J, Werth N, Schnatzer P, Diederichs S, et al. Regulation of H19 and its encoded microRNA-675 in osteoarthritis and under anabolic and catabolic in vitro conditions. J Mol Med (Berl). 2012;90:1185–95.

31. Adkins RM, Somes G, Morrison JC, Hill JB, Watson EM, Magann EF, et al. Association of birth weight with polymorphisms in the IGF2, H19, and IGF2R genes. Pediatr Res. 2010;68:429–34.

32. Gao W, Zhu M, Wang H, Zhao S, Zhao D, Yang Y, et al. Association of polymorphisms in long non-coding RNA H19 with coronary artery disease risk in a Chinese population. Mutat Res. 2015;772:15–22.

33. Li X, Liu R, Yang J, Sun L, Zhang L, Jiang Z, et al. The role of long noncoding RNA H19 in gender disparity of cholestatic liver injury in multidrug resistance 2 gene knockout mice. Hepatology. 2017;66:869–84.

34. Su W, Xie W, Shang Q, Su B. The long noncoding RNA MEG3 is downregulated and inversely associated with VEGF levels in osteoarthritis. Biomed Res Int. 2015;2015:356893.

35. Xu J, Xu Y. The lncRNA MEG3 downregulation leads to osteoarthritis progression via miR-16/SMAD7 axis. Cell & bioscience. 2017;7:69.

36. Kim D, Song J, Han J, Kim Y, Chun CH, Jin EJ. Two non-coding RNAs, MicroRNA-101 and HOTTIP contribute cartilage integrity by epigenetic and homeotic regulation of integrin-alpha1. Cell Signal. 2013;25:2878–87.

17

The acceptance of the clinical photographic posture assessment tool (CPPAT)

Carole Fortin[1,2][*] (iD), Paul van Schaik[3], Jean-François Aubin-Fournier[2], Josette Bettany-Saltikov[4], Jean-Claude Bernard[5] and Debbie Ehrmann Feldman[1,6]

Abstract

Background: There is a lack of evidence-based quantitative clinical methods to adequately assess posture. Our team developed a clinical photographic posture assessment tool (CPPAT) and implemented this tool in clinical practice to standardize posture assessment. The objectives were to determine the level of acceptance of the CPPAT and to document predictors as well as facilitators of and barriers to the acceptance of this tool by clinicians doing posture re-education.

Methods: This is a prospective study focussing on technology acceptance. Thirty-two clinician participants (physical therapists and sport therapists) received a 3–5 h training workshop explaining how to use the CPPAT. Over a three-month trial, they recorded time-on-task for a complete posture evaluation (photo - and photo-processing). Subsequently, participants rated their acceptance of the tool and commented on facilitators and barriers of the clinical method.

Results: Twenty-three clinician participants completed the trial. They took 22 (mean) ± 10 min (SD) for photo acquisition and 36 min ± 19 min for photo-processing. Acceptance of the CPPAT was high. Perceived ease of use was an indirect predictor of intention to use, mediated by perceived usefulness. Analysis time was an indirect predictor, mediated by perceived usefulness, and a marginally significant direct predictor. Principal facilitators were objective measurements, visualization, utility, and ease of use. Barriers were time to do a complete analysis of posture, quality of human-computer interaction, non-automation of posture index calculation and photo transfer, and lack of versatility.

Conclusion: The CPPAT is perceived as useful and easy to use by clinicians and may facilitate the quantitative analysis of posture. Adapting the user-interface and functionality to quantify posture may facilitate a wider adoption of the tool.

Keywords: Posture, Posture assessment, Musculoskeletal disorders, Technology acceptance, Innovation adoption

Background

Physiotherapists are often consulted to assess and correct posture for persons with various musculoskeletal conditions [1, 2]. Presently, there is a lack of high-quality evidence regarding the effectiveness of physiotherapy interventions on posture [3–5]. This may be due to the lack of evidence-based quantitative clinical methods to adequately assess the outcomes of therapeutic interventions [3, 6, 7]. Currently, quantitative methods for posture assessment require elaborate 3D analysis systems such as Motion Analysis and surface topography [8, 9]. However, these systems are not easily accessible for most clinicians since they are expensive and require specialized trained technicians. Physiotherapists and physicians commonly assess posture by descriptive visual inspections that lack scientific validation [1, 10, 11]. There is a growing field of interest in using clinical tools to quantitatively assess posture. A promising technique to assess posture clinically is a method that calculates body angles and distances on photographs reflecting posture in all planes [12–15]. In recent years, different non-invasive computer-based methods as well as mobile applications (APPs) have been proposed to assess posture in a clinical setting [15–20]. Boland et al. [16] reported good intra and inter-rater agreement (ICCs ≥0.75) for seven out of 13 posture indices in ten young healthy adults using a mobile APP. Posture deviations of the head, trunk and pelvis were also measured using an iPhone APP in a large group of healthy collegiate students but the reliability and validity of such measurements are not provided. Aroeira et al. [15]

* Correspondence: carole.fortin@umontreal.ca
[1]École de réadaptation, Faculté de médecine, Université de Montréal, C.P. 6128, succursale Centre-ville, Montréal, Québec H3C 3J7, Canada
[2]Research center, CHU Sainte-Justine, Montreal, Quebec, Canada
Full list of author information is available at the end of the article

reported that most of the new computer-based methods proposed in the literature to assess posture in adolescents with idiopathic scoliosis (four on 2D photogrammetry and 11 on laser or structured light, ultrasound and moiré scanner projection) focussed only on the back view and that the methodology of these studies was of low quality. These authors pointed out the importance of measuring posture of the whole body in patients with idiopathic scoliosis because the posture alterations may be extended to the whole body. Our team has developed a software program for quantitative analysis of whole body posture from digital photographs in youth with idiopathic scoliosis [18, 19]. Measures obtained using this software-based method showed excellent test-retest and inter-rater reliability for marker placement as well as good concurrent validity with spinal angles measured on radiographs and 3D trunk posture indices measured from a topography system in adolescents with idiopathic scoliosis [18, 19]. According to Aroeira et al. [15], this innovative clinical photographic posture assessment tool (CPPAT) is the only validated clinical tool offering assessment of the full body posture. The CPPAT could be used to standardize posture assessment in persons with scoliosis or other musculoskeletal pathologies.

The acceptance of rehabilitation technology by clinicians [21, 22] and patients [23] is essential for its successful uptake to both improve clinical practice as well as outcomes for patients. Previous research [22] established that drivers of the use of a low-cost portable system for postural assessment include training/skills, clinical use, quality of human-computer interaction, visualization and time-on-task; barriers to use include time-on-task, costs, quality of human-computer interaction, training/skills, clinical use, IT/equipment required and technical measurement issues.

Furthermore, it is essential to develop an understanding of how different factors influence technology acceptance. Highly influential has been Davis's [24] technology acceptance model (TAM; see Fig. 1) and its further development [25–27]. Our study uses TAM and focuses on three core model variables: intention to use the CPPAT, perceived usefulness and perceived ease of use of the CPPAT. According to TAM, the intention to use a product (system) is the major factor influencing the extent to which

potential users will employ the product (actual system use). In turn, intention to use is influenced by perceived usefulness and perceived ease of use. Perceived ease of use also indirectly influences intention to use through its direct effect on perceived usefulness. Product characteristics (system design features) directly influence both perceived usefulness and perceived ease of use and thereby indirectly influence intention to use and actual system use.

Research has also examined the relationship between task performance and perceived ease of use. Specifically, Venkatesh and Bala [25] measured 'objective usability' as novice-to-expert ratio of time-on-task and showed that objective usability predicts both perceived ease of use and perceived usefulness. Moreover, Chiou et al. [28] established that time-on-task predicts perceived usefulness. As task performance predicts perceived usefulness and perceived usefulness predicts intention to use, perceived usefulness may be a mediator of the effect of task performance on intention.

In our study, we address the following research questions: (1) what is the level of acceptance of this CPPAT by clinicians doing posture re-education, (2) what are the predictors of acceptance and (3) what are the drivers of and the barriers to acceptance of CCPAT for the evidence-based measurement of posture?

Method
Design

In a prospective mixed design study using quantitative and qualitative methods, we measured perceived ease of use, perceived usefulness and intention to use the software-based CPPAT (see Material and apparatus) for posture measurement as well as time-on-task for photo acquisition and photo-processing with the CPPAT.

Participants

We recruited 32 clinicians (22 physical therapists and ten sports therapists) working in public (35%) or private institutions in Canada (Montreal [MTL] and Quebec city [QC]), France (Lyon) and United Kingdom (UK – London, Middlesbrough, Chesterfield). Therapists working in public centers and private clinics were invited by e-mail in order to allow the clinician participants to attend the training and the focus group discussion. Collaborators affiliated with our

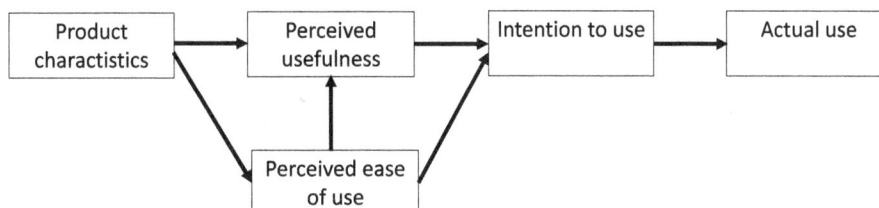

Fig. 1 Technology acceptance model (after Davis & Venkatesh, 1996 [38])

research teams were responsible to recruit a total of 30 therapists in the three countries. The inclusion criteria were clinicians assessing posture of persons with musculoskeletal disorders within their clinical practice and having access to a dedicated space for photo acquisitions. Eight participants did not complete the trial because they had changed their workplace and one for unknown reasons. Clinician-participants (18 women) had an average of 19.6 years (SD = 9.7) of experience in clinical practice and 12.6 years (SD = 7.7) of experience in posture assessment. In terms of computer use, ten participants had a low level, seven a moderate level, two a high level and four participants did not answer this question (see Additional file 1 for description of levels of computer use [29, 30]). The project was approved by the Institutional Ethics Committee of Sainte-Justine university hospital centre (approval reference number: 2015–691, 3905) and all clinician-participants signed a consent form.

Materials and apparatus

Description of the clinical photographic posture assessment tool (CPPAT)

CPPAT is a software-based program with a graphical interface for the analysis of four to six photographs of a patient's posture (front, back, left and right) acquired in standing using a standard procedure (see Fortin et al., [18, 19] for more details). We have shown excellent test-retest and inter-rater reliability for marker placement among a senior and novice physical therapists (reliability coefficients between 0.90 and 1.00 and standard error of measurement ranging from 0.5° to 3.0° and 3 to 6 mm) [18].

The software uses interactive click-on markers with the computer mouse. The user selects each specific marker from the graphical interface and places it directly on the corresponding anatomical landmark or anatomical reference points (e.g. eyes, upper end, lower end and center of the waist) on the person's photographs (see Fig. 2). The program allows zooming in on a marker for more accuracy. Different sets of markers are available according to each view (anterior, posterior or lateral). Following the selection of the markers associated with the calculation of an angle, its value can be displayed. All measurements can be exported in Excel- or Word formats. We thus choose to study the acceptance of the CPPAT because this tool has good demonstrated reliability and validity, allows posture assessment of the whole body, was designed to be user-friendly and follows a standardized procedure.

Procedure

The first part of the project involved the training of clinicians. The principal investigator (CF) and a research physical therapist (J-F A-F) trained clinician-participants. Participants received a tool kit including a detailed procedure for standardization of photo acquisition (following Fortin et al.'s study [18]) and of photo-processing with the software program and markers. The training consisted of a three- to five-hour workshop in each centre. The workshop was divided into three parts: 1) rationale and explanation of the software program, 2) equipment requirements (simple digital camera on a tripod) and demonstration of posture assessment with the placement of markers and

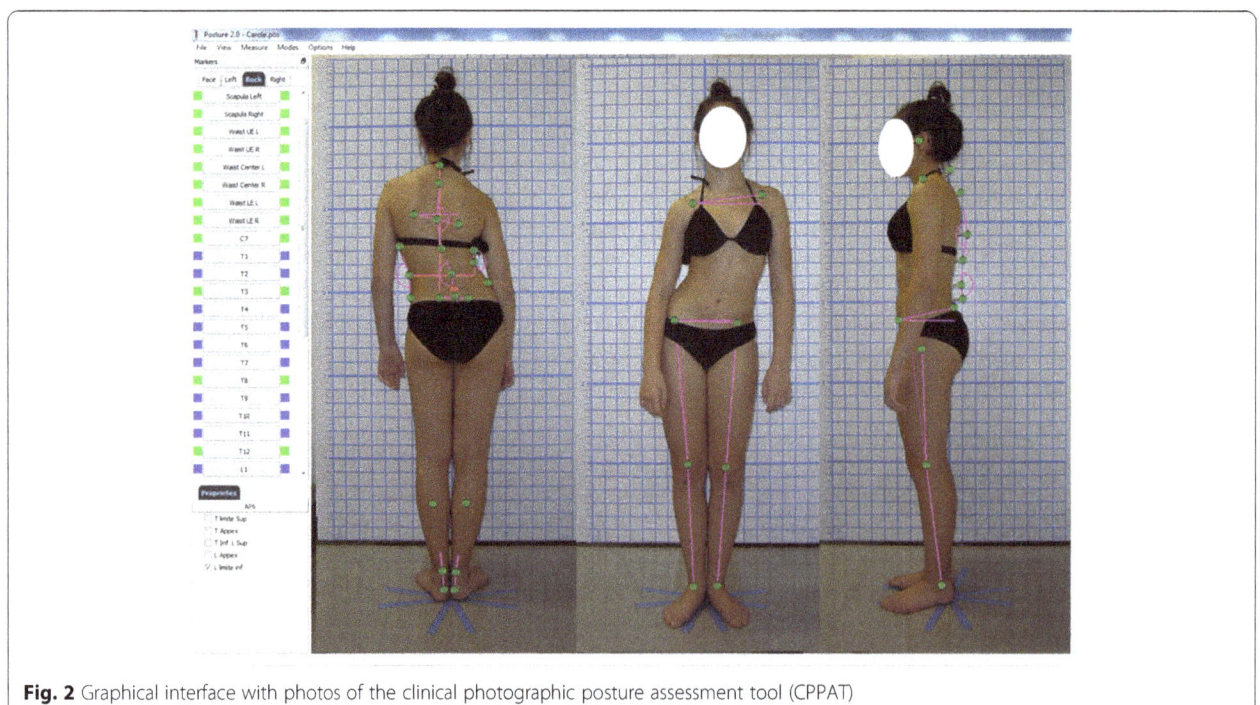

Fig. 2 Graphical interface with photos of the clinical photographic posture assessment tool (CPPAT)

photo acquisition and 3) instruction and practice using the software for photo-processing. As part of their training, clinician-participants had to use the software program to assess posture of three persons (patients or colleagues) before beginning the trial, to ensure they were familiar with the posture assessment procedure. Following the training period, participants were asked to collect the number of patients assessed with the tool and time spent for photo acquisition and for photo-processing with the software program on a data sheet for three months.

The second part consisted of a post-trial focus group discussion in small groups of up to six participants. Before beginning the discussion, participants submitted their data sheet with the number of patients analysed with the tool, together with the time for photo acquisition and photo-processing. Subsequently, van Schaik et al.'s [22] questionnaire was used to measure technology acceptance in terms of perceived ease of use, perceived usefulness and intention to use (see Additional file 2). The focus group discussion was conducted by the researchers in UK (J B-S) and in France (CF) and a physical therapist research assistant (J-F A-F) in Quebec (Canada). We used a semi-structured procedure with specific questions regarding general positive and negative aspects of the tool, its utility, utilization and patients' feedback. Participants were also asked to comment on the advantages/disadvantages they experienced of the clinical method, drivers/barriers of system use and other possible applications of the method.

Statistical analysis

Descriptive statistics (mean and *SD*), confidence intervals and *t*-tests were used to characterize the number of patients assessed with the method and time for photo acquisition and photo-processing with the CPPAT. The data were examined for normality; skew and kurtosis were not extreme ($|z[skew]|$ < 1.8; z[kurtosis] < 1.1) and the distributions were not significantly different from the normal distribution(Komolgorov-S-mirnov test: $p > .05$). t-tests were used to determine if scores obtained for each sub-scale differed from the neutral score (represented by a value of 4 on a seven-point Likert scale). We assessed reliability of each acceptance measure scale by calculating Cronbach's alpha. Correlation analysis examined the association between the three acceptance variables. A first mediation analysis was conducted to test perceived usefulness as a potential mediator of perceived ease of use to predict intention to use the system; a second analysis tested mediation of the predictor average photo-processing time (see mediation models in Figs. 3 and 4)[1].

A qualitative analysis was achieved using van Schaik et al.'s [22] procedure to document drivers and barriers to the acceptance of the CPPAT. The research physical therapist (J-F A-F) read all comments and initially categorised each comment into themes. He reviewed the themes again and created more general (higher-order) categories on top of the initial categories. He and the senior researcher (CF) then discussed and agreed a higher-order list of themes/categories. Both researchers independently coded all comments using the higher-order categories and recorded their codings. Finally, they compared their results, noted the number of disagreements out of the total number of codings, and discussed and resolved any disagreements.

Results
System use

During the course of the trial, participants assessed a mean of 7.7 patients ($SD = 4.17$, $CI(95\%) = [6.14; 9.29]$). The most frequent medical diagnosis were respectively idiopathic scoliosis, back pain and hyper-kyphosis. At their first evaluation, clinician-participants took 36 min (mean, $SD = 19$, $CI(95\%) = [29; 43])$[2] for photo acquisition and 54 min (mean, $SD = 29$, $CI(95\%) = [43; 66]$) for photo-processing with CPPAT. At their last evaluation, the time-on-task with the CPPAT decreased significantly, to 22 min (mean, $SD = 10$, $CI(95\%) = [18; 27]$, $t(20) = 3.99$, $p = .001$, $d = 0.88$) for photo acquisition and to 36 min (mean, $SD = 19$, $CI(95\%) = [29; 44]$, $t(20) = 5.29$, $p < .001$, $d = 0.74$) for photo-processing.

Level of acceptance

Perceived usefulness, perceived ease of use and intention to use were measured reliably (Cronbach's alpha = 0.89, 0.92 and 0.87, respectively).[3] Descriptive statistics indicated that

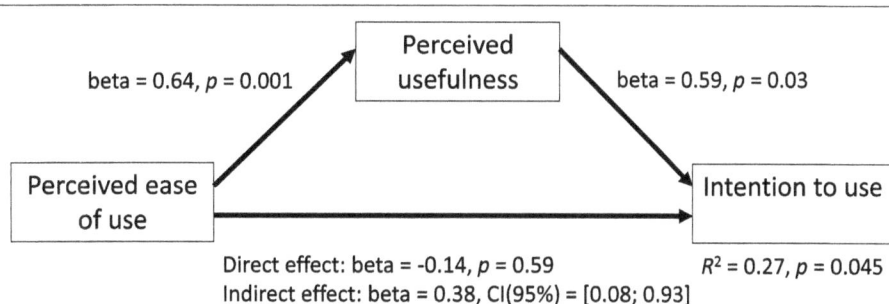

Fig. 3 Mediation analysis (perceived ease of use)

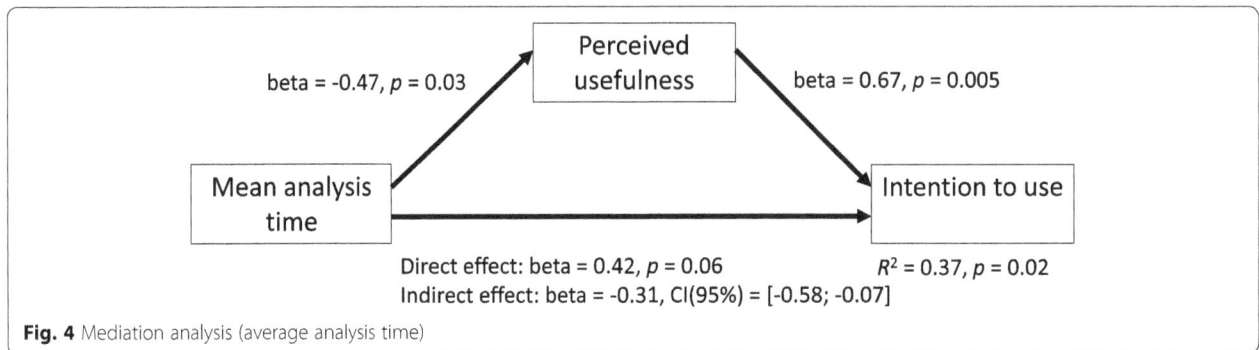

Fig. 4 Mediation analysis (average analysis time)

respondents believed the CPPAT was useful (mean = 5.09, $SD = 1.05$, $CI(95\%) = [4.66; 5.52]$), easy to use (mean = 4.83, $SD = 1.29$, $CI(95\%) = [4.32; 5.30]$) and had the intention to use the tool (mean = 4.42 ($SD = 1.27$, $CI(95\%) = [3.90; 4.98]$). Perceived usefulness, perceived ease of use and intention to use were significantly higher than neutral, with a large effect size ($d = 1.04$), medium effect size ($d = 0.64$) and small effect size ($d = 0.31$), respectively.[4]

Mediation model of technology acceptance

Correlations among the variables showed that perceived usefulness was strongly correlated with perceived ease of use ($r = .64$, $p = .001$) and intention to use ($r = .51$, $p = .01$). Therefore, as perceived usefulness and perceived ease of use increased, intention to use also increased. The correlation between perceived ease of use and intention to use was small ($r = .24$, $p = .26$). In addition, mean analysis time was strongly negatively correlated with perceived usefulness ($r = -.47$, $p = .03$) and moderately negatively correlated with perceived ease of use ($r = -.39$, $p = .08$). Therefore, as time increased, perceived usefulness and perceived ease of use decreased. The positive correlation between intention to use and analysis time was small ($r = .11$, $p = .64$).

Mediation analyses were conducted to test perceived usefulness as a mediator of the predictors (1) perceived ease of use and (2) analysis time for intention to use. In the first analysis, the mediation model was statistically significant, explaining 27% of variance in intention to use (see Fig. 3). Perceived ease of use was significant as an indirect positive predictor of intention to use, mediated by perceived usefulness. Therefore, the reason why intention to use was higher when the system was perceived to be easier to use was that it was perceived to be more useful. However, perceived ease of use was not significant as a direct predictor. According to Zhao et al.'s [31] decision tree, the pattern of results can be interpreted as indirect-only mediation: the mediator fully mediated[5] and explained the prediction of intention to use by perceived ease of use. Apart from its function as a mediator, its significant regression coefficient on intention to use (see Fig. 3) shows that perceived usefulness was also a predictor of intention to use, independent of perceived ease of use.

The mediation model in the second analysis was also significant, explaining 37% of variance in intention to use (see Fig. 4). Analysis time was significant as an indirect negative predictor of the intention to use, mediated by perceived usefulness. Therefore, the reason why intention to use was reduced when analysis time was longer was that the system was perceived to be less useful. Analysis time was significant as a direct predictor, so mediation was partial: the prediction of intention to use by analysis time was partially mediated by perceived usefulness. According to Zhao et al.'s [31] decision tree, the pattern of results showing partial mediation can be interpreted as indicative of an incomplete theoretical framework. In other words, although part of the prediction of intention to use by analysis time was explained by the mediator perceived usefulness, in future research one or more other further mediators that were not included here may explain the significant direct prediction that was found. Apart from its function as a mediator, its significant regression coefficient on intention to use (see Fig. 4) shows that perceived usefulness also was a predictor of intention to use, independent of analysis time.

Drivers and barriers

Our clinician-participants indicated four principal facilitators/advantages and four principal barriers/disadvantages. Frequencies of advantages and disadvantages are presented in Figs. 5 and 6.

Facilitators/advantages

Principal advantages were objective measures (17), visualization for both patients and therapists (17), utility (16), and ease of use (12). Within objective measures, accuracy of measurements and ability to document quantitative changes of posture were the most frequent answers. Regarding visualization, answers showed advantages in helping patients' adherence to treatment, as well as guiding the therapists in seeing posture compensation. For utility, most frequent answers were useful for clinical research, as an x-ray substitute, screening tool, for patient education, treatment justification, and discussion with physicians. In terms of ease of use, the advantages were stated to be as

Advantages

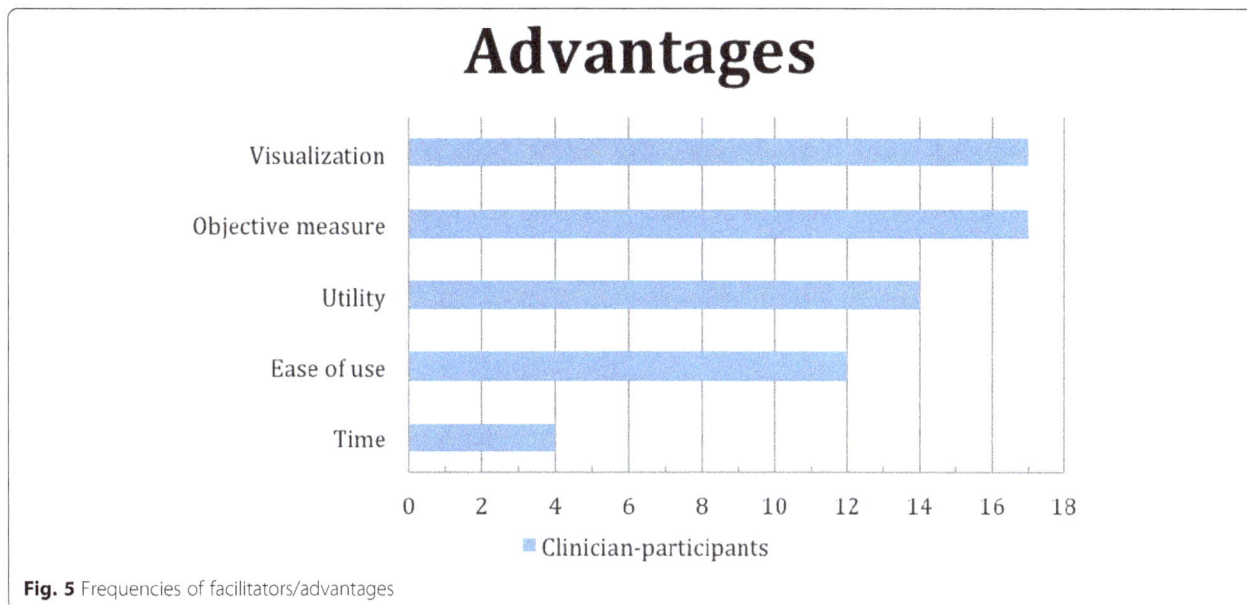

Fig. 5 Frequencies of facilitators/advantages

follows: manipulation of images in the graphical interface and image processing. Four clinician-participants considered time as an advantage since they were able to achieve a complete evaluation of posture within an hour.

Barriers/disadvantages

The principal barriers stated were time to do a complete analysis of posture (19), the quality of human-computer interaction (18), non-automation of posture index calculation and photo transfer (18) and lack of versatility (14). Within the time category, participants included the time to take the photo, to transfer the photo into the software program, as well as processing the photo. For human-computer interaction, participants indicated that it was hard to print or copy the processed photo, the software program was only functioning on Windows systems (not on tablet, iPhone or MAC computer), it was complex to export data and the technology was complex in general for older therapists. Regarding non-automation, the most frequent answers were manual processing of the photo, a few software bugs, manual importation of photo, and manual conversion from pixels to cm for linear posture indices. In terms of versatility, being limited to four photos, all in standing and the lack of some posture indices such as head protraction in cm or not being able to add other posture indices were the most frequent comments reported. Some clinician-participants stated the absence of normative data (5) as well as the patients' discomfort with removing clothing (7) or therapists' comfort in terms of positioning themselves while putting the markers on anatomical landmarks of the lower extremities (3) as further disadvantages.

Disadvantages

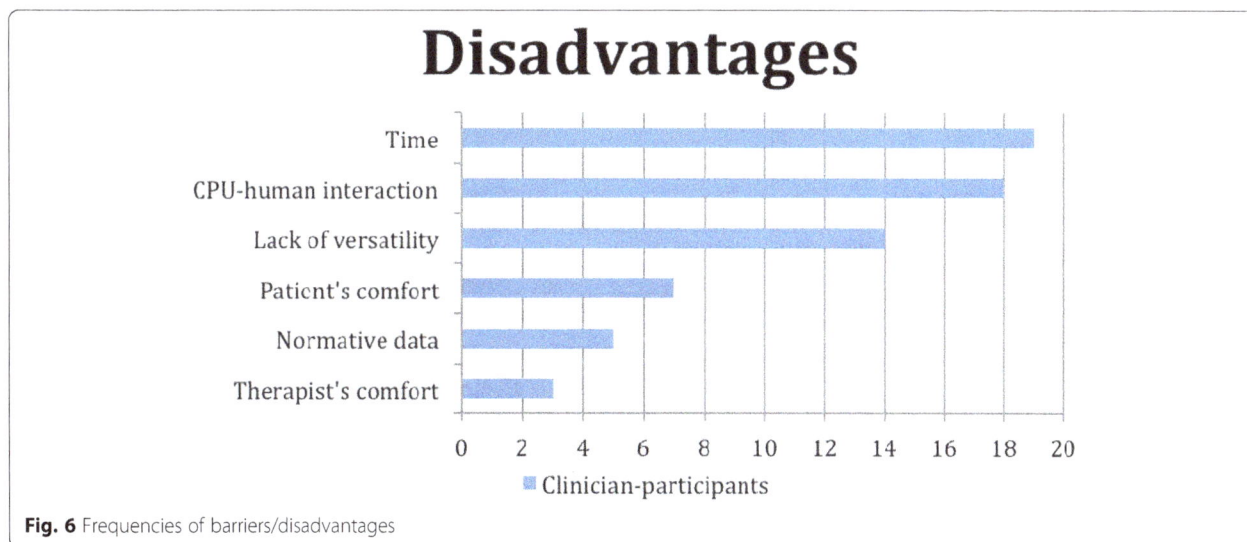

Fig. 6 Frequencies of barriers/disadvantages

Discussion

The aim of this study was to assess the acceptance of a new CPPAT among therapists who frequently assess posture as part of their clinical practice. We found strong and moderate acceptance of the CPPAT respectively in terms of usefulness and ease of use with a slightly positive intention to use the CPPAT. Our mediation analysis revealed that perceived usefulness and perceived ease of use as well as analysis time were indirect predictors of intention to use. This is in agreement with previous studies that showed the importance of these components in technology acceptance [22, 26, 27, 32].

According to Rogers [33], a new technology is more easily adopted if it is compatible with current practice, is seen as more advantageous than current practice and is easy to use (low complexity). Posture assessment was an integral part of the current practice of our participants. However, their perception of performing better in their job was divided: some saw an advantage to use the tool while others did not.

Other factors such as attitudes towards the new innovation, measurement properties of a tool, perception of self-efficacy, being able to observe its use by others and having the possibility to try it out are important for innovation adoption [33–35]. In our study, participants agreed with the good measurement properties of the tool and with the usefulness of the tool for quantifying body posture but their intention to use the tool was only slightly positive. In his model, Davis [24] pointed out that ease of use is often associated with the notion of no effort. For some participants, learning to use the tool seemed to be a greater effort than for other participants and may have led to a perception of poor self-efficacy. Indeed, several participants ($n = 10$) mentioned having a low level of computer use. Human-computer interaction and time to do a complete analysis of posture (photo acquisition and photo-processing with the CPPAT) were the most important barriers to acceptance.

In our laboratory, our research physical therapist takes on average 15 to 20 min for photo acquisition and our trained-students (same training offered to our clinician-participants) take ten to 12 min for photo-processing with the CPPAT for one complete trial. At the end of the three-month trial, 15 out of 23 (65%) and 11 out of 23 (48%) participants achieved this performance, respectively, for photo acquisition and for photo-processing with the CPPAT. With the exception of two participants, the better performance for photo acquisition was found in those participants who were used to take photos as part of their routine posture assessment of their patients.

Furthermore, some participants worked more specifically with children. It was therefore expected that it would take them more time to conduct the photo acquisition because children have more difficulty in maintaining a quiet standing posture [36]. Regarding photo-processing time, all

participants conducted at least three complete evaluations of posture following their practice trial. This suggests that they had the minimal requirements to develop new skills and to achieve a good performance with the CPPAT.

Factors such as clinician-participants' age or level of computer use may have affected task performance [34, 37]. Kaya [37] reported a negative effect of age and of low computer experience on attitudes toward computers in healthcare practitioners. Our clinician-participants had a mean of 20 years of experience in clinical practice and eight out of the ten participants who had taken a longer time for photo-processing with the CPPAT had a low level of computer use, which may explain their difficulty in performing better as well as their low level of interest to use the tool. This may also explain why for half of our participants the graphical interface of the software program was seen as user-friendly while not for the others.

Other barriers for the CPPAT acceptance were the lack of automation of posture index calculation and photo transfer, and the lack of versatility of the tool in terms of positions of posture acquisition and computer operating system. Further development of the tool focusing on automation of photo transfer and posture index analysis would contribute to a substantially decreased time for photo-processing and may thus promote an increased adoption of the tool. Some participants mentioned that they could not take photos in other positions apart from standing or could not add new posture indices. In the present study, they were asked to take photos in a standing position but we showed in a previous study that it is also possible to take and analyse photos in a sitting position [17]. Moreover, new posture indices would be easy to implement in a new version of the tool.

Limitations

The main limitation of our study was the small number of participants that completed the trial. However, this sample size was large enough to demonstrate a high level of perceived ease of use and perceived usefulness and demonstrate statistical mediation, and identify the main barriers for the CPPAT acceptance. Moreover, the sample size in each country was too small to formally compare the results between countries. The two participants in France were familiar with sophisticated systems to measure static and dynamic posture. Hence, they both found the tool easy to use and user-friendly. Participants from UK and Quebec (Canada) were more heterogeneous and tend to show similar results in the acceptance of the tool.

We also acknowledge that some participants did not have easy access to a dedicated space for photo acquisitions even though this was an inclusion criterion. Moreover, a non-facilitating environment including the absence of local champions is an important barrier and may affect innovation adoption [33, 35]. Although we had identified champions in several centres before the study began, for several reasons, these persons could not act as champion in their respective centre. A local champion might have helped in resolving problems such as the accessibility to a dedicated space for photo acquisitions or minor bugs with the software program. Attitudes towards the new technology and self-efficacy are also important factors for innovation adoption [32, 34]. In this study, we did not directly measure these factors and we did not use a validated questionnaire to measure the level of computer use. This will need to be done in a future study. Selection bias may have occurred since some clinician-participants knew the researchers and the physician leading this project. However, the answers of the clinician-participants seem to objectively reflect their 'true' acceptance of the tool.

Clinical implications

This study highlights the usefulness of the CPPAT for quantifying posture in a clinical setting. The majority of our participants found this tool useful to document quantitative changes of posture, for a complete or partial evaluation of posture, as a screening tool, for patient education as well as for treatment justification and for discussion with physicians. According to our participants, photos allow visualization of posture, which is perceived as a good means to help patients' adherence to treatment and guiding therapists in seeing posture compensation. Participants used the tool among persons presenting with spinal deformities such as scoliosis, hyper-kyphosis or hyper-lordosis, with back pain and lower-limb impairments. Taking photos facilitated the measurement of several body angles at a time and is more accurate and rapid than measuring direct body angles on a person, especially in those with back pain [13]. Few participants mentioned the need to have the software program functioning on Windows systems as well as on tablet, iPhone or MAC computer. Other mobile APPs have been developed to measure posture and showed promising results, but posture indices measurement errors of these APPs and their validity still need to be documented [16, 20]. Some participants also indicated that less than 30 min should be taken for a complete assessment of posture. Being able to integrate automation of photo transfer and of posture index calculation into the CPPAT should allow clinicians to have a more efficient tool and may promote adherence to this tool. To be more cost- and time-effective, clinicians may also select a set of relevant posture indices according to a patient's condition to document change in posture over time. However, clinicians should interpret changes in posture over time with caution since reliability and validity of posture indices measurements of the CPPAT have been reported only in adolescents with idiopathic scoliosis and sensitivity to change of these posture indices measurements is not yet determined.

Conclusion

Our results indicate that the CPPAT is perceived to be useful and easy to use by clinicians. The CPPAT tool contributes to clinical practice by facilitating the quantitative analysis of posture and by enhancing the education of patients presenting with different musculoskeletal impairments. The principal barriers for the acceptance of CPPAT were the time to conduct a complete postural analysis and difficulties in interacting with the system. Adapting the software-human interface and automation for posture index calculation may facilitate the wider adoption of the tool.

Endnotes

[1]In a mediation model, the followings effects are analysed: (1) the effect of the mediator (e.g., perceived usefulness) on the outcome (e.g., intention to use), with the predictor (e.g., perceived ease of use) held constant, (2) the direct effect of the predictor on the outcome with the mediator held constant and (3) the indirect effect of the predictor on the outcome through the mediator.

[2]Bias-corrected accelerated confidence intervals are presented, with $N = 1000$ bootstrap samples.

[3]For ease of interpretation of the results, average scores on each scale were calculated, reverse-scored and then used in subsequent analysis.

[4]Cohen's (1988) conventions for effect size were used for d (small: ± 0.2; medium: ± 0.5; large: ± 0.8) and r (small: ± 0.1; medium: ± 0.3; large: ± 0.5).

[5]Full mediation occurs when the regression coefficient of the predictor (e.g. perceived ease of use) on the outcome variable (e.g. intention to use) becomes non-significant when the mediator (e.g., perceived usefulness) is introduced.

Abbreviations
CPPAT: Clinical Photographic Posture Assessment Tool; TAM: technology acceptance model

Acknowledgements
The authors acknowledge Julie Deceuninck for her contribution in the training of clinician-participants in Lyon (France) and the clinician participants.

Funding
This project was supported by the Planning and Dissemination Grants program of the Canadian Institutes of Health Research (CIHR # 201306DMH – 309711). C.Fortin is currently funded by a Junior 1 salary award from the Fonds de Recherche du Québec – Santé (FRQ-S).

Authors' contribution
CF, JB-S and DEF designed the study. CF, J-FA-F and J-CB were responsible for data collection. CF, PvS and J-FA-F were responsible for data analysis and interpretation. CF and PvS drafted the manuscript. JB-S and DEF critically revised the manuscript. All authors revised and approved the final version of the manuscript.

Competing interests

The authors declare that they have no competing interest.

Author details

[1]École de réadaptation, Faculté de médecine, Université de Montréal, C.P. 6128, succursale Centre-ville, Montréal, Québec H3C 3J7, Canada. [2]Research center, CHU Sainte-Justine, Montreal, Quebec, Canada. [3]Department of Psychology, Teesside University, Middlesbrough, UK. [4]Institute of Health and Social Care, Teesside University, Middlesbrough, UK. [5]Centre Médico-Chirurgical de Réadaptation des Massues, Croix Rouge française, Lyon, France. [6]Institut de Recherche en santé publique de l'Université de Montréal and Centre for interdisciplinary research in rehabilitation, Montreal, Quebec, Canada.

References

1. Kendall Peterson F, McCreary Kendall E, Provance Geise P, McIntyre R, Romani WA. Muscles: testing and function, with posture and pain. 5th ed. Baltimore, MD: Lippincott Williams & Wilkins; 2005.
2. Sahrmann SA. Diagnosis and treatment of movement impairment syndromes. Mosby Inc: St.Louis, MO; 2002.
3. Negrini S, Fusco C, Minozzi S, Atanasio S, Zaina F, Romano M. Exercises reduce the progression rate of adolescent idiopathic scoliosis: results of a comprehensive systematic review of the literature. Disabil Rehabil. 2008; 30(10):772–85.
4. Romano M, Minozzi S, Bettany-Saltikov J, Zaina F, Chockalingam N, Kotwicki T, Maier-Hennes A, Negrini S. Exercises for adolescent idiopathic scoliosis. Cochrane Database Syst Rev. 2012;8 CD007837.
5. Weinstein SL, Dolan LA, Cheng JCY, Danielsson A, Morcuende JA. Adolescent idiopathic scoliosis. Lancet. 2008;371:1527–37.
6. Lensinck MLB, Frijlink AC, Berger MY, Bierma-Zeinstra SMA, Verkerk K, Verhagen AP. Effect of bracing and other conservative interventions in the treatment of idiopathic scoliosis in adolescents: a systematic review of clinical trials. Phys Ther. 2005;85(12):1329–39.
7. Wong MS, Liu WC. Critical review on non-operative management of adolescent idiopathic scoliosis. Prosthetics Orthot Int. 2003;27:242–53.
8. Pazos V, Cheriet F, Dansereau J, Ronsky J, Zernicke RF, Labelle H. Reliability of trunk shape measurements based on 3-D surface reconstruction. Eur Spine J. 2007;16:1882–91.
9. Zabjek KF, Leroux MA, Coillard C, Rivard CH, Prince F. Evaluation of segmental postural characteristics during quiet standing in control and idiopathic scoliosis patients. Clin Biomech. 2005;20:483–90.
10. Carr EK, Kenney FD, Wilson-Barrett J, Newham DJ. Inter-rater reliability of postural observation after stroke. Clin Rehabil. 1999;13:229–42.
11. Tyson SF, DeSouza LH. A clinical model for the assessment of posture and balance in people with stroke. Disabil Rehabil. 2003;25(3):120–6.
12. Canhadas Belli JF, Chaves TC, de Oliveira AS, Grossi DB. Analysis of body posture in children with mild to moderate asthma. Eur J Pediatr. 2009;168: 1207–16.
13. Fortin C, Feldman DE, Cheriet F, Labelle H. Clinical methods for quantifying body segment posture: a literature review. Disabil Rehabil. 2011;33(5):367–83.
14. McEvoy MP, Grimmer K. Reliability of upright posture measurements in primary school children. BMC Musculoskelet Disord. 2005;6:35.
15. Aroeira RM, de Las Casas EB, Pertence AE, Greco M, Tavares JM. Non-invasive methods of computer vision in the posture evaluation of adolescent idiopathic scoliosis. J Bodyw Mov Ther. 2016;20(4):832–43.
16. Boland DM, Neufeld EV, Ruddell J, Dolezal BA, Cooper CB. Inter- and intra-rater agreement of static posture analysis using a mobile application. J Phys Ther Sci. 2016;28(12):3398–402.
17. Fortin C, Ehrmann Feldman D, Cheriet F, Labelle H. Differences in standing and sitting postures of youth with idiopathic scoliosis from quantitative analysis of digital photographs. Phys Occup Ther Pediatr. 2013;33(3):313–26.
18. Fortin C, Feldman Ehrmann D, Cheriet F, Gravel D, Gauthier F, Labelle H. Reliability of a quantitative clinical posture assessment tool among persons with idiopathic scoliosis. Physiotherapy. 2012;98:64–75.
19. Fortin C, Feldman Ehrmann D, Cheriet F, Labelle H. Validity of a quantitative clinical measurement tool of trunk posture in idiopathic scoliosis. Spine. 2010;35(19):E988–94.
20. Thiyagarajan S, Tanna T. Posture analysis by using iPhone app (posture zone) in collegiate – a pilot study. Ann Yoga Phys Ther. 2016;1(1):1002.
21. Strudwick G. Predicting nurses' use of healthcare technology using the technology acceptance model: an integrative review. Comput Inform Nurs. 2015, 33(5):189–198; quiz E181.
22. Van Schaick P, Bettany-Saltikov JA, Jg W. Clinical acceptance of a low cost portable system for postural assessmen. Behav Inf Technol 2002, 219(1):47–57.
23. Robinson J, Dixon J, Macsween A, van Schaik P, Martin D. The effects of exergaming on balance, gait, technology acceptance and flow experience in people with multiple sclerosis: a randomized controlled trial. BMC Sports Sci Med Rehabil. 2015;7:8.
24. Davis FD. User acceptance of information technology: system characteristics, user perceptions and behavioral impacts. Int J Man Mach Stud. 1993;38(3): 475–87.
25. Venkatesh V, Bala H. Technology acceptance model 3 and a research agenda on interventions. Decis Sci. 2008;39(2):273–315.
26. Venkatesh V, Davis FD. Theoretical extension of the technology acceptance model: four longitudinal field studies. Manag Sci. 2000;46(2):186–204.
27. Venkatesh V, Morris MG, Davis GB, Davis FD. User acceptance of information technology: toward a unified view. MIS Quarterly: Management Information Systems. 2003;27(3):425–78.
28. Chiou W, Perng C, Lin C. The relationship between technology acceptance model and usability test - case of performing E-learning task with PDA. 2009 WASE International Conference on Information Engineering, ICIE 2009, Taiyuan, Shanxi 2009:579–582.
29. Northstar basic computer skills certificate. https://www.digitalliteracyassessment.org/standards.
30. Illinois Valley Community College. Basic Computer Skills Self-Assessment. https://www.ivcc.edu/forms/Practice_Skills_Assessment.aspx?ekfrm=11574.
31. Zhao X, Lynch Jr. JG, Chen Q. Reconsidering baron and Kenny: myths and truths about mediation analysis. J Consum Res 2010, 37(2):197–206.
32. Park SY. An analysis of the technology acceptance model in Understanding University students' behavioral intention to use e-learning. Educational Technology & Society. 2009;12(3):150–62.
33. Rogers EM. Diffusion of innovations. New York: Free Press; 2003.
34. Cork RD, Detmer WM, Friedman CP. Development and initial validation of an instrument to measure physicians' use of, knowledge about, and attitudes toward computers. J Am Med Inform Assoc. 1998;5(2):164–76.
35. Graham ID, Logan J. Innovations in knowledge transfer and continuity of care. Can J Nurs Res. 2004;36(2):89–103.
36. Oba N, Sasagawa S, Yamamoto A, Nakazawa K. Difference in postural control during quiet standing between young children and adults: assessment with Center of Mass Acceleration. PLoS One. 2015;10(10): e0140235.
37. Kaya N. Factors affecting nurses' attitudes toward computers in healthcare. Comput Inform Nurs. 2011;29(2):121–9.
38. Davis FD, Venkatesh V. A critical assessment of potential measurement biases in the technology acceptance model : three experiments. Int J Human – Computer Studies. 1996;45:19–45.

18

Periprosthetic infection is the major indication for TKA revision – experiences from a university referral arthroplasty center

S. P. Boelch, A. Jakuscheit, S. Doerries, L. Fraissler, M. Hoberg, J. Arnholdt[*†]◉ and M. Rudert[†]

Abstract

Background: We hypothesized, that periprosthetic joint infection (PJI) accounts for the major proportion of first (primary) and repeated (secondary) Total Knee Arthroplasty revisions at our university referral arthroplasty center.

Methods: One thousand one hundred forty-three revisions, performed between 2008 and 2016 were grouped into primary (55%) and secondary (45%) revisions. The rate of revision indications was calculated and indications were categorized by time after index operation. The odds ratios of the indications for primary versus secondary revision were calculated.

Results: In the primary revision group PJI accounted for 22.3%, instability for 20.0%, aseptic loosening for 14.9% and retropatellar arthrosis for 14.2%. PJI (25.6%) was the most common indication up to 1 year after implantation, retropatellar arthrosis (26.8%) 1–3 years and aseptic loosening (25.6%) more than 3 years after implantation.
In the secondary revision group PJI accounted for 39.7%, aseptic loosening for 16.2% and instability for 13.2%. PJI was the most common indication at any time of revision with 43.8% up to one, 35.4% 1–3 years and 39.4% more the 3 years after index operation.
The odds ratios in repeated revision were 2.32 times higher ($p = 0.000$) for PJI. For instability and retropatellar arthrosis the odds ratios were 0.60 times ($p = 0.006$) and 0.22 times ($p = 0.000$) lower.

Conclusions: PJI is the most common indication for secondary TKA revision and within one year after primary TKA. Aseptical failures such as instability, retropatellar arthrosis and aseptical loosening are the predominant reasons for revision more than one year after primary TKA.

Keywords: Knee arthroplasty, Revision, Periprosthetic infection, Failure

Background

Total knee arthroplasty (TKA) is the treatment of choice for symptomatic arthrosis. Patient satisfaction with TKA has improved from 81.2% between the years 1990 and 1999 to 85% between the years 2000 and 2012 [1], but still absolute revision numbers are increasing. Although revision rates after TKA remain constantly low, data from the Nationwide Inpatient Sample (NIS) showed an increase of TKA revisions of 39% from 48,260 in 2006 to 67,534 in 2010 in the US [2]. In the first annual report of the German joint registry an increase of 144% was demonstrated from 7238 in 2004 to 17,658 in 2014 [3]. Recent clinical studies focusing solely on primary revisions found aseptic reasons such as instability with 19 and 22%, and aseptic loosening with 31 and 22% the two most common indications [4, 5]. The analysis of the Swedish, Norwegian, Finnish, Danish, Australian and the New Zealand registry by Sadoghi et al. stated, that the two most common reasons for TKA revisions between 1979 and 2009 were aseptic and septic loosening with 29.8% and 14.8%, respectively [6]. In contrast to aseptical revisions, management of periprosthetic joint infections

* Correspondence: j-arnholdt.klh@uni-wuerzburg.de
†J. Arnholdt and M. Rudert contributed equally to this work.
Department of Orthopaedic Surgery, Julius-Maximilians University Wuerzburg, Koenig-Ludwig-Haus, 11 Brettreichstrasse, 97074 Wuerzburg, Germany

(PJI) necessitates an interdisciplinary setting and special care [7]. This peculiarity of PJI management leads to a pooling of the affected patients at specialized referral arthroplasty centers, as the study institution is.

That is why we hypothesized, that PJI accounts for the major proportion of primary and secondary revisions at our institution. Additionally, we hypothesized that, in contrast to primary revision, the frequency of PJI is not related to time of revision for secondary revision.

Methods
Study design
This observational study was performed at the Department of Orthopaedic Surgery, University of Wuerzburg in Germany. Approval was waived by the University's ethics committee (approval number 20180613 01).

Setting
In August 2016, our department's electronic data was scanned for all TKA revisions, that were performed since the introduction of our electronic database in December 2008. Only procedures involving an arthrotomy were considered a revision. The failure mechanism described by the operating surgeon as decisive for revision strategy was defined as indication for revision. Indications were categorized into polyethylene (PE)-wear, aseptic loosening, PJI, instability, periprosthetic fracture, malalignment, extensor mechanism deficiency, arthrofibrosis, retropatellar arthrosis and other.

The authors acknowledge that diagnostic algorithms of the painful TKA are discussed controversial and are still under investigation [8–12]. Thus, the predominant indications for revision are described in brief: PE-wear was diagnosed by radiographs showing osteolysis or progressive joint space narrowing under load, by intraoperatively macroscopic visible wear and by histopathologic evaluation of intraoperative samples according to Krenn and Morawietz [13].

PJI was evaluated in accordance with the guidelines of the Infection Disease Society of America [14]. Two stage exchanges were regarded as one event.

Instability was assessed based on the patient's history for example with swelling and giving way events. Additionally, coronal and sagittal instability was evaluated by clinical examination and on radiographs as described elsewhere [10]. In cases of concomitant loosening or PE-wear, these were the primary diagnosis.

Arthrofibrosis was diagnosed by painful restriction of range of motion that was refractory to intensified physiotherapy, without any other underlying reason.

For alignment evaluation, we routinely used the alignment parameters based on The Knee Society Total Knee Arthroplasty Roentgenographic Evaluation and Scoring System [15, 16]. CT-scans were added on the bases of clinical and radiologic work up.

Patients
One thousand one hundred forty-three revisions were identified. Revisions were performed in 36.4% in male and in 63.6% in female patients with a mean age of 67.9 years (21–93). First revisions after the primary TKA (index operation) were assigned to the primary revision group (55.0%). In case of any previous revision, which was not the primary implantation, this was regarded the index operation for the secondary revision group (45.0%).

The mean duration from index operation to revision was 42.1 months (0–279). 55.5% of the primary revision cases and 38.9% of the secondary revision cases were transferred to our institution for further operation.

To support a unification of the time to failure categorization we subdivided the time from index operation to revision in accordance with the recently published study by Thiele et al. into 1 year, 1–3 years and more than 3 years [5].

Statistics
Means were compared with the t-Test. Odds ratios for the indications were calculated depending on primary or secondary revision and tested for significant differences with the Pearson chi square test. Statistics were performed with SPSS 24 (SPSS Inc. Chicago, USA).

Results
Primary revision group
In the primary revision group the major proportion (71.4%) of revisions was due to the four indications: PJI (22.3%), instability (20.0%), aseptic loosening (14.9%) and retropatellar arthrosis (14.2%) (Fig. 1).

26.7% were revised within 1 year after the implantation. In this group, the most common indication was PJI (25.6%), followed by instability (19.0%) and retropatellar arthrosis (13.1%). 31.5% of TKAs failed 1–3 years after implantation. Of these 26.8% were due to retropatellar arthrosis, 24.7% due to instability and 20.7% due to PJI. 41.0% were revised more than three after index operation. 25.6% of these revisions were because of aseptic loosening, 20.2% because of PJI, 18.2% because of PE-wear and 17.4% because of instability. The complete distributions are shown in Fig. 2.

Secondary revision group
In the secondary revision group 68.1% of the revisions were due to three indications: PJI (39.7%), aseptic loosening (16.2%) and instability (13.2%) (Fig. 3).

The most common indication of the 37.7% revisions within 1 year from index operation was PJI (43.8%), followed by aseptic loosening (13.9%) and instability

Periprosthetic infection is the major indication for TKA revision – experiences from a university referral...

139

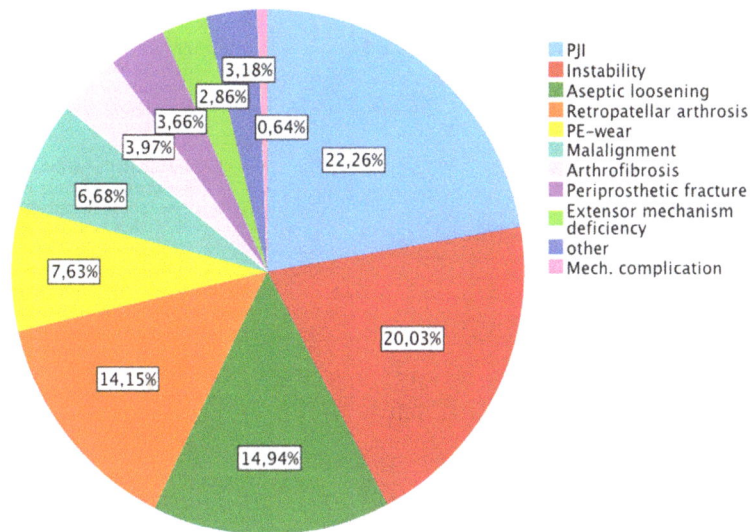

Fig. 1 Indications for primary revision

(11.3%). A comparable distribution was found for the 36.8% revisions between 1 and 3 years with 35.4, 15.9 and 14.8% and for the remaining 25.5% revision after more than 3 years with 39.4, 21.3 and 12.6%. The detailed distributions are depicted in Fig. 4.

Comparison of primary and secondary revisions

The odds of being revised for PJI were 2.5 times higher ($p < 0.000$) for secondary revisions. However, the odds of being revised for instability or retropatellar arthrosis were significantly lower for secondary revisions (Table 1).

The mean duration to revision because of PJI and because of aseptic loosening was significantly ($p = 0.000$) shorter in the secondary revision group (Table 2).

Discussion

We found PJI to be the most common indication for both, primary and secondary TKA revision at a university referral arthroplasty center. This result is in accordance with the numbers published from the NIS for knee arthroplasty revisions, without discriminating primary from secondary revisions [17]. The odds ratio from the current study demonstrates, that PJI is particularly the major revision indication for secondary revisions. The few other available studies on reasons for re-revisions report comparable rates of PJI as revision indication for secondary revisions. Suarez et al. had a re-revision rate of 46% for PJI in their 68 knees that underwent secondary revision [18]. Mortazavi et al. described this rate to be 44% in their study of 102 knees [19]. However, in contrast to previous publications, we found PJI to be the

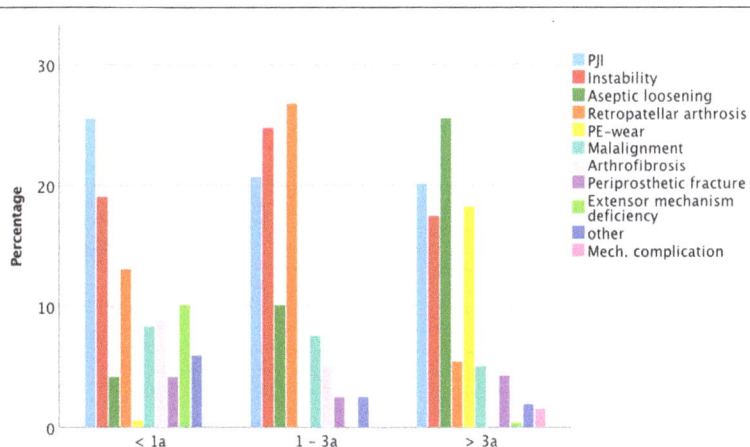

Fig. 2 Distributions of indications for primary revision

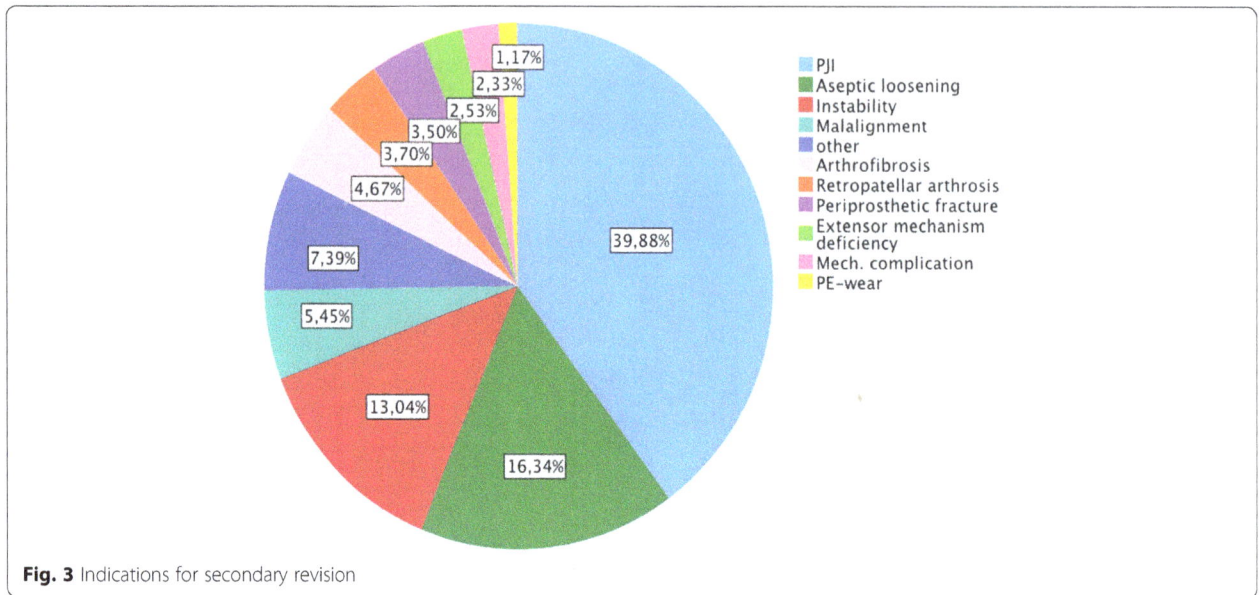

Fig. 3 Indications for secondary revision

most common indication for primary revisions, too. In the study of 358 primary revisions by Thiele et al. PJI was the fourth most common indication with a proportion of 15% [5]. In their study, revisions with component retention were excluded. However, debridement and irrigation with retention of the fixed components is a warranted treatment regime for early postoperative or acute periprosthetic infection [14, 20]. These cases are included in our study and are represented by the finding, that PJI was predominantly found for primary revision within 1 year after index operation. Schroer et al. described PJI the third most common reason with a proportion of 16.2% of 844 patients treated at six different institutions [4]. However, we present monocentric results based on standardized diagnostic algorithms.

In contrast to PJI, retropatellar arthrosis and instability are specific issues of primary TKA. In accordance with our results, instability is consistently reported a major failure mechanism after primary TKA [4, 5, 21]. However, retropatellar arthrosis was the most common revision reason 1–3 years after the implantation, what reflects the development of clinically relevant and radiographically obvious retropatellar wear.

This study has limitations because of its retrospective design and the complexity of TKA revision.

If the treatment of PJI failed and the patient was readmitted, the following revision was considered a new

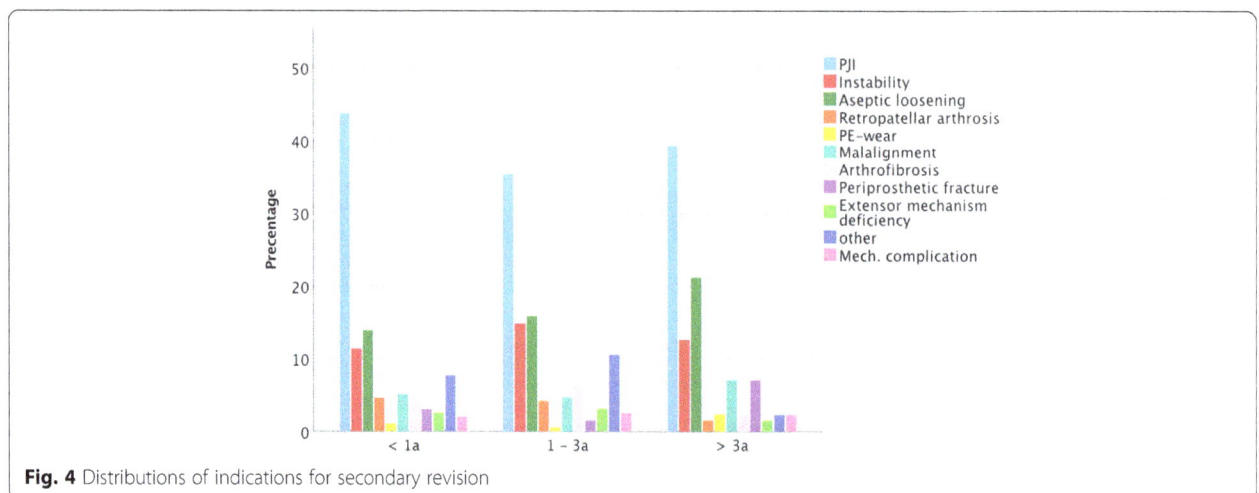

Fig. 4 Distributions of indications for secondary revision

Table 1 Odds ratios depending on secondary revision/primary revision of the 4 major indications for revision

Indication for revision	Odds ratio (95% CI)	Pearson chi square test p
PJI	2.32 (1.79–3.00)	0.000
Instability	0.60 (0.43–0.83)	0.002
Aseptic loosening	1.11 (0.81–1.53)	0.517
Retropat. arthrosis	0.22 (0.13–0.36)	0.000

case. In this study with 345 primary and secondary revisions, about 10% were repeatedly revised for reinfection. Thus, the proportion of PJI might be biased by patient specific characteristics.

Further, we did not investigate the proportion of resurfaced patellae before revision. These cases were not excluded from the analysis because the proportion of failures due to patellar arthrosis is clinically relevant and the discussion of the best treatment is still going on [22]. The significantly higher proportion of retropatellar arthrosis in the primary revision group is highly likely to be owed to the fact, that the secondary revisions had a higher rate of resurfaced patella before re-revision.

The 14th NJR annual reported aseptical failure mechanisms the most frequent reasons for primary revision [23]. The current monocenter study at a university referral arthroplasty center found PJI the leading failure mechanism irrespectively whether after primary or revised TKA. This discrepancy is owed the pooling of patients. It displays the enormous challenge of referral arthroplasty centers to especially ensure the management of PJI as a potentially life threating TKA failure with the danger of devastating sequela.

Conclusion

PJI is the most common indication for secondary TKA revision and within one year after primary TKA. Aseptical failures such as instability, retropatellar arthrosis and aseptical loosening are the predominant reasons for revision more than one year after primary TKA.

Table 2 Mean duration and range from index operation to revision in months

Indication for revision	Duration to primary revision in months (range)	Duration to secondary revision in months (range)	p
PJI	49.00 (0–279)	28.11 (0–198)	0.000
Instability	37.67 (2–226)	31.48 (4–153)	0.301
Aseptic loosening	94.68 (5–242)	31.05 (1–163)	0.000
Retropatellar arthrosis	24.54 (3–106)	19.53 (3–58)	0.677

Abbreviations
CT: Computed tomography; NIS: Nationwide Inpatient Sample; PE: Polyethylene; PJI: Periprosthetic joint infection; TKA: Total knee arthroplasty

Acknowledgments
None.

Funding
This publication was supported by the Open Access Publication Fund of the University of Wuerzburg. The study was funded by internal sources of the Department of Orthopaedic Surgery, Koenig-Ludwig-Haus. The funding body had no role in the design of the study and collection, analysis, and interpretation of data and in writing the manuscript.

Authors' contributions
SB were responsible for the design and coordination of this study and wrote the manuscript. AJ and SD were responsible for the acquisition of data, interpretation of data and performed the statistical analysis. LF made substantial contributions to conception and design of the study and to analysis and interpretation of data. MH and JA supervised the project and helped to draft the manuscript. MR and JA revised the manuscript and gave final approval for publication. MR made substantial contributions to conception and design of the study. All authors read and approved the final manuscript.

Competing interests
The authors declare that they have no competing interests.

References
1. Choi YJ, Ra HJ. Patient satisfaction after total knee arthroplasty. Knee Surg Relat Res. 2016;28(1):1–15. https://doi.org/10.5792/ksrr.2016.28.1.1.
2. Bozic KJ, Kamath AF, Ong K, Lau E, Kurtz S, Chan V, et al. Comparative epidemiology of revision arthroplasty: failed THA poses greater clinical and economic burdens than failed TKA. Clin Orthop Relat Res. 2015;473(6):2131–8. https://doi.org/10.1007/s11999-014-4078-8.
3. EPRD Jahresbericht 2015 [database on the Internet]. Endoprothesenregister Deutschland. 2015. Accessed: 07/05/2017.
4. Schroer WC, Berend KR, Lombardi AV, Barnes CL, Bolognesi MP, Berend ME, et al. Why are total knees failing today? Etiology of total knee revision in 2010 and 2011. J Arthroplast. 2013;28(8 Suppl):116–9. https://doi.org/10.1016/j.arth.2013.04.056.
5. Thiele K, Perka C, Matziolis G, Mayr HO, Sostheim M, Hube R. Current failure mechanisms after knee arthroplasty have changed: polyethylene wear is less common in revision surgery. J Bone Joint Surg Am. 2015;97(9):715–20. https://doi.org/10.2106/JBJS.M.01534.
6. Sadoghi P, Liebensteiner M, Agreiter M, Leithner A, Bohler N, Labek G. Revision surgery after total joint arthroplasty: a complication-based analysis using worldwide arthroplasty registers. J Arthroplast. 2013;28(8):1329–32. https://doi.org/10.1016/j.arth.2013.01.012.
7. Tande AJ, Gomez-Urena EO, Berbari EF, Osmon DR. Management of prosthetic joint infection. Infect Dis Clin N Am. 2017;31(2):237–52. https://doi.org/10.1016/j.idc.2017.01.009.
8. Thiele K, Fussi J, Perka C, Pfitzner T. The Berlin diagnostic algorithm for painful knee TKA. Orthopade. 2016;45(1):38–46. https://doi.org/10.1007/s00132-015-3196-7.
9. Ahmad SS, Becker R, Chen AF, Kohl S. EKA survey: diagnosis of prosthetic knee joint infection. Knee Surg Sports Traumatol Arthrosc. 2016;24(10):3050–5. https://doi.org/10.1007/s00167-016-4303-y.
10. Chang MJ, Lim H, Lee NR, Moon YW. Diagnosis, causes and treatments of instability following total knee arthroplasty. Knee Surg Relat Res. 2014;26(2):61–7. https://doi.org/10.5792/ksrr.2014.26.2.61.
11. De Valk EJ, Noorduyn JC, Mutsaerts EL. How to assess femoral and tibial component rotation after total knee arthroplasty with computed tomography: a systematic review. Knee Surg Sports Traumatol Arthrosc. 2016;24(11):3517–28. https://doi.org/10.1007/s00167-016-4325-5.
12. Hofmann S, Seitlinger G, Djahani O, Pietsch M. The painful knee after TKA: a diagnostic algorithm for failure analysis. Knee Surg Sports Traumatol Arthrosc. 2011;19(9):1442–52. https://doi.org/10.1007/s00167-011-1634-6.

13. Krenn V, Morawietz L, Perino G, Kienapfel H, Ascherl R, Hassenpflug GJ, et al. Revised histopathological consensus classification of joint implant related pathology. Pathol Res Pract. 2014;210(12):779–86. https://doi.org/10.1016/j.prp.2014.09.017.

14. Osmon DRBE, Berendt AR, Lew D, Zimmerli W, Steckelberg JM, Rao N, Hanssen A, Wilson WR, Infectious Diseases Society of America. Executive summary: diagnosis and management of prosthetic joint infection: clinical practice guidelines by the Infectious Diseases Society of America. Clin Infect Dis. 2013;56(1):1–10.

15. Ewald FC. The knee society total knee arthroplasty roentgenographic evaluation and scoring system. Clin Orthop Relat Res. 1989;(248):9–12.

16. Hadi M, Barlow T, Ahmed I, Dunbar M, McCulloch P, Griffin D. Does malalignment affect patient reported outcomes following total knee arthroplasty: a systematic review of the literature. Springerplus. 2016;5(1): 1201. https://doi.org/10.1186/s40064-016-2790-4.

17. Bozic KJ, Kurtz SM, Lau E, Ong K, Chiu V, Vail TP, et al. The epidemiology of revision total knee arthroplasty in the United States. Clin Orthop Relat Res. 2010;468(1):45–51. https://doi.org/10.1007/s11999-009-0945-0.

18. Suarez J, Griffin W, Springer B, Fehring T, Mason JB, Odum S. Why do revision knee arthroplasties fail? J Arthroplast. 2008;23(6 Suppl 1):99–103. https://doi.org/10.1016/j.arth.2008.04.020.

19. Mortazavi SM, Molligan J, Austin MS, Purtill JJ, Hozack WJ, Parvizi J. Failure following revision total knee arthroplasty: infection is the major cause. Int Orthop. 2011;35(8):1157–64. https://doi.org/10.1007/s00264-010-1134-1.

20. Parvizi J, Gehrke T, Chen AF. Proceedings of the international consensus on periprosthetic joint infection. Bone Joint J. 2013;95-B(11):1450–2. https://doi.org/10.1302/0301-620X.95B11.33135.

21. Fehring TK, Odum S, Griffin WL, Mason JB, Nadaud M. Early failures in total knee arthroplasty. Clin Orthop Relat Res. 2001;392:315–8.

22. Sandiford NA, Alao U, Salamut W, Weitzel S, Skinner JA. Patella resurfacing during total knee arthroplasty: have we got the issue covered? Clin Orthop Surg. 2014;6(4):373–8. https://doi.org/10.4055/cios.2014.6.4.373.

23. 14 Anual Report 2017 National Joint Registry for England, Wales, Northern Ireland and the Isle of Man [database on the Internet] 2017. Available from: http://www.njrreports.org.uk/Portals/0/PDFdownloads/NJR%2014th%20Annual%20Report%202017.pdf. Accessed: 2017/10/07.

19

Thymol turbidity test is associated with the risk of cyclops syndrome following anterior cruciate ligament reconstruction

Yuya Kodama, Takayuki Furumatsu*, Tomohito Hino, Yusuke Kamatsuki, Yoshiki Okazaki, Shin Masuda, Yuki Okazaki and Toshifumi Ozaki

Abstract

Background: Cyclops nodule formation is a serious complication after anterior cruciate ligament (ACL) reconstruction. The purpose of our study was to investigate whether an increase in thymol turbidity test (TTT) values is involved in the development of cyclops nodule formation or cyclopoid scar formation following ACL reconstruction.

Methods: Between 2011 and 2014, 120 cases underwent outside-in ACL reconstruction. Forty-seven patients who had high TTT values were individually matched for age, sex, body mass index, and meniscus injury to a low TTT value group of 47 patients. The primary outcome was the occurrence of cyclops nodule formation or cyclopoid scar formation. All 94 patients were divided into 3 groups using surgical records and intra-operative video to enable a sub-analysis. The groups were a no-cyclops group, a cyclopoid group, and a cyclops group. Blood examinations, including TTT, and knee range of motion evaluations were performed before surgery, 3 months after surgery, and 1 year after surgery.

Results: There were no differences in preoperative demographic data between the two groups. TTT values did not significantly influence cyclopoid scar formation (OR, 1.67; 95% CI, 0.62 to 4.66; $p = 0.362$). However, patients with cyclops nodule formation showed significantly higher TTT values than the control patients. (OR, 9.34; 95% CI, 1.94 to 90.3; $p = 0.002$). Knee extension loss was observed in the cyclopoid and cyclops groups 3 months after reconstruction. In the cyclops group, arthroscopic resection of the cyclops nodule was performed 3 months after reconstruction. Eventually, almost full range of motion was restored in all patients.

Conclusions: High TTT values before ACL reconstruction were an indicator of cyclops nodule formation. Furthermore, cyclopoid scar formations may not be the result of an individual's immune reaction but that of extension loss in the early post-reconstruction phase.

Keywords: Cyclops syndrome, Anterior cruciate ligament, Thymol turbidity test, Cyclops nodule, Knee extension, Range of motion, Cyclopoid scar

Background

Cyclops nodule formation is a serious complication after anterior cruciate ligament (ACL) reconstruction, and it is characterized by loss of terminal knee extension due to proliferative fibrous nodule formation in the intercondylar notch [1]. The incidence of post-operative cyclops nodule formation ranges from 1.9 to 10.6% [2, 3], whereas the incidence of cyclops lesions without extension loss varies from 2.2 to 46.8% [4, 5]. This distinction of symptoms is due to 2 distinct types of cyclops lesions, a true cyclops nodule and a cyclopoid scar [6]. Although there are several hypotheses regarding the pathogenesis of cyclops nodule formation, including bone and cartilage residue in the joint following tibial tunnel drilling and preparation for graft passage [1, 6], repeated graft impingement on the notch [1], post-operative hamstring contracture [7], and narrowing of the femoral intercondylar notch [8], histologically, a cyclops nodule formation is composed of disorganized

* Correspondence: matino@md.okayama-u.ac.jp
Department of Orthopaedic Surgery, Okayama University Graduate School of Medicine, Dentistry, and Pharmaceutical Sciences, 2-5-1 Shikatacho, Kitaku, Okayama 700-8558, Japan

fibrous connective tissue with a central region of granulation tissue and newly formed vessels [1, 5, 6]. Cyclopoid scar formations are composed of a build-up of fibrous tissue showing elements of granulation tissue [6]. However, the same symptoms, along with similar arthroscopic and histologic findings, also occur in acute ACL injury without reconstruction [9, 10]. Therefore, the reparative processes occurring as an immune reaction of the vital tissue may be the main triggering factors for the process of cyclops nodule formation.

The thymol turbidity test (TTT) is a type of colloidal reaction test that reflects immunoglobulin M [11]. TTT is considered a marker of inflammatory conditions such as chronic hepatitis, chronic infection, or collagen disease [12, 13]. Before ACL reconstruction surgery, we routinely perform blood examination, including the TTT. By chance, we discovered that TTT results tended to be higher in patients with cyclops nodule formation, whereas there were no other blood examination abnormalities. To the best of our knowledge, a relationship between an immune reaction of the vital tissue and cyclops or cyclopoid development has been proposed, but not yet proven [6, 9]. In addition, there are no reports on blood examinations in patients with cyclops syndrome. The purpose of our study was to investigate whether an increase in TTT value was involved in the occurrence of cyclops nodule formation or cyclopoid scar formation. Furthermore, in order to investigate this in detail, a comparison between 3 groups (a no-cyclops group, a cyclopoid group, and a cyclops group) was performed using blood test results and knee range of motion measurements.

Methods
Study subjects
This retrospective study was performed with the approval of the institutional review board, and all patients signed the consent form drafted for the study. Between 2011 and 2014, 120 consecutive patients underwent outside-in ACL reconstruction [14] performed by two surgeons at our hospital. Exclusion criteria were patients who had previous ligament injury, and those who had a concomitant medial collateral ligament injury classified as greater than grade III. Patients who had undergone revision ACL reconstruction were also excluded. Finally, 47 patients with TTT ≥ 4 and 58 patients with TTT < 4 were included. The 47 patients in the TTT ≥ 4 group were matched for age, sex, and body mass index (BMI) with 47 patients in the TTT < 4 group (Fig. 1). In order to conduct case-control research, the research design was set as follows. The population included patients for whom final assessments could be made after reconstruction following an ACL tear. Exposure was defined as a TTT value ≥4 and control was defined as a TTT value < 4. Outcomes included the occurrence of cyclops nodule formation or cyclopoid scar formation. Cyclops and cyclopoid lesions were diagnosed using arthroscopic video based on a previous report [6].

All 94 patients were divided into 3 groups using surgical records and intra-operative video to perform a sub-analysis (Fig. 2). These groups were a cyclops group (case) ($n = 16$), a no-cyclops group (control 1) ($n = 51$), and a cyclopoid group (control 2) ($n = 27$). In addition to the TTT, aspartate transaminase (AST), alanine transaminase (ALT), and C-reactive protein (CRP) levels were evaluated 1 week before reconstruction. The same inspection was performed after cyclops resection (3 months after reconstruction) and 1 week before second-look arthroscopy. The knee range of motion at 3 different time points was determined from clinical records.

Surgical procedure
A double-bundle, outside-in, arthroscopic ACL reconstruction was performed in all patients, using the semitendinosus tendon (ST) and, if necessary, the gracilis tendon. The harvested tendons were double-looped over an Endobutton fixation device (Smith & Nephew, Andover, MA), with the distal ends anchored using a Krackow suture, thus recreating the anteromedial (AM) and posterolateral (PL) bundles of the ACL. To prevent elongation of the grafts, a continuous 30-s loading with 70 N was applied twice to the graft (70 N-1 min), and then the same loading was applied repeatedly (70 N-2 min) [15]. The femoral tunnel was created using an outside-in technique. The longitudinal linear resident's ridge [16] and the posterior cartilage, used as landmarks for the ACL femoral footprint, were identified. Two 2.4-mm guide pins were then inserted separately from the outside into the ACL footprints behind the resident's ridge and just anterior to the articular margin, using an anterolateral entry femoral aimer (Smith & Nephew). A 5.5-mm to 6.5-mm tunnel was then created for the AM and PL grafts by over-drilling via the guide pins. The autogenous tendon was harvested and transected into 2 double-looped grafts. Two Endobutton-CLs® (Smith & Nephew) were connected to the end of each loop graft. The appropriate graft length was determined from the length of the femoral tunnel to allow the introduction of sufficient graft materials (> 13 mm) into the bone tunnels. After creation of the femoral tunnel, the ACL tibial tunnel was created. The AM tunnel was created using the following intra-articular landmarks: just lateral to the medial intercondylar ridge and just posterior to the anterior ridge so as not to damage the lateral meniscus anterior insertion [17, 18]. The PL tunnel was created posterior to the AM tunnel, just lateral to the medial intercondylar ridge. In all cases, tibial fixation of the graft was performed using double-spike plates (Meira, Aichi, Japan), with the knee flexed at 20°, and an initial

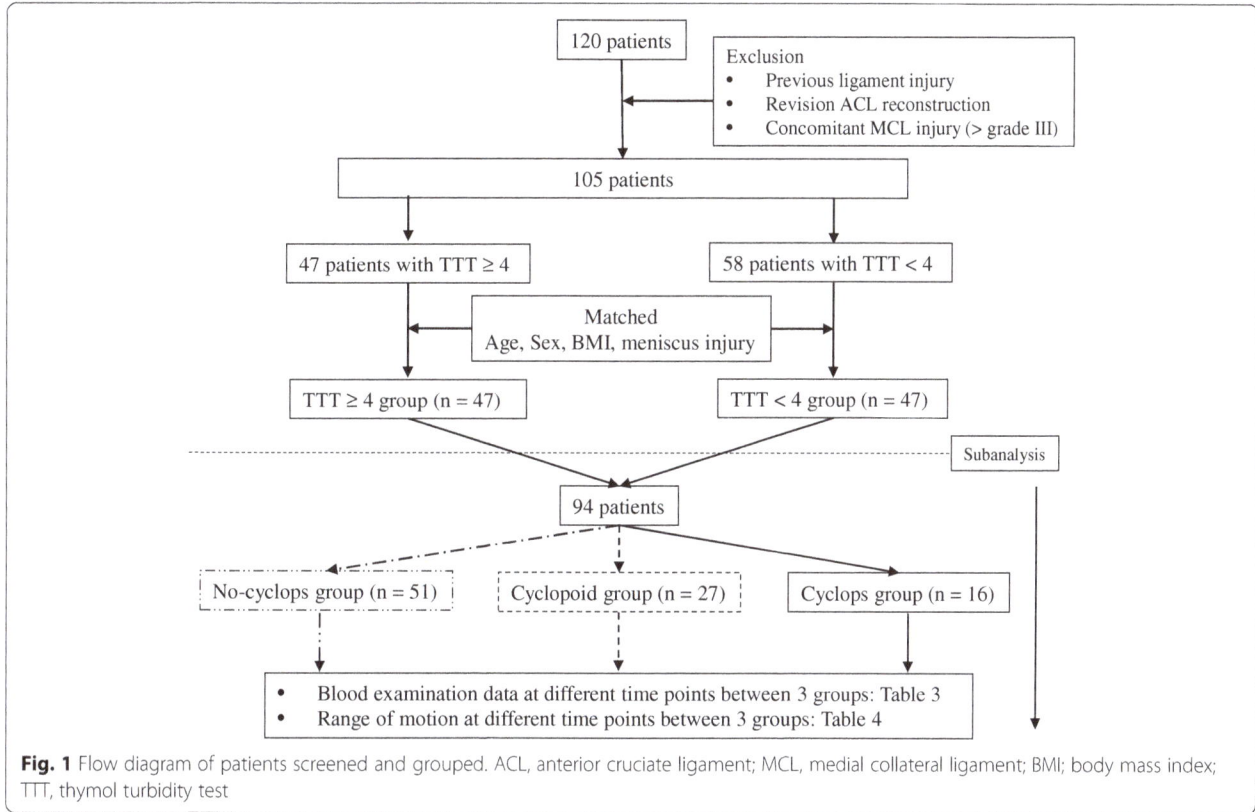

Fig. 1 Flow diagram of patients screened and grouped. ACL, anterior cruciate ligament; MCL, medial collateral ligament; BMI; body mass index; TTT, thymol turbidity test

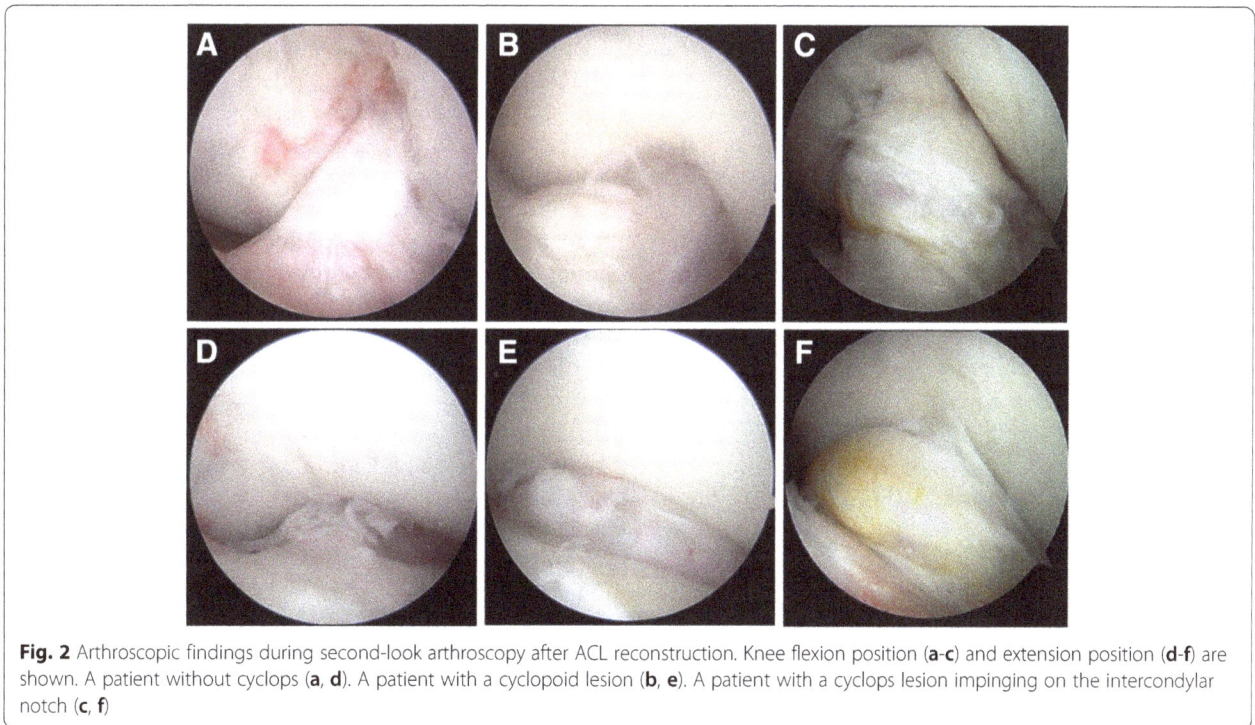

Fig. 2 Arthroscopic findings during second-look arthroscopy after ACL reconstruction. Knee flexion position (**a-c**) and extension position (**d-f**) are shown. A patient without cyclops (**a**, **d**). A patient with a cyclopoid lesion (**b**, **e**). A patient with a cyclops lesion impinging on the intercondylar notch (**c**, **f**)

tension of 20 N was applied to the PL bundle and 30 N to the AM bundle. The tension in each bundle was measured independently using a tensiometer. Finally, we checked for impingement to the notch at full extension. In all cases, there was no impingement to the notch at full extension. Thus, femoral notchplasty was not performed in all cases.

Second-look arthroscopic examination, clinical evaluations, and post-operative management

Second-look arthroscopy was performed approximately 1 year after reconstruction for the removal of the 2 double-spike plates, fixed with screws into the tibia, which were used for tibial fixation of the ACL graft. Knee range of motion was evaluated with a goniometer before reconstruction, 3 months after reconstruction, and after second-look arthroscopy. Extension loss was measured in degrees and compared with the normal contralateral extremity. For post-operative rehabilitation, knees without associated meniscal tears were maintained in a brace for 1 week, and knees with meniscus sutures were immobilized for 2 weeks. After immobilization, all patients followed the same rehabilitation protocol including isometric exercises, range of motion exercises, and proprioceptive rehabilitation.

Blood examination

Blood examination, including TTT, was performed in all patients automatically using a reagent (Clinimate TTT reagent, Sekisui Medical, Japan) that does not require adjustment. This reagent can be used in an automatic analyzer. The reference standard range was set to 4 McLagan units or less.

Statistical analysis

Descriptive data were presented as the mean ± standard deviation (SD). We first performed a Fisher's exact test to obtain odds ratios (ORs) of the occurrence of cyclops nodule formation and cyclopoid scar formation in the control and exposure groups. An independent-samples Student's t test was used to compare group differences for normally distributed variables. The Mann-Whitney U test was used for non-normally distributed variables and a one-way analysis of variance with the Fisher protected least significant difference test for post hoc multiple comparisons. All analyses were performed using SPSS 11.0. Statistical significance was set at $p < 0.05$, a priori.

Results

As mentioned above, 47 patients were included in each group in this retrospective study. There were no differences in preoperative patient characteristics between the two groups (Table 1). TTT values did not significantly

Table 1 Preoperative patient characteristics

	TTT ≥ 4 (n = 47)	TTT < 4 (n = 47)	P value
Mean age, years	24.0 ± 7.4	24.0 ± 6.4	0.989
Gender (Male/Female)	26/21	26/21	1.000
BMI, kg/m^2	23.7 ± 3.3	23.2 ± 3.0	0.488
Meniscal injury, n, %	33 (70.2%)	25 (53.2%)	0.137

Data are expressed as the mean ± SD
TTT thymol turbidity test, *BMI* body mass index

influence cyclopoid scar formation (OR, 1.67; 95% CI, 0.62 to 4.66; $p = 0.362$). However, patients with cyclops nodule formation showed significantly higher TTT values than the control patients. (OR, 9.34; 95% CI, 1.94 to 90.3; $p = 0.002$) (Table 2).

Cyclops nodule formation was found in 16 of the 94 patients (14.9%) and cyclopoid lesions were found in 27 patients (28.7%) during second-look arthroscopy. Blood examination data before ACL reconstruction showed that the cyclops group (case) had a significant highly TTT value compared to the no-cyclops (control 1) and cyclopoid group (control 2) (6.3 ± 3.6, 3.3 ± 2.0, and 3.8 ± 2.4, respectively; $p < 0.05$) (Table 3). There was no difference in TTT values in the no-cyclops group (control 1) and the cyclopoid group (control 2). When comparing the different time point blood examinations, TTT values were significantly lower after resection of the cyclops lesion (3 months after reconstruction) and before second-look arthroscopy compared to before reconstruction. After cyclops nodule resection, TTT values increased slightly until before second-look arthroscopy, but did not return to pre-reconstruction TTT values.

Range of motion was compared in the 3 groups (Table 4). There was no significant difference in the 3 groups before reconstruction. Extension loss was observed in the cyclopoid (control 2) and cyclops groups (case) 3 months after reconstruction. In addition, knee flexion was also restricted in the cyclops group (case) compared to that in the no-cyclops group (control 1). In the cyclops group (case), arthroscopic resection of the cyclops nodule was performed 3 months after reconstruction. Eventually, almost full range of motion was restored in all patients and there were no dissatisfied patients.

Discussion

The most important finding of this study was that high TTT values before ACL reconstruction may be a potential risk factor for developing cyclops nodule formation. Many researchers have reported that the cause of cyclops syndrome (due to an impinged cyclops nodule) is multi-factorial, and therefore, the pathological condition is not completely understood [1, 7, 8]. In fact, although surgical procedures corresponding to the causative disease condition have been reported [19, 20], surgical procedures still fail to prevent the

Table 2 Odds of cyclops nodule and cyclopoid scar following TTT value

	TTT ≥ 4 ($n = 47$)	TTT < 4 ($n = 47$)	OR (95% CI)	P value
Cyclops nodule, n, %	14 (29.8%)	2 (4.26%)	9.34 (1.94–90.3)	0.002*
Cyclopoid scar, n, %	16 (34.0%)	11 (23.4%)	1.67 (0.62–4.66)	0.362

Data are expressed as the mean ± SD
*Statistically significant difference ($P < 0.05$)
TTT thymol turbidity test

occurrence of cyclops lesions. We believe the cyclops nodule formation that occurs after surgery is related to the individual's immune response. This is because the patterns observed during cyclops nodule formation cannot be explained by the potential causes that have been reported so far. The clinical problem of cyclops syndrome (due to an impinged cyclops nodule) is to cause loss of irreversible knee extension that does not improve without surgery. Furthermore, nodule formation is considered to be completed by about 6 weeks after surgery [7]. On the other hand, it has been reported that resection of cyclops nodule formation improves symptoms without recurrence. This suggests that acute vital tissue reactions occurring after ACL injury or in the early phase after reconstruction may be involved in development of cyclops nodules. The continuous contact between the graft and intercondylar notch may produce an irritating stimulus, which may induce an inflammatory response with the production of granulation tissue, which would be transformed into fibrocartilaginous and cartilaginous tissue [21]. However, because all knees in our cohort achieved full extension at the end of surgery, failure to regain full extension may be due the wound healing process after surgery. Intra-

or post-operative factors may promote the process, but they are not the key factors. Injury to the ligament and the reparative processes occurring as a result of vital tissue reactions are the main triggering factors for cyclops nodule formation [9]. The response of living tissue in this reparative process varies from individual to individual, and it is possible that an immune response is involved.

We discovered that TTT values associated with the risk of developing cyclops nodule formation following ACL reconstruction. TTT was reported as an indicator of hepatic injury in the mid-twentieth century [13]. Basically, this examination reflects a decrease in serum albumin and an increase in globulin. γ globulin has a tendency to precipitate, and this increases the amount of sedimentation; however, if hydrophilic albumin increases, γ globulin does not precipitate. The TTT value is relatively high even with lower albumin levels associated with chronic hepatitis and chronic inflammation. Although, we did evaluate AST, ALT, and CRP, and there were no differences at the different time points (before reconstruction, at 3 months, and 1 year after reconstruction) (Table 3). Previous reports have shown that TTT is

Table 3 Blood examination data at different time points between 3 groups

Blood examination (mean value)	Control 1 ($n = 51$)	Control 2 ($n = 27$)	Case ($n = 16$)	F value
Before ACL reconstruction				
TTT	3.3 ± 2.0	3.8 ± 2.4	6.3 ± 3.6[a]	8.86
AST	19.2 ± 3.7	19.1 ± 4.9	20.9 ± 5.8	2.25
ALT	20.6 ± 6.3	20.6 ± 8.3	22.7 ± 13.1	3.65
CRP	0.1 ± 0.1	0.1 ± 0.2	0.1 ± 0.1	0.88
3 months after reconstruction (after cyclops resection)				
TTT	–	–	3.5 ± 1.3[b]	
AST	–	–	20.4 ± 4.9	
ALT	–	–	22.5 ± 10.5	
CRP	–	–	0.10 ± 0.1	
Before second-look arthroscopy				
TTT	3.4 ± 1.9	3.4 ± 1.5	4.5 ± 1.2[a/b]	9.86
AST	21.2 ± 4.5	20.4 ± 3.9	21.6 ± 6.7	2.21
ALT	20.5 ± 5.8	19.1 ± 8.3	22.7 ± 11	3.75
CRP	0.1 ± 0.5	0.2 ± 0.6	0.1 ± 0.3	1.25

Data are expressed as the mean ± SD
ACL anterior cruciate ligament, *TTT* thymol turbidity test, *AST* aspartate transaminase, *ALT* alanine transaminase, *CRP* C-reactive protein
[a]$P < 0.05$ when compared with control 1 and control 2 group, using post hoc multiple comparisons
[b]$P < 0.05$ when compared with before reconstruction, using Student's t test

Table 4 Range of motion at different time points

Range of motion	Control 1 (n = 51)	Control 2 (n = 27)	Case (n = 16)	F value
Before reconstruction				
Extension (°)	1.3 ± 2.6	1.0 ± 2.8	1.2 ± 2.6	2.08
Flexion (°)	135.5 ± 9.8	136.2 ± 6.8	135.2 ± 8.5	1.37
3 months after reconstruction				
Extension (°)	1.3 ± 2.6	−6.9 ± 3.8*	− 10.2 ± 4.8*	18.9
Flexion (°)	130.5 ± 7.2	131.2 ± 5.8	118 ± 5.5*	12.5
After second-look arthroscopy				
Extension (°)	1.3 ± 2.6	− 1.2 ± 1.8	−1.8 ± 3.2	2.23
Flexion (°)	135.5 ± 9.8	136.2 ± 6.8	134.0 ± 5.5	1.28

Data are expressed as the mean ± SD
*Statistically significant difference (P < 0.05)

associated with immune reaction [11, 21, 22]. Our findings are clinically relevant, since the pathophysiological effect of the presence of a cyclops nodule formation is not fully understood to date.

We performed cyclops resection in the cyclops group 3 months after reconstruction. Interestingly, the high pre-operative TTT values were reduced following cyclops resection. Furthermore, the TTT values did not return to the pre-reconstruction values before second-look arthroscopy, but they were higher than the no-cyclops group (Table 3). It may be suggested that resection of the cyclops using the arthroscope suppressed the reaction that occurs in the body of a living organism when the body rejects something. Furthermore, the gradually increasing TTT values after nodule resection may indicate that the patients who developed cyclops nodule formation originally had high immunoglobulin levels.

There was no difference in TTT values in the group that developed cyclopoids and the no-cyclops group. The cyclopoid is the displaced portion of the ACL with an angulated fold at the anterior end, giving it a tongue-like appearance [1, 23]. Histologically, cyclopoid scar formations are made up of fibrous tissue, showing elements of granulation tissue [6]. Similar to these reports, the cyclopoid scars observed during second-look arthroscopy in our study were recognized as soft, scar-like tissue in front of the ACL graft impinging on the intercondylar region during knee extension (Fig. 2). Regarding range of motion in the cyclopoid group, extension loss was observed at 3 months (Table 4), and 10 patients showed extension loss of more than 10 degrees 3 months after reconstruction. However, due to no palpable "clunk" with terminal extension, we did not perform surgery on the cyclopoid group. As a result, in the cyclopoid group, range of motion recovered to that of the contralateral knee 1 year after reconstruction in all cases. Extension loss in the early phase after reconstruction prevents closure of the intercondylar notch and allows local organization of the post-operative hemarthrosis [24]. Soft tissues such as cyclopoid scars may not be the result of an individual's immune reaction, but due to extension loss in the early post-reconstruction phase.

Given that this was a retrospective case control study, we did not examine other joint abnormalities. Given that flexion was also limited in the cyclops group, we further believe that the development of this nodulous scar formation is merely the expression of a generalized inclination to fibrotic healing. We showed that the occurrence of cyclops nodule formation may be involved in the response of living tissue, which is a potential factor that varies between individuals. Given this, low-dose steroids administered for the treatment of arthrofibrosis may be effective for patients with high TTT values.

Limitations

Although we have shown that the development of cyclops nodule formation depends on TTT values, TTT values are said to vary depending on the amount of immunoglobulin; however, we did not evaluate antibody-producing lymphocytes or antigen-presenting dendritic cells. Further evaluations using immunostaining of cyclops tissue are necessary. In addition, further studies are required to investigate the secretion of cytokines, growth factors, chemokines, inflammatory mediators, and matrix molecules and proteins that contribute to motility, proliferation, and differentiation of fibroblasts and myofibroblasts involved in the growth phase during wound healing.

Conclusions

High TTT values before ACL reconstruction were a potential risk factor for developing cyclops nodule formation. Furthermore, cyclopoid scar formations may not be the result of an individual's immune reaction, but due to extension loss in the early post-reconstruction phase.

Abbreviations
ACL: Anterior cruciate ligament; ALT: Alanine transaminase;
AM: Anteromedial; AST: Aspartate transaminase; BMI: Body mass index;
CRP: C-reactive protein; CT: Computed tomography; MR: Magnetic
resonance; PL: Posterolateral; ST: Semitendinosus tendon; TTT: Thymol
turbidity test

Acknowledgements

We would like to thank Editage (http://www.editage.jp) for English language editing.

Authors' contributions

YKo designed the study and wrote the manuscript. TF performed surgery and designed the study. TH and YKa performed the radiological measurements. YoO and SM performed the arthroscopic evaluations. YuO performed the statistical analyses. TO organized the laboratory works. All authors have read and approved the final version of the manuscript submitted.

Competing interests

The authors declare that they have no competing interests.

References

1. Jackson DW, Schaefer RK. Cyclops syndrome: loss of extension following intra-articular anterior cruciate ligament reconstruction. Arthroscopy. 1990;6: 171–8.
2. Ahn JH, Yoo JC, Yang HS, Kim JH, Wang JH. Second-look arthroscopic findings of 208 patients after ACL reconstruction. Knee Surg Sports Traumatol Arthrosc. 2007;15:242–8.
3. Sonnery-Cottet B, Lavoie F, Ogassawara R, Kasmaoui H, Scussiato RG, Kidder JF, et al. Clinical and operative characteristics of cyclops syndrome after double-bundle anterior cruciate ligament reconstruction. Arthroscopy. 2010; 26:1483–8.
4. Dandy DJ, Edwards DJ. Problems in regaining full extension of the knee after anterior cruciate ligament reconstruction: does arthrofibrosis exist? Knee Surg Sports Traumatol Arthrosc. 1994;2:76–9.
5. Delcogliano A, Franzese S, Branca A, Magi M, Fabbriciani C. Light and scan electron microscopic analysis of Cyclops syndrome: etiopathogenic hypothesis and technical solutions. Knee Surg Sports Traumatol Arthrosc. 1996;4:194–9.
6. Muellner T, Kdolsky R, Groschmidt K, Schabus R, Kwasny O, Plenk H Jr. Cyclops and cyclopoid formation after anterior cruciate ligament reconstruction: clinical and histomorphological differences. Knee Surg Sports Traumatol Arthrosc. 1999;7:284–9.
7. Guerra-Pinto F, Thaunat M, Daggett M, Kajetanek C, Marques T, Guimares T, et al. Hamstring contracture after ACL reconstruction is associated with an increased risk of Cyclops syndrome. Orthop J Sport Med. 2017;5: 232596711668412.
8. Fujii M, Furumatsu T, Miyazawa S, Okada Y, Tanaka T, Ozaki T, et al. Intercondylar notch size influences cyclops formation after anterior cruciate ligament reconstruction. Knee Surg Sports Traumatol Arthrosc. 2015;23:1092–9.
9. Tonin M, Saciri V, Veselko M, Rotter A. Progressive loss of knee extension after injury. Cyclops syndrome due to a lesion of anterior cruciate ligament. Am J Sports Med. 2001;29:545–9.
10. Veselko M, Rotter A, Tonin M. Cyclops syndrome occurring after partial rupture of the anterior cruciate ligament not treated by surgical reconstruction. Arthroscopy. 2000;16:328–31.
11. Ohwada H, Nakayama T, Tomono Y, Yamanaka K. Predictors, including blood, urine, anthropometry, and nutritional indices, of all-cause mortality among institutionalized individuals with intellectual disability. Res Dev Disabil. 2013 Jan;34(1):650–5.
12. Ohwada H, Nakayama T, Nara N, Tomono Y, Yamanaka K. An epidemiological study on anemia among institutionalized people with intellectual and/ or motor disability with special reference to its frequency, severity and predictors. BMC Public Health. 2006;6:85.
13. Kunkel HG, Hoagland CL. Mechanism and significance of the thymol turbidity test for liver disease. J Clin Investigation. 1947;26:1060–71.
14. Lubowitz JH, Konicek J. Anterior cruciate ligament femoral tunnel length: cadaveric analysis comparing anteromedial portal versus outside-in technique. Arthroscopy. 2010;26:1357–62.
15. Fujii M, Furumatsu T, Miyazawa S, Tanaka T, Inoue H, Kodama Y, et al. Features of human autologous hamstring graft elongation after pre-tensioning in anterior cruciate ligament reconstruction. Int Orthop. 2016;40: 2553–8.
16. Shino K, Suzuki T, Iwahashi T, Mae T, Nakamura N, Nakata K, et al. The resident's ridge as an arthroscopic landmark for anatomical femoral tunnel drilling in ACL reconstruction. Knee Surg Sports Traumatol Arthrosc. 2010;18: 1164–8.
17. Kodama Y, Furumatsu T, Miyazawa S, Fujii M, Tanaka T, Inoue H, et al. Location of the tibial tunnel aperture affects extrusion of the lateral meniscus following reconstruction of the anterior cruciate ligament. J Orthop Res. 2017;35:1625–33.
18. Furumatsu T, Ozaki T. Iatrogenic injury of the lateral meniscus anterior insertion following anterior cruciate ligament reconstruction: a case report. J Orthop Sci. 2018;23:197–201.
19. Delince P, Krallis P, Descamps PY, Fabeck L, Hardy D. Different aspects of the cyclops lesion following anterior cruciate ligament reconstruction: a multifactorial etiopathogenesis. Arthroscopy. 1998;14:869–76.
20. Imam MA, Abdelkafy A, Dinah F, Adhikari A. Does bone debris in anterior cruciate ligament reconstruction really matter? A cohort study of a protocol for bone debris debridement. SICOT J. 2015;1:4.
21. Van Der Sluis JJ, Menke HE. Role of IgG fractions with high isoelectric points in the thymol turbidity test in syphilis. Evidence for an increase in basic IgG in early syphilis. Br J Vener Dis. 1975;51(3):158–60.
22. Franklin EC. The role of the basic fraction of γ-globulin in the flocculation tests. Clin Chim Acta. 1959;4:259–64.
23. Plotkin BE, Agarwal VK, Varma R. Stump entrapment of the torn anterior cruciate ligament. Radiol Case Rep. 2016;4:268.
24. Wang J, Ao Y. Analysis of different kinds of cyclops lesions with or without extension loss. Arthroscopy. 2009;25:626–31.

20

Early referral and control of disease's flares prevent Orthopedic and Hand Surgery Indication (OHSI) in a dynamic cohort of Hispanic early rheumatoid arthritis patients

Irazú Contreras-Yáñez[1], G. Guaracha-Basáñez[1], E. Díaz-Borjón[2], M. Iglesias[3] and V. Pascual-Ramos[1]* ⓘ

Abstract

Background: Reconstructive joint surgery is an indicator of poor prognosis in rheumatoid arthritis (RA). Objectives of this study were to describe the incidence rate of orthopedic and hand surgery indication (OHSI) in an ongoing cohort of Hispanic early RA patients treated according to a T2T strategy and to investigate predictors.

Methods: Through February 2018, the cohort comprised 185 patients recruited from 2004 onwards, with variable follow-up, and rheumatic assessments at fixed intervals that included prospective determination of OHSI. Charts were reviewed by a single data abstractor. OHSI incidence rate was calculated. A case-control study nested within a cohort investigated the predictors; cases (OHSI patients) were paired with controls (1:4) according to age, sex and autoantibodies. A logistic regression model included baseline and cumulative (up to OHSI or equivalent) variables related to disease activity, treatment and to persistence with therapy. The IRB approved the study.

Results: Patients from the cohort were predominantly middle-aged (mean ± SD age: 38.5 ± 12.9 years) females (87. 6%) with 5.4 ± 2.6 months of disease duration. The cohort contributed to 1538 patient-years of follow-up. Twelve patients received incidental OHSI at a follow-up of 85 ± 44.5 months. The OHSI incident global rate was 8/1000 patient-years. Longer symptom duration at cohort referral (OR: 1.313, 95%CI: 1.02–1.68, $p = 0.032$) and a higher number of flares/patient (OR: 1.608, 95%CI: 1.05–1.61, $p = 0.015$) predicted OHSI. OHSI patients had more severe flares than their counterparts, and the opposite figure was true for mild flares.

Conclusion: Early referral for appropriate management and flare control may prevent OHSI in Hispanic recent-onset RA patients.

Keywords: Rheumatoid arthritis, Orthopedic surgery predictors, Disease flares, Early referral

Background

Rheumatoid arthritis (RA) patients from Latin-America present distinctive epidemiological, serological and phenotypic characteristics when compared to Caucasians patients, and these are known to impact patient outcomes [1–3]. In addition, treating RA to target (T2T) has become an internationally agreed standard of good practice [4] although the implementation of such strategy may be restricted in developing countries and non-universal health care systems where adherence to treatment may be dramatically compromised [5, 6].

Despite early and more aggressive treatment guidelines adopted in the last decades, some patients present progressive joint destruction and eventually require a surgical solution. Joint surgery is generally considered an indicator of medical therapy failure and of poor prognosis. In addition, the appropriate orchestration and selection of joint surgical interventions are controversial and problematic for the rheumatologist [7, 8]. Recognition of predictive and reversible factors for RA patients in whom a reconstructive procedure and joint surgery may

---

* Correspondence: virtichu@gmail.com
[1]Department of Immunology and Rheumatology, Instituto Nacional de Ciencias Médicas y Nutrición Salvador Zubirán, Vasco de Quiroga 15, Colonia Sección XVI, Belisario Domínguez, 14500 Ciudad de México, CP, Mexico
Full list of author information is available at the end of the article

be needed seems imperative. Few studies have addressed the topic in the T2T era and in the context of early RA patients, with conflicting results. None had been performed in Latin-American patients in whom the disease has unique characteristics. Most often, studies have focused on predictors at disease presentation and identified relevant, clinical and laboratory markers of disease activity and severity [9–12], number of copies of the shared epitope present in the patient [9, 12], radiographic damage [9, 10], demographic variables [9, 11] and short disease duration [9]. In addition, the most important time-varying factors associated with a reduced risk of joint surgery have been early treatment with conventional DMARDS during the first 2 years [10], good response to treatment during the first years of follow-up [10, 13, 14], lower annual radiographic progression rate [10, 12] and lower HAQ score at the beginning of a follow-up window [11] or in the early course of the disease [12]. Finally, the intensity of RA-specific treatment during the first year of disease diagnosis has also been associated with longer time to joint replacement surgery [13].

The objectives of the study were to describe the incidence rate of orthopedic and hand surgery indication (OHSI) in a cohort of Mexican Mestizo early RA patients treated with conventional DMARDs according to a T2T strategy (objective 1) and to investigate OHSI predictors (objective 2).

Methods

Setting and study population

Patients with RA were identified from the Early Arthritis Clinic (EAC) of the Instituto Nacional de Ciencias Médicas y Nutrición "Salvador Zubirán," located in México City. When first evaluated in the clinic, patients had disease duration of less than a year and no specific rheumatic diagnosis except RA. Once enrolled, the patients were evaluated every 2 months during the first 2 years of follow-up and every 2, 4 or 6 months, thereafter. Treatment prescribed was T2T oriented; traditional DMARDs were used in 98% of the patients with/without corticosteroids (up to 55% of the patients received low doses of oral corticosteroids) during their follow-up.

At baseline evaluation, a complete medical history and demographic data were recorded along with rheumatoid factor (RF) and antibodies to cyclic citrullinated peptides (ACCP). Follow-up evaluations were standardized and included prospective assessments of swollen and tender joint counts, patient- and physician-reported outcomes [2, 3], extensive disease activity evaluation, comorbidity, treatment and persistence with therapy; complete laboratory parameters were also determined. Hand and feet X-rays were performed at baseline and thereafter every year. In addition, at follow-ups, indication of joint surgery (yes/no and date of the indication) and, when

appropriate, identification of the joint(s) candidate(s) for surgery, of the intervention recommended and of the surgery date were prospectively recorded.

Study design

Through February 2018, the cohort comprised 198 RA patients recruited from 2004 onwards; among them, 185 patients had at least fourteen months of follow-up that was required due to the case-control nested within a cohort design (the first OHSI was at 14 months of follow-up); 5 out of 185 patients (2.7%) were deceased and 43 (23.3%) were lost to follow-up while 137 (74%) had active follow-up. Charts up to the last follow-up or death, were retrospectively reviewed.

A case-control study nested within a cohort was designed to accomplish objective 2. Cases were defined as RA patients with (incidental) OHSI (see definition below). Controls (RA patients without OHSI) were paired to cases (4 controls: 1 case) according to age (± 5 years), sex, baseline RF and ACCP (absent vs. present).

Definitions

- (Incidental) **OHSI** was corroborated by either the orthopedic surgeon or the hand surgeon, for the first time, after at least 6 months of follow-up. All of the cases had rheumatic and surgical evaluations. Surgical indication (instead of surgery) was considered due to the following reasons: Patient's desire to delay the surgery due to costs or fears, surgical waiting list that may last up to 6-12 months, and a prosthesis donation program waiting list that may last up to 1 year. OHSI were, in all the cases, indicated for joint damage secondary to RA.

- At each follow-up evaluation, **disease activity** was graded as remission, mild, moderate and high disease activity, based on DAS28 cut-offs [15]. **Sustained remission (SR)** was defined if the patient's DAS28-ESR was maintained at < 2.6 for at least 6 months of continuous follow-up; **time in SR** was computed from the first visit (time) that SR was achieved to the last follow-up with SR. **Flare** was arbitrarily defined as any increase in EULAR disease activity category.

- **Cumulative disease activity** was computed from baseline evaluation up to OHSI for cases or equivalent time for controls, as the mean of DAS28 at each follow-up assessment; **number of flares** was similarly computed (one patient had persistent high disease activity and the maximum number of flares/patient was arbitrarily assigned: 14 flares). Finally, **follow-up time in remission** was computed as the percentage of the entire follow-up the patient had periods of at least 6 months of follow-up with DAS28 < 2.6, either continuous or not.

- At each assessment, **persistent patients** were identified as previously published [2]. **Persistence** was defined (within each patient) as the percentage of the patient's entire follow-up (up to OHSI for cases or equivalent for controls) that he/she was persistent with therapy.

Finally, for each patient, a precise description of cumulative DAS28, sustained remission, time in sustained remission, number flares/patient, patient category regarding being persistent (vs. not persistent) and patient's persistence during the follow-up period was provided; treatment was also provided.

Statistical analysis

Descriptive statistics was used. Student t test and X^2 were used for normally distributed variables and Mann-Whitney U for non-normally distributed variables.

To achieve objective 2, baseline characteristics were first compared between OHSI patients (N = 12) and their counterpart (N = 173). In addition, a case-control study nested in the cohort was designed to compare cumulative disease activity, treatment and persistence between cases and controls. Finally, a logistic regression model was used to identify predictors of first OHSI. The selection of variables was based on their statistical significance in the bivariate analysis ($p \leq 0.06$); variables a priori considered were disease duration (at baseline),

cumulative disease activity and persistence related variables. Based on the number of outcomes of interest (N = 12), 3 to 4 variables were included.

All statistical tests were 2-sided and evaluated at the 0.05 significance level. Statistical analysis was performed using the SPSS/PC program (v.17.0; Chicago, IL).

Ethics approval and consent to participate

The study was approved by the Institution's Internal Review board "Comité de Ética del Instituto Nacional de Ciencias Médicas y Nutrición Salvador Zubirán" with reference number IRE-274-10/ 11-1. Written informed consent was obtained from all of the patients to have their charts reviewed and data presented in scientific forums or published.

Results

Study population characteristics (Table 1)

Patients entering the EAC were predominantly middle-aged (mean ± SD age of 38.5 ± 12.9 years) and female (87.6%), with (median, 25th–75th IQR) 5.3 (3. 3-7.0) months of symptom duration. As expected, patients had high disease activity, high disability and poor function. The majority of

Table 1 Population characteristics at baseline and comparison between patients with/without OHSI, and between OHSI patients and their paired controls

	Population (N = 185)	Patients with OHSI (N = 12)	Patients without OHSI (N = 173)	OHSI-paired controls (N = 48)	p_1	p_2
Female sex, N° (%) of patients	162 (87.6)	11 (91.7)	151 (87.3)	44 (99.7)	1	1
(Mean ± SD) Age at cohort inclusion, years	38.5 ± 12.9	42 ± 15.6	38.3 ± 12.7	42 ± 14.9	0.33	1
Medium-low socioeconomic level, N° (%) of patients	165 (89.2)	11 (91.7)	154 (89)	43 (89.6)	1	1
(Mean ± SD) Years of formal education	11.2 ± 3.9	10.2 ± 4.3	11.3 ± 3.9	10.8 ± 4.2	0.32	0.66
Disease duration, months	5.3 (3. 3-7.0)	7.5 (6. 2-9.3)	5 (2. 9-7.4)	5 (2. 9-7.4)	0.02	0.02
N° (%) of patients with RF	152 (82.8)	11 (91.7)	141 (81.5)	44 (99)	0.7	1
N° (%) of patients with ACCP	158 (85.9)	12 (100)	146 (84.9)	43 (91.5)	0.22	0.6
N° (%) of patients with erosions	18 (9.7)	2 (16.7)	16 (9.2)	5 (10.4)	0.33	0.62
DAS28	5.9 (4.8-6.9)	7 (5.4-7.7)	6.3 (4.9-7.5)	6.3 (4.9-7.5)	0.27	0.27
Physician-VAS	36 (36–49)	51 (31-68)	41 (30-52)	41 (30-51.5)	0.23	0.23
CRP, mg/dL	0.7 (0.3-2.5)	3.6 (0.5-7.1)	1.2 (0.3-2.3)	1.2 (0.3-2.3)	0.06	0.06
ESR, mm/H	11 (12-39)	42 (19-74)	26 (15-49)	26 (15. 3-49)	0.14	0.14
Charlson Score	1 (1-1)	1 (1-1)	1 (1-1)	1 (1-1)	0.18	0.12
HAQ (0–3)	1.4 (0.9-2.1)	1.4 (1-2.3)	1.4 (0.9-2)	1.4 (0.9-2)	0.73	0.73
SF-36 (0–100)	38 (27-55)	33 (24-56)	34 (26-57)	33.8 (26.4-57.4)	0.94	0.94
Patient-overall disease-VAS	53 (33-76)	71 (41–92)	62 (34-78)	62 (34-78)	0.29	0.29
Pain-VAS	50 (31-73)	61 (46–98)	52 (33-78)	52 (33.3-77.8)	0.48	0.48
N° (%) of patients with DMARDs	101 (54.6)	7 (58.3)	94 (54.3)	19 (39.6)	1	1
N° (%) of patients with corticosteroids	72 (38.9)	4 (33.3)	68 (39.3)	15 (31.3)	0.77	1

OHSI orthopaedic and hand surgery indication, *N* number, *SD* standard deviation, *RF* rheumatoid factor, *ACCP* antibodies to cyclic citrullinated peptides, *DAS* disease activity score (28 joints evaluated), *VAS* visual analogue scale, *CRP* C reactive protein, *ESR* erythrocyte sedimentation rate, *HAQ* health assessment questionnaire, *SF-36* short form 36, P_1 Comparison between patients with vs. without OHSI, P_2 Comparison between patients with OHSI vs. paired controls
Data presented as median (25th–75th IQR) unless otherwise indicated

the patients had RF and ACCP while a few (9.7%) had erosive disease. (Median, 25th–75th IQR) Charlson score was 1 (1-1). Regarding treatment at referral to the clinic, 54.6% of the patients were indicated at least one DMARD and 38.9% low doses of oral corticosteroids (Table 1).

Description of the patients with OHSI

Through February 2018, the cohort contributed to 1538 patient-years of follow-up. There were 12 patients with incidental OHSI, 11 of them were female, their range of age was 20-66 years old and OHSI was at a follow-up of 85 ± 44.5 months; 8 patients (66.7%) received orthopedic surgery indication while 4 (33.3%) received hand surgery indication; the incident global rate was 8/1000 patient-years. Figure 1 summarizes the OHSI annual incident rate that progressively increased after the 2nd year of follow-up.

Patient description and surgery indication are summarized in Table 2, which also identifies patients already intervened, 8 patients (66.7%). Half of the patients ($N = 6$) received a surgical indication between 5 and 10 years of follow-up, and 3 (25%) patients each, before 5 years of follow-up and after 10 years of follow-up.

Comparison of baseline characteristics from patients with/without OHSI

Table 1 summarizes the results; OHSI patients had longer symptom duration and tended to have higher CRP levels than their counterparts.

OHSI predictors (objective 2)

Data from 12 cases paired with 48 controls (1:4) are summarized in Table 1 (comparison of baseline characteristics) and Table 3 (comparison of cumulative variables). Regarding baseline characteristics, similar results

as those described when OHSI were compared to their counterparts were found. Regarding cumulative variables (Table 3), OHSI patients had a significantly higher cumulative number of flares and had a lower percentage of their follow-ups in remission status. In addition, OHSI patients were less frequently persistent with therapy during follow-up and had a lower percentage of their follow-up with treatment persistence. Cumulative treatment was similar between cases and controls.

The different multiple regression models tested included baseline variables (months of symptom disease duration) and cumulative variables (N° of flares/patient, % of follow-up in remission status, N° of patients persistent and % of follow-up patients were persistent with therapy) and yielded similar results: Longer symptom duration at referral to the EAC (OR: 1.31, 95%CI: 1.02–1.68, $p = 0.032$) and a higher number of flares (OR: 1.61, 95%CI: 1.05–1.61, $p = 0.015$) were the only predictors of OHSI.

Finally, we used ROC to define the best cut-off for symptom duration and cumulative number of flares to predict OHSI and identified 6 months (sensitivity: 0.833; specificity: 0.665; AUC: 0.746, 95% CI: 0.593–0.899) and 5 flares/patient (sensitivity: 0.750; specificity: 0.625; AUC: 0.702, 95% CI: 0.522–0.882), respectively.

Flare distribution

Flares were divided into six categories: (1) Patients who had increased disease activity from remission status to low disease activity; (2) from remission to moderate disease activity; (3) from remission to high disease activity; (4) from low disease activity to moderate disease activity; (5) from low disease activity to high disease activity and (6) from moderate disease activity to high disease activity. Eleven patients with OHSI (one patient did not present flares

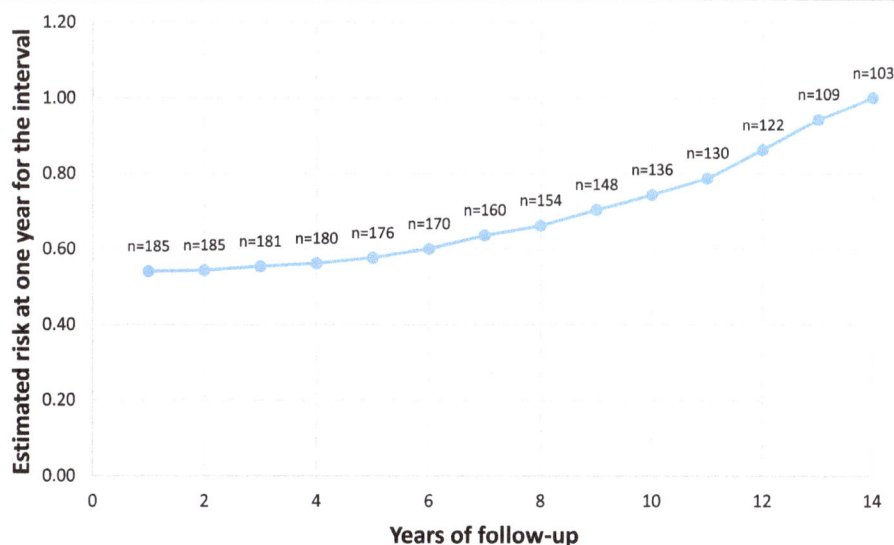

Fig. 1 OHSI annual incident rate according to cohort follow-up. *Per 100 person years*

Table 2 OHSI patient's description

Number of patient	DR months	Baseline DAS28	OHSI DAS28	Follow-up to OHSI, months	Treatment at OHSI	Surgical indication
1[a]	7.3	5.6	3.4	110	MTX + SUL + LEF + PDN	Left hip arthroplasty
2[a]	4.7	7.2	2.4	114	MTX + PDN	Right knee arthroplasty
3[a]	7.6	8.7	6.4	68	MTX + PDN	Left hip arthroplasty
4[a]	1	7.1	3.0	132	MTX + PDN	Hemi-resection of the distal ulna and extensor tendon's reconstruction (right hand)
5	8.8	7.8	2.4	146	MTX + PDN	Extensor tendon's reconstruction (left hand)
6	6	5.8	3.4	124	CLQ + SUL + PDN	Right hip arthroplasty
7	10.5	5.3	2.5	72	MTX + CLQ + PDN	Right knee arthroplasty
8[a]	6.7	4.6	5.2	114	AZA + PDN	Extensor tendon's reconstruction (left hand)
9[a]	9.5	8.0	2.3	66	MTX + PDN	Left shoulder arthroplasty
10[a]	7.2	7.1	2.6	52	MTX + CLQ + SUL + PDN	Right hand synovectomy
11	12.1	5.3	2.2	14	MTX + CLQ + SUL	Right knee arthroplasty
12[a]	8.5	6.8	2.5	14	MTX + CLQ + SUL + PDN	Left hip arthroplasty

DAS28 Disease activity score (28 joints evaluated), MTX methotrexate, SUL sulphasalazine, LEF leflunomide, PDN prednisone, CLQ chloroquine, AZA azathioprine, F female, M male, DR months of symptom's disease duration up to cohort baseline evaluation, DAS28 disease activity
[a]Patients already intervened

during follow-up) had 81 flares while 41 controls (7 were flare-free) had 177 flares. Figure 2 summarizes the comparison of the flare-category distribution between both groups. Interestingly, the controls showed a higher number of category (1) flares compared to cases while the opposite figure was true regarding category (6) flares. At the patient level, similar tendencies were observed but differences did not reached statistical significance (data not shown).

Discussion

The present study was developed in a dynamic cohort of Hispanic early RA patients, in whom comprehensive rheumatologic follow-up evaluations were performed from 2004 onwards. The main purpose of the study was to prospectively assess the occurrence of and predictive factors for joint surgery indication; surgical indication (instead of surgery) was chosen due to intrinsic and extrinsic sources of vulnerability from our patients, who may delay or even halt interventions because of costs [16, 17].

We found a low incident global rate of OHSI (8/1000 patient-years) after a mean follow-up of 7 years. The OHSI annual incidental rate progressively increased after the second year. In the literature, few inception cohorts of early RA had assessed rates of orthopedic and small joint surgery, with conflicting results [9–14, 18, 19]; prevalence ranged from 5.3% at a mean follow-up of 4.6 years [13] to 58% after a mean follow-up of 16 years [12]; variations may be explained by a lack of a uniform definition of "early disease" [9–14, 19], a wide spectrum of follow-ups that may last up to 25 years [19],

Table 3 Comparison of cumulative disease activity, treatment and persistence with therapy between OHSI and paired controls

	Cases (N = 12)	Controls (N = 48)	p
DAS28	3.1 (2.5-3.5)	2.6 (2.3-3.2)	0.09
N° (%) of patients who achieved a 1st SR	8 (66.7)	40 (83.3)	0.23
Months in 1st SR	12 (0–28.5)	27 (10-41.5)	0.12
N° of flares/patient	6 (3.5-9.5)	3 (1-6)	0.03
% of follow-up in remission status	50.7 (19-65.6)	71.4 (50.3-80.6)	0.02
N° DMARD/patient	1.5 (1-3)	2 (1-2.5)	0.88
N° of patients with corticosteroids	11 (91.7)	42 (87.5)	1
Dose of corticosteroids	7.5 (5-7.5)	5 (5-7.5)	0.32
N° (%) of patients persistent	2 (16.7)	24 (50)	0.05
N° (%) of patients always persistent	2 (16.7)	22 (45.8)	0.06
% of patients follow-up persistent with therapy	75 (50–82.5)	92.5 (75–100)	0.04

Data presented as median (Q25-Q75) unless otherwise indicated
OHSI orthopaedic and hand surgery indication, N number

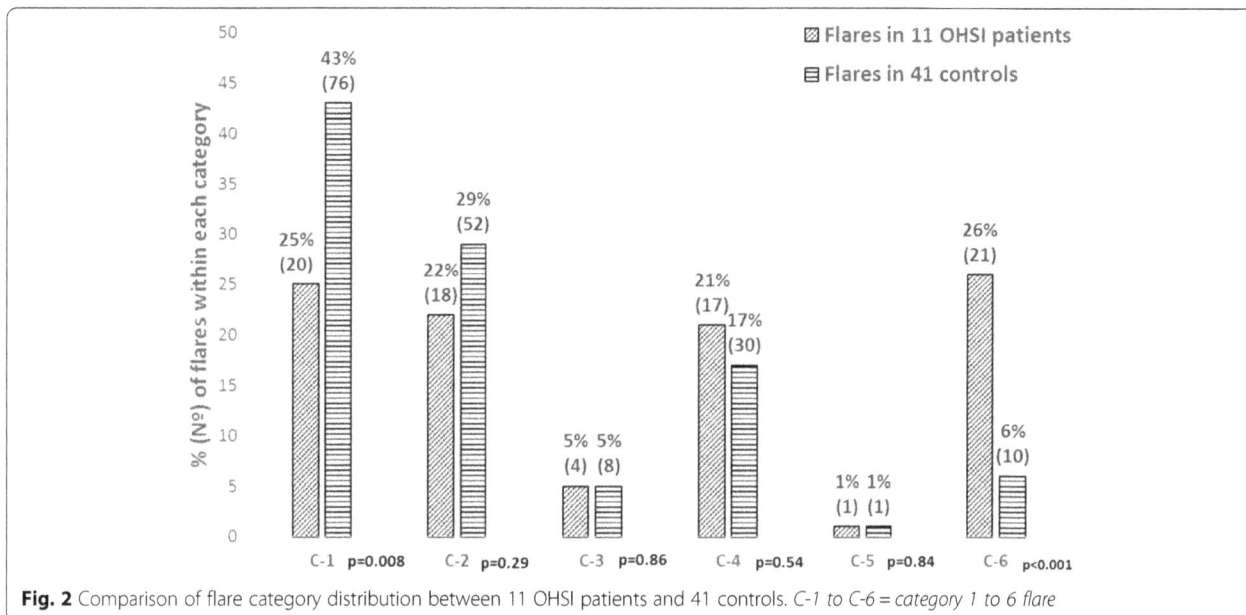

Fig. 2 Comparison of flare category distribution between 11 OHSI patients and 41 controls. *C-1 to C-6 = category 1 to 6 flare*

differences in the genetic background of the populations in whom surgery was assessed (from the UK [9, 11, 14], Sweden [12, 18], Canada [13], the Netherlands [10] and Finland [19]) and the year of patient's inclusion, which may have affected the current standard of care. Our cohort had distinctive characteristics which may additionally explain our low OHSI prevalence, estimated as 2.2% at 5 years and reaching 11.7% at last follow-up (13 years); all of our patients were of Hispanic origin and there is only one study which evaluated 355 major joint surgeries performed in Brazilian patients, although only 8 patients had RA diagnosis, which precludes any comparison [20]; also, mean symptom's duration from our patients was close to 5 months, the cohort had a limited follow-up and included patients from 2004 onwards; finally, our patients received a T2T strategy, primarily with combined traditional DMARDs meanwhile only 4 patients had access to biologics. Of note, Moura et al. [13] identified new-onset RA patients in the Québec Health Insurance Program databases from 2002 to 2011, which is close to our cohort initiation date, and described 10.9 joint replacements during 1000 person-years, similar to our finding. Published recent-onset cohorts with a higher prevalence of joint surgery included patients one or more decades previous to our inclusion date [9–12, 14, 18, 19]. These data suggest a decline in orthopedic surgery utilization and might be explained by earlier, more aggressive and better treatment strategies [21–24]. Nonetheless, it should be mentioned that there are conflicting results regarding benefits of biological DMARDs on the need for joint replacement surgery [25, 26].

Longer symptom duration at referral and a higher number of flares/patient during follow-up were the only

predictors of incidental OHSI. Early RA cohorts identified additional predictors, and the variability of the results may be explained by the cohort's heterogeneity (as previously described), the selection of variables to be included and how the models were built. Baseline and comprehensive cumulative variables related to disease activity, to treatment and to adherence were both included in the model as a unique characteristics of our study design. Two groups of investigators, Gwinnith et al. [11] and Kapetanovic et al. [12], also assessed baseline and time varying predictors of orthopedic surgery in recent-onset RA cohorts; the former found that functional disability at time-points was the strongest predictor of future major surgery while acute reactant-phase determinations, baseline HAQ, and early radiological changes were identified as predictors of future need for large joint replacements in the second cohort. In addition, disease activity, radiographic damage, acute reactant-phase determinations, female sex and genotyping were identified as predictors of joint surgery in recent-onset RA, when only baseline variables were considered [9, 11].

In our study, the disease activity construct was extensively assessed during follow-up. Our results highlight that in order to prevent joint surgery, the number of flares must be controlled. Interestingly, we also found differences between patients with/without OHSI in the distribution of category-1 and -6 flares. The former represents a surrogate of adequate disease activity control and mild flares and was the predominant category of flares in patients without OHSI; meanwhile, category-6 flares indicate unsatisfactory disease activity control and were predominant in patients who ultimately received OHSI. Markusse et al. [27] followed up 508 RA patients from the BeSt study, who were T2T for 10 years. The authors formulated 3 definitions of disease flare based on the original DAS; patients who suffered a minor flare B showed more joint damage progression when compared with their counterpart. A higher number of flares was associated with higher disease activity [28] that, if uncontrolled, may progress to severe joint destruction, unremitting pain and joint deformity; in such clinical context, joint arthroplasty has proven to be a successful intervention to improve physical function [29–31].

In addition to flare control, symptom duration at referral was also found to prevent joint surgery and could be considered a surrogate of early use of DMARDs. Moura et al. [13] found that longer exposure to methotrexate or DMARDs during the first year of follow-up after RA diagnosis was associated with longer time to joint replacement surgery, in a new-onset cohort of 11,333 RA patients. Our patients were indicated DMARDs at first evaluation and symptom duration at referral cut-off of 6 months may be considered an early referral, which is an evidence-based recommendation in newly diagnosed RA patients who improves long-term outcomes and patient quality of life [32].

The study has limitations that must be addressed. First, the study was conducted at a single center which limits the generalization of the results. Second, it was also conducted in an observational cohort and therefore has the limitations of such cohorts, particularly follow-up losses and lack of standardization and control with respect to certain variables and outcomes [33]. Third, we arbitrarily defined and classified flares into 6 categories; it should be emphasized that at the patient level, the six categories may be present and it is unknown if a predominant category may eventually have the greatest impact; also, flare was arbitrarily defined based on a change in EULAR categories, although there is no consensus on flare's definition, as recently published [34]; nonetheless, we performed a sensitivity analysis defining flare as DAS28 > 3.2 [34] and same patients were identified. Fourth, access to biologics was restricted and it may have impacted disease activity control. Finally, the number of OHSI patients was limited and results should be interpreted with caution.

Conclusions

Our study complements the existing literature related to predictors of joint surgery in real world early RA patients. A delay/prevention of joint surgery may be added to the list of benefits when patients are referred early to a rheumatologist. In addition, flare attenuation should also be considered a target to impact joint interventions, particularly those flares that translate into high disease activity.

Abbreviations
RA: Rheumatoid Arthritis; OHSI: Orthopedic and hand surgery indication; T2T: Treat-to-Target; IRB: Institutional Review Board; OR: Odds Ratio; CI: Confidence Interval; EULAR: European League Against Rheumatism; DMARDs: Disease Modifying Anti-rheumatic Drugs; HAQ: Health Assessment Questionnaire; EAC: Early Arthritis Clinic; RF: Rheumatoid Factor; ACCP: Antibodies to Cyclic Citrullinated Peptides; DAS28: Disease Activity Score on 28 Joints; ESR: Erythrocyte Sedimentation Rate; SR: Sustained Remission; SPSS/PC: Statistical Package for the Social Sciences; CRP: C Reactive Protein; ROC: Receiver Operating Characteristic; AUC: Area Under Curve

Acknowledgements
None

Funding
No funding was received for this research.

Authors' contributions
ICY: Participated in the conception and design of the study, performed the statistical analysis, in charge of databases integrity of the early arthritis clinic. GGB: Participated in the conception and design of the study, performed patient's clinical evaluations, and reviewed the manuscript. EDB: Participated in the conception of the study, assessed surgical indication and reviewed the manuscript. MI: Participated in the conception of the study, assessed surgical indication and reviewed the manuscript. VPR: Participated in the conception and design of the study, performed patient's clinical evaluations; performed the statistical analysis and drafted the manuscript. In charge of the early arthritis clinic. All authors read and approved the final manuscript.

Authors' information
All authors read and approved this manuscript.

Competing interests
The authors declare that they have no financial interests, which could create a potential conflict of interest with regard to the work.

Author details
[1]Department of Immunology and Rheumatology, Instituto Nacional de Ciencias Médicas y Nutrición Salvador Zubirán, Vasco de Quiroga 15, Colonia Sección XVI, Belisario Domínguez, 14500 Ciudad de México, CP, Mexico. [2]Department of Surgery, Orthopedic Unit, Instituto Nacional de Ciencias Médicas y Nutrición Salvador Zubirán, Mexico City, Mexico. [3]Department of Surgery, Plastic Surgery Unit, Instituto Nacional de Ciencias Médicas y Nutrición Salvador Zubirán, Mexico City, Mexico.

References
1. Mody GM, Cardiel MH. Challenges in the management of rheumatoid arthritis in developing countries. Best Pract Res Clin Rheumatol. 2008;22: 621–41.
2. Pascual Ramos V, Contreras-Yáñez I, Villa AR, Cabiedes Jt, Rull-Gabayet M. Medication persistence over two years of follow-up in a cohort of early rheumatoid arthritis patients: Associated factors and relationship with disease activity and disability. Arthritis Res Ther. 2009;11:R26.
3. Contreras-Yáñez I, Pascual-Ramos V. Predictors of health care drop-out in an inception cohort of patients with early onset rheumatoid arthritis. BMC Musculoskelet Disord. 2017;18:321.
4. Smolen JS, Breevedl FC, Burmester GR, Bykerk V, Dougados M, Emery P, et al. Treating rheumatoid arthritis to target: 2014 update of the recommendations of an international task force. Ann Rheum Dis. 2016;75:3–15.
5. Curkendall S, Patel V, Gleeson M, Campbell RS, Zagari M, Dubois R. Compliance with biologics therapies for rheumatoid arthritis: do patients out-of-pocket payments matter? Arthritis Rheum. 2008;59:1519–26.

6. Pascual-Ramos V, Conteras-Yáñez I. Motivations for inadequate persistence with disease modifying anti-rheumatic drugs in early rheumatoid arthritis: the patient's perspective. BMC Musculoskelet Disord. 2013;14:336.

7. Anderson RJ. Controversy in the surgical treatment of the rheumatoid hand. Hand Clinic. 2011;27:21–5.

8. Alderman AK, Ubel PA, Kim HM, Fox DA, Chung KC. Surgical management of the rheumatoid hand: consensus and controversy among rheumatologists and hand surgeon. J Rheumatol. 2003;30:1464–72.

9. James D, Young A, Kulinskaya E, Knight E, Thompson W, Ollier W, et al. On behalf of the early rheumatoid arthritis study group (ERAS), UK. Orthopaedic intervention in early rheumatoid arthritis. Occurrence and predictive factors in an inception cohort of 1064 patients followed for 5 years. Rheumatology. 2004;53:369–76.

10. Verstappen SM, Hoes JN, Ter Borg EJ, Bijlsma JW, Blaauw AA, Van Albada-Kuipers GA, on behalf of the Utrecht rheumatoid arthritis cohort study group, et al. Joint surgery in the Utrecht rheumatoid arthritis cohort: the effect of treatment strategy. Ann Rheum Dis. 2006;65:1506–11.

11. Gwinnutt JM, Symmons DPM, MacGregor AJ, Chipping JR, Lapraik C, Marshall T, et al. Predictors of and outcomes following orthopaedic joint surgery in patients with early rheumatoid arthritis followed for 20 years. Rheumatology. 2017;56:1510–7.

12. Kapetanovic MC, Lindqvist E, Saxne T, Eberhardt K. Orthopaedic surgery in patients with rheumatoid arthritis over 20 years: prevalence and predictive factors of large joint replacement. Ann Rheum Dis. 2008;67:1412–6.

13. Moura CS, Abrahamowicz M, Beauchamp ME, Lacaille D, Wang Y, Boire G, et al. Early medication use in new-onset rheumatoid arthritis may delay joint replacement: results of a large population-based study. Arthritis Res Ther. 2015;17:197.

14. Nikiphorou E, Norton S, Young A, Carpenter L, Dixey J, Walsh DA, et al. On behalf of ERAS and ERAN: association between rheumatoid arthritis disease activity, progression of functional limitation and long-term risk of orthopedic surgery. Combined analysis of two prospective cohort supports EULAR treat to target DAS thresholds. Ann Rheum Dis. 2016;75:2080–6.

15. van Gestel AM, Prevoo ML, Van't Hof MA, van Rijswijk MH, Van de putte LB, van Riel PL. Development and validation of the European league against rheumatism response criteria for rheumatoid arthritis. Arthritis Rheum. 1996;39:34–40.

16. Rogers W, Ballantyne A. Special populations: vulnerability and protection. RECIIS. 2008. https://doi.org/10.3395/reciis.v2.Sup1.207en.

17. Pérez-Román DI, Ortiz-Haro AB, Ruiz-Medrano E, Contreras-Yáñez I, Pascual-Ramos V. Outcomes after rheumatoid arthritis patients complete their participation in a long-term observational study with tofacitinib combined with methotrexate: practical and ethical implications in vulnerable populations after tofacitinib discontinuation. Rheumatol Intl. 2018;38:599–606.

18. Eberhardt K, Fex E, Johnson U, Wollheim FA. Association of HLA-DRB and – DQ genes with 2 and 5 year outcome in rheumatoid arthritis. Ann Rheum Dis. 1996;55:34–9.

19. Palm TM, Kaarela K, Hakala MS, Kautiainen HJ, Kröger HP, Belt EA. Need and sequence of large joint replacements in rheumatoid arthritis. A 25-year follow-up. Clin Exp Rheumatol. 2002;20:392–4.

20. De Piano LP, Golmia RP, Scheinberg MA. Decreased need of large joint replacement in patients with rheumatoid arthritis in a specialized Brazilian center. Clin Rheumatol. 2011;30:549–50.

21. da Silva E, Doran MF, Crowson CS, O'Fallon WM, Matteson EL. Declining use of orthopedic surgery in patients with rheumatoid arthritis? Results of a long-term, population-based assessment. Arthritis Rheum. 2003;49:216–20.

22. Weiss RJ, Ehlin A, Montgomery SM, Wick MC, Stark A, Wretenberg P. Decrease of RA-related orthopedic surgery of the upper limbs between 1998 and 2004: data from 54579 Swedish RA inpatients. Rheumatol. 2008;47:491–4.

23. Nikiphorou E, Carpenter L, Morris S, McGregor AJ, Dixey J, Kiely P, et al. Hand and foot surgery decline rates in rheumatoid arthritis have declined from 1986 to 2011, but large joint replacement rates remain unchanged: results from the UK inception cohort. Arthritis Rheumatol. 2014;66:1081–9.

24. Sokka T, Kautiainen H, Hannonen P. Stable occurrence of knee and hip total joint replacement in Central Finland between 1986 and 2003; an indication of improved long-term outcomes of rheumatoid arthritis. Ann Rheum Dis. 2007;66:341–4.

25. Aaltonen KJ, Virkki LM, Jamsen E, Sokka T, Konttinen YT, Peltomaa R, et al. Do biologic drugs affect the need for and outcome of joint replacements in patients with rheumatoid arthritis? A register-based study. Sem Arthritis Rheum. 2013;43:55–62.

26. Asai S, Takahashi N, Funahashi K, Yoshioka Y, Takemoto T, Terabe K, et al. Concomitant methotrexate protects against total knee arthroplasty in patients with rheumatoid arthritis treated with tumor necrosis factor inhibitor. J Rheumatol. 2015;42:2255–60.

27. Markusse IM, Dirven L, Gerards AH, van Groenendael JH, Ronday HK, Kerstens PJ, et al. Disease flares in rheumatoid arthritis are associated with joint damage progression and disability: 10-year results from the BeSt study. Arthtitis Res Ther. 2015;17:232.

28. Bykerk VP, Shadick N, Frits M, Bingham CO 3rd, Jeffery I, Iannaccone C, Weinblatt M, et al. Flares in rheumatoid arthritis: frequency and management. A report from the BRASS registry. J Rheumatol. 2014;41:227–34.

29. Lee JK, Choi CH. Total knee arthroplasty in rheumatoid arthritis. Review article. Knee Surg Relat Res. 2012;24:1–6.

30. Wolfe F, Zwillich SH. The long-term outcomes of rheumatoid arthritis. 23 year prospective, longitudinal study of total joint replacement and its predictors in 1600 patients with rheumatoid arthritis. Arthritis Rheum. 1998;41:1072–82.

31. Loza E, Abásolo L, Clemente D, López-González R, Rodríguez L, Vadillo C, et al. Variability in the use of orthopedic surgery in patients with rheumatoid arthritis in Spain. J Rheumatol. 2007;34:1484–90.

32. Emery P, Breedveld FC, Dougados M, Kalden JR, Schiff MH, Smolen JS. Early referral recommendation for newly diagnosed rheumatoid arthritis: evidence based development of a clinical guide. Ann Rheum Dis. 2002;61:290–7.

33. Inanc M. Very early 'rheumatoid' arthritis cohorts: limited by selection. Editorial. Rheumatology. 2007;46:185–7.

34. Kuijper TM, Lamers-Karnebeeck FB, Jacobs JW, Hazes JM, Luime JJ. Flare rate in patients with rheumatoid arthritis in low disease activity or remission when tapering or stopping synthetics or biologic DMARD: a systematic review. J Rheumatol. 2015;42:2012–22.

21

The association between multisite musculoskeletal pain and cardiac autonomic modulation during work, leisure and sleep – a cross-sectional study

Tatiana de Oliveira Sato[1]*[iD], David M. Hallman[2], Jesper Kristiansen[3] and Andreas Holtermann[3,4]

Abstract

Background: The prevention and rehabilitation of multisite musculoskeletal pain would benefit from studies aiming to understand its underlying mechanism. Autonomic imbalance is a suggested mechanism for multisite pain, but hardly been studied during normal daily living. Therefore, the aim of the study is to investigate the association between multisite musculoskeletal pain and cardiac autonomic modulation during work, leisure and sleep.

Methods: This study is based on data from the "Danish Physical activity cohort with objective measurements" among 568 blue-collar workers. Pain intensity scales were dichotomized according to the median of each scale, and the number of pain sites was calculated. No site was regarded as the pain-free, one site was considered as single-site musculoskeletal pain and pain in two or more sites was regarded as multisite musculoskeletal pain. Heart rate variability (HRV) was measured by an electrocardiogram system (ActiHeart) and physical activity using accelerometers (Actigraph). Crude and adjusted linear mixed models were applied to investigate the association between groups and cardiac autonomic regulation during work, leisure and sleep.

Results: There was no significant difference between groups and no significant interaction between groups and domains in the crude or adjusted models for any HRV index. Significant differences between domains were found in the crude and adjusted model for all indices, except SDNN; sleep time showed higher values than leisure and work time, except for LF and LF/HF, which were higher during work.

Conclusion: This cross-sectional study showed that multisite musculoskeletal pain is not associated with imbalanced cardiac autonomic regulation during work, leisure and sleep time.

Keywords: Heart rate variability, Autonomic nervous system, Chronic pain, Physical activity

Background

Chronic musculoskeletal pain has high prevalence and large consequences for the society [12, 34]. Although most studies focus on pain localized in a particular body region (single-site pain), such as low back pain or neck/shoulder pain [41], musculoskeletal pain usually occurs concurrently in several anatomical sites [4, 7]. This condition is called multisite pain [31] and has been shown to be associated with increased healthcare utilization,

sick leave, early retirement, sickness and social welfare benefit [11, 13, 17].

In contrast to single-site pain, which is considered to be due to overload or insufficient use of a particular body region [7], multisite pain may be driven by more generalized mechanisms, such as an imbalance in autonomic cardiac modulation [42].

Autonomic cardiac modulation can be assessed by heart rate variability (HRV) reflecting parasympathetic and sympathetic regulation of beat-to-beat heart rate. Recent systematic reviews show moderate evidence supporting a decrease in parasympathetic modulation in chronic pain patients [20, 40]. However, we are aware of

---

* Correspondence: tatisato@ufscar.br
[1]Physical Therapy Department, Federal University of São Carlos (UFSCar), Rodovia Washington Luís, km 235, São Carlos, SP 13565-905, Brazil
Full list of author information is available at the end of the article

only one study (the Netherlands Study of Depression and Anxiety - NESDA) investigating the association between multisite musculoskeletal pain and HRV, finding no relationship between HRV and pain onset [14] or recovery [15]. However, more studies on the association between multisite musculoskeletal pain and HRV are required before any conclusion can be drawn.

For better prevention and rehabilitation of multisite musculoskeletal pain, it is important to understand the underlying mechanism [8], e.g., if it is related to an imbalanced autonomic regulation. It is also relevant to investigate large populations with a wide variation in the number of pain sites, and the variation of autonomic activity throughout daily living (not only artificial conditions). Moreover, because physical activity and body postures influence HRV in ambulatory recordings [2, 5, 33], it is important to use valid technical information of physical activity and body postures during the measurement of HRV. Also, a previous study of HRV in a working population showed differences between work and leisure time only for the sitting posture [35]. None of the previous studies on multisite musculoskeletal pain and HRV has taken all these factors into account. Thus, the aim of this study was to investigate the association between multisite musculoskeletal pain and cardiac autonomic modulation during work, leisure and sleep, and the interaction between multisite musculoskeletal pain and time domains.

Methods

Study population and exclusion criteria

This is a cross-sectional study based on data from "The Danish Physical activity cohort with objective measurements" (DPhacto) cohort, conducted on blue-collar workers recruited in the cleaning in public and private sector (i.e. hospitals, schools, municipalities, and private firms), manufacturing and production companies in metal, plastic, and food industries, and transportation (i.e. mail, and parcel service companies). The recruitment was performed in collaboration with a labor union and the data were collected between 2012 and 2013. The inclusion criteria were: to be allowed to participate during the paid working time, to be employed for more than 20 h per week and being between 18 and 65 years. Exclusion criteria were declining to sign the informed consent, pregnancy, fever on the testing day, and allergy to adhesives.

Among 2107 potentially eligible workers in the DPhacto cohort, objective measurement data from 759 blue-collar workers were available for analysis. Workers having less than 4 h of valid HRV recordings during work, leisure and sleep time ($n = 163$) and with no information about pain intensity ($n = 3$) were excluded, resulting in a final sample of 568 blue-collar workers

(Fig. 1). The response rate was 63%. Detailed information about the DPhacto cohort can be found elsewhere [18].

Multisite musculoskeletal pain

Musculoskeletal pain was assessed by modified questions from the validated Nordic Musculoskeletal Questionnaire [23] with questions on pain intensity in seven anatomical areas (neck/shoulders; elbows; hands/wrists; low back; hips; knees and feet/ankles) during the past three months using a scale from 0 (no pain) to 10 (worst pain). Pain intensity scales were dichotomized from the median, i.e. less than median = 'no pain', more than median = 'pain' [31]. The cut-off values were 3 points for neck/shoulder and low back, and 0 points for elbows, hands/wrists, hips, knees, feet/ankles. The elbows and hands/wrists were grouped to represent the upper limbs and the hips; knees and feet/ankles represented the lower limbs. The four regions were summed to provide information about the number of pain sites (0 = none to 4 = 4 pain sites). Pain in none of the regions was regarded as 'pain-free', one pain site was regarded as 'single-site pain', while the pain in two or more sites was defined as 'multisite musculoskeletal pain'.

Technical measurements of heart rate variability and physical activity

HRV was measured by the ActiHeart system (Camntech Ltd., Cambridge, UK) with electrocardiography sensitivity of 0.250 mV. The sensor was attached by a two-led configuration at the recommended position [3]. The analogue signal was band-pass filtered (10–35 Hz), sampled with a frequency of 128 Hz, and processed by a real-time QRS-detection algorithm to achieve a 1 ms time resolution of the RR intervals. Since data was collected during daily living conditions, respiratory rate was not controlled. Abnormal beats were removed using an automatic algorithm before analyzing HRV [22].

HRV data were analyzed using a robust method [37] from 5-min windows with less than 10% erroneous interbeat intervals (IBI). For time domain, the measures obtained were the standard deviation of R-R intervals (SDNN), which is a measure of overall variability; and the root mean square of successive differences of R-R intervals (RMSSD), a measure of beat-to-beat variability, which is related to the vagal modulation. For frequency domain, the low (LF, 0.04–0.15 Hz) and high frequency (HF, 0.15–0.40 Hz) components were analyzed, as well as the sympathovagal balance (LF/HF ratio). HF indicates the parasympathetic modulation of the cardiac rhythm, while LF is an indicator of both sympathetic and parasympathetic cardiac modulations [26, 28].

Physical activity and body posture were objectively measured using multiple accelerometers (ActiGraph

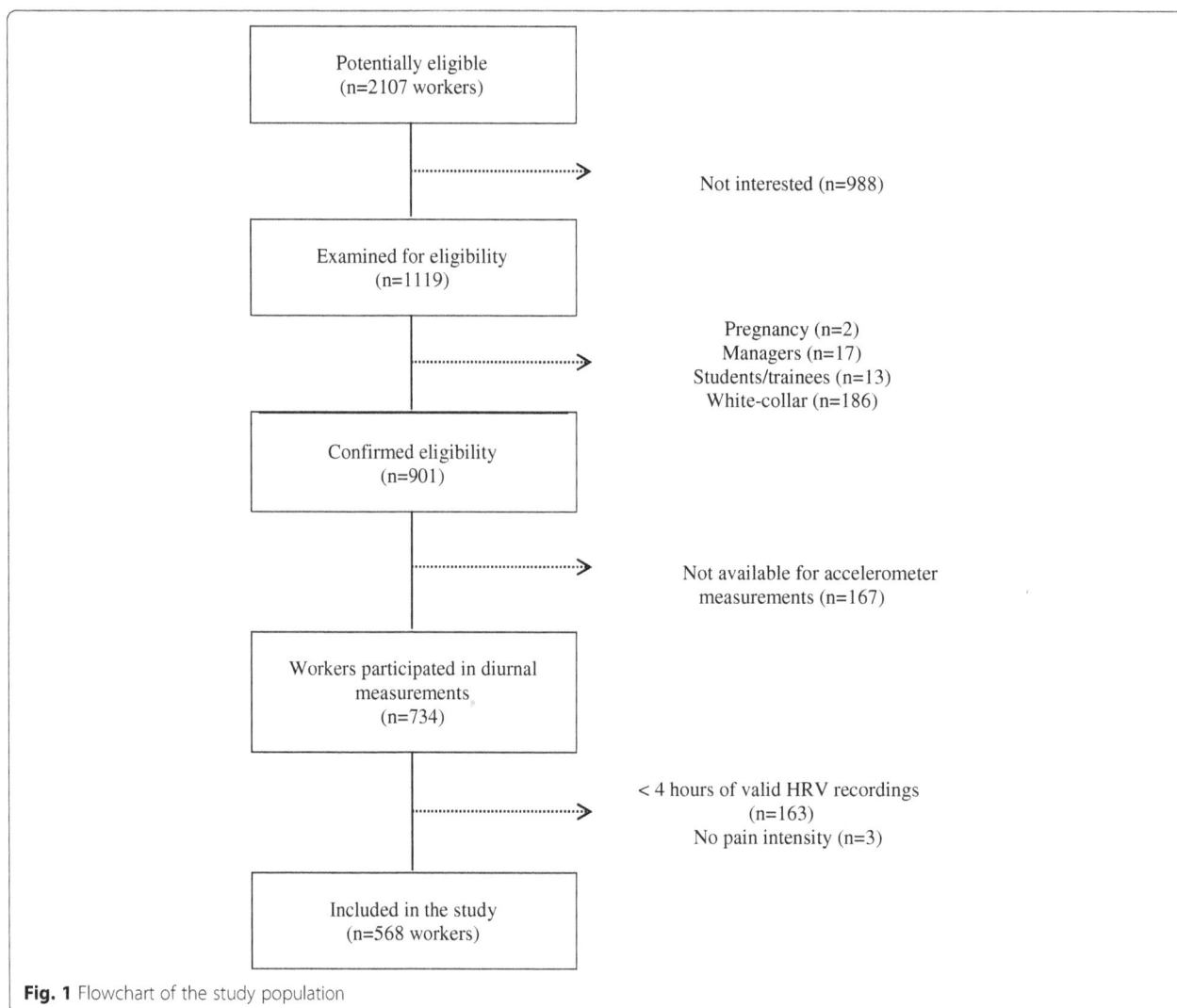

Fig. 1 Flowchart of the study population

GT3X+, Actigraph, Florida, USA). The accelerometers were attached to the thigh and upper back for several days, including work, leisure and sleep time. A diary was also filled out by the workers, including information about times getting up in the morning, starting and finishing work, and going to bed, as well as times of the reference position (upright stance) for calibration of the accelerometer records [18].

Physical activity and HRV data were processed using the Acti4 software (The National Research Centre for the Working Environment, Copenhagen, Denmark and BAuA, Berlin, Germany). The Acti4 software classifies different physical activities (walking, moving, cycling and running) and body postures (sitting, standing, and lying down) with high sensitivity and specificity [36]. The HRV indices obtained during 5-min non-overlap intervals in sitting posture at work and leisure were analyzed, as well as three periods with the lowest R-R intervals during nocturnal sleep without movement [16].

Assessment of individual and occupational factors

A self-reported questionnaire was administered to the workers including age, gender, alcohol and tobacco use, medication prescription, job seniority, lifting and carrying during work. Height (cm) was measured using a scale (Seca, model 123) and weight (kg) was measured by a digital scale (Tanita model BC 418 MA). Body mass index (BMI) was calculated according to the formulae BMI = weight (kg)/height^2 (m).

Statistical analysis

Groups were compared for the characterization variables using one-way ANOVA and Tukey's post hoc tests for continuous variables and Chi-square test for categorical variables. The HRV indices, except IBI, showed a non-normal distribution (Kolmogorov Smirnov test; see Additional file 1: Figures S1, S2 and S3). Thus a natural logarithm (ln) transformation was applied.

Linear mixed models with two fixed factors were applied to verify the association between groups (pain-free, single-site pain, multisite pain), domains (work, leisure, sleep), and interaction of groups and domains. Linear mixed models were chosen because it includes fixed and random effects and increase the study power including in the analysis subjects with missing data. Subject and intercept were included as random effects. The covariance type was unstructured, and the restricted maximum likelihood (REML) estimation method was chosen. When the interaction was significant, the mean difference (MD), standard error (SE) and P value for the pairwise comparison, based on estimated marginal means, were reported.

Crude and adjusted models were tested. In the adjusted model, age, sex, BMI, tobacco use, objectively measured moderate and vigorous physical activity (i.e. fast walking, running, stair climbing and cycling) at work and leisure, and sitting time at work and leisure were included as covariates since these factors may affect both multisite pain and HRV [1, 10, 19, 21, 29, 32]. Sensitivity analyses, excluding workers reporting prescribed medication in the last three months and considering the cut-off point of zero to dichotomize the pain intensity scales, were also performed. Stratified analyses were applied to explore possible effect modification of age (< 50 years; ≥50 years) and sex (male; female). All analyses were performed using SPSS software (version 24.0), and the significance level was set at 1% to control for type I error in multiple comparison tests.

Results

About 44% of the sample was composed of females, the mean age was 45 years and mean BMI was 27 kg/m^2. About 29% of the workers smoked daily or occasionally; 19% reported to use analgesic medication, 12% antihypertensive, 3% heart medication and 3% antidepressants. Most of the workers were from the manufacturing sector (72%), and 41% reported to carry and lift for at least half of the work time. The prevalence of single-site pain was 23% (CI 95%, 20–27%), and the prevalence of multisite pain was 63% (CI 95%, 58–66%). In both groups, the most affected body parts were knees (single-site pain: 32%; multisite pain: 67%), lower back (single-site pain: 13%; multisite pain: 65%) and neck/shoulder (single-site pain: 15%; multisite pain: 65%).

The three groups were similar in most of the sociodemographic variables, except for a larger proportion of lifting and carrying almost all the time to ¼ of the time in the multisite pain group. Pain intensity, the number of pain sites and the proportion of workers with prescribed analgesic medication were also higher in the multisite pain group compared with the pain-free and single-site pain groups. There were no differences

between the groups for the other types of medication (Table 1).

Table 2 shows the mean and interquartile range for the HRV indices during work, leisure and sleep time for each group. The between groups comparison showed similar values for all indices during work, leisure and sleep time.

The results from the linear mixed models showed no significant differences between groups and no significant interaction between groups and domains in the crude or adjusted models for any HRV index (Table 3). Significant differences between domains were found in the crude and adjusted model for all indices, except SDNN; sleep time showed higher values than leisure and work time, except for LF and LF/HF, which were higher during work.

The sensitivity analysis, excluding workers with prescribed medication in the last three months ($n = 234$), showed no significant differences between groups and significant differences among domains for all indices in the crude and adjusted model, except for SDNN. The interaction between groups and domains was not significant for all indices. When using a more restrictive definition of a pain-free group, i.e., including in the pain-free group workers reporting no pain in all body parts (cut-off point = 0), the sensitivity analysis also showed no significant differences between groups, significant differences between domains (except for SDNN) and no significant interaction between groups and domains for all indices (Additional file 1: Table S1). The same results were found in the stratified analyses for age (Additional file 1: Table S2) and sex (Additional file 1: Table S3).

Discussion

This cross-sectional study showed no association between multisite musculoskeletal pain and cardiac autonomic modulation during work, leisure and sleep.

Previous systematic reviews indicated that chronic pain is associated with a decrease in parasympathetic modulation [20, 40]. However, in agreement with our findings, Generaal et al. [14, 15] showed that autonomic cardiac modulation was not impaired with chronic multisite pain. One possible explanation for this divergence between the systematic reviews and the MSP studies could be that the results from the systematic reviews showing an autonomic imbalance in chronic pain are mainly based on studies with fibromyalgia patients. So, the autonomic imbalance involved in the pathophysiology of fibromyalgia [27] does not necessarily extend to active workers with multisite pain.

Another possible explanation for our findings can be related to the study population and data collection conditions. Most studies are based on patient samples

Table 1 Characteristics of the blue-collar workers in DPhacto according to the pain groups. Continuous data are present as [mean (SD)], and frequencies are presented as [n (%)]

Characteristics	All (n = 568)	Pain-free (n = 74)	Single-site pain (n = 136)	Multisite pain (n = 358)	P value
Female	247 (43.5%)	25 (33.8%)	57 (41.9%)	165 (46.1%)	0.13
Age, years	45.3 (9.8)	46.8 (10.3)	45.0 (9.3)	45.1 (9.8)	0.39
Body mass index, kg/m^2	27.3 (4.7)	27.2 (4.8)	26.9 (4.8)	27.5 (4.7)	0.43
Smokers	161 (29.1%)	18 (24.3%)	40 (31.0%)	103 (29.4%)	0.58
Alcohol, units/week	4.5 (5.9)	5.6 (7.2)	3.9 (4.7)	4.6 (6.0)	0.15
Use of medication	234 (41.2%)	25 (33.8%)	42 (30.9%)	167 (46.6%)	< 0.01
Antihypertensive	70 (12.3%)	9 (12.2%)	14 (10.3%)	47 (13.1%)	0.69
Heart	19 (3.3%)	3 (4.1%)	4 (2.9%)	12 (3.4%)	0.91
Antidepressants	18 (3.2%)	0 (0.0%)	2 (1.5%)	16 (4.5%)	0.06
Analgesic	108 (19.0%)	7 (9.5%)	14 (10.3%)	87 (24.3%)	< 0.01
Other	128 (22.5%)	14 (18.9%)	28 (20.6%)	86 (24.0%)	0.52
Occupational sector					0.44
Cleaning	109 (19.2%)	11 (14.9%)	31 (22.8%)	67 (18.7%)	
Manufacturing	410 (72.2%)	57 (77.0%)	97 (71.3%)	256 (71.5%)	
Transportation	49 (8.6%)	6 (8.1%)	8 (5.9%)	35 (9.8%)	
MVPA work time, h/day	1.3 (0.5)	1.3 (0.5)	1.3 (0.5)	1.3 (0.5)	0.95
MVPA leisure time, h/day	0.9 (0.3)	0.9 (0.4)	0.9 (0.4)	0.8 (0.3)	0.40
Sitting work time, h/day	2.5 (1.7)	2.5 (1.7)	2.5 (1.6)	2.5 (1.8)	0.95
Sitting leisure time, h/day	4.7 (1.3)	4.7 (1.5)	4.6 (1.3)	4.7 (1.3)	0.93
Seniority, months	13.4 (10.4)	12.9 (10.2)	13.1 (9.7)	13.6 (10.7)	0.80
Lifting and carrying					0.01
Almost all the time	75 (13.3%)	8 (10.8%)	15 (11.1%)	52 (14.6%)	
3/4 of the time	53 (9.4%)	1 (1.4%)	9 (6.7%)	43 (12.0%)	
1/2 of the time	102 (18.0%)	13 (17.6%)	22 (16.3%)	67 (18.8%)	
1/4 of the time	151 (26.7%)	16 (21.6%)	42 (31.1%)	93 (26.1%)	
Rarely/very little	157 (27.7%)	32 (43.2%)	37 (27.4%)	88 (24.6%)	
Never	28 (4.9%)	4 (5.4%)	10 (7.4%)	14 (3.9%)	
Highest pain intensity, 0–10	5.5 (2.9)	1.0 (1.2)	4.2 (2.1)	6.9 (2.1)	< 0.01
Number of pain sites	2.0 (1.2)	0.0 (0.0)	1.0 (0.0)	2.8 (0.8)	< 0.01

DPhacto Danish Physical activity cohort with objective measurements, *MVPA* Moderate to vigorous physical activity

evaluated in artificial conditions which can differ from active workers concerning physical, cognitive and psychosocial characteristics. Thus, it is possible that people with pain who is still at work are healthier, more physically active and have better coping mechanisms with their pain compared to clinical samples with pain [9, 24], which may be reflected in better autonomic function throughout daily living conditions, including work, leisure and sleep time. It is still possible that there are sub-groups of people with other features of multisite pain not captured in our study. Likewise, other factors like sleep disturbance, depressed mood, somatising tendency and psychosocial aspects of work may be involved in chronic multisite pain [6, 38]. These factors were not

examined in our study, which is a limitation. Our findings may also suggest publication bias of positive results in previous studies [39].

The sensitivity analysis for medication yielded the same findings as the main analysis, including workers with prescribed medication. Additionally, the adoption of a more restrictive definition of pain-free resulted in the same findings. Also, stratified analysis on sex and age did not show association between multisite musculoskeletal pain and cardiac autonomic modulation during work, leisure and sleep.

The prevalence of multisite pain was very high in our sample, as it affected 63% of the DPhacto blue-collar workers, with the mean peak pain intensity of 6.9 points

Table 2 Heart rate variability indices during work, leisure and sleep time for each group among the blue-collar participants in DPhacto. Data are presented as mean (interquartile range - IQR)

Variables	Work			Leisure			Sleep		
	Pain-free (n = 74)	Single-site pain (n = 136)	Multisite pain (n = 357)	Pain-free (n = 74)	Single-site pain (n = 136)	Multisite pain (n = 358)	Pain-free (n = 72)	Single-site pain (n = 135)	Multisite pain (n = 354)
IBI, ms	793.8 (136)	786.1 (130)	781.3 (136)	820.6 (132)	824.0 (133)	820.6 (132)	1068.3 (211)	1079.5 (212)	1075.7 (173)
SDNN, ms	53.5 (26)	54.7 (22)	54.7 (23)	52.4 (23)	53.0 (23)	53.6 (22)	54.2 (34)	52.9 (27)	56.8 (31)
ln SDNN	3.92 (0.51)	3.95 (0.40)	3.95 (0.43)	3.90 (0.46)	3.92 (0.45)	3.93 (0.42)	3.89 (0.66)	3.90 (0.52)	3.95 (0.58)
RMSSD, ms	26.9 (16)	26.2 (14)	26.6 (14)	27.6 (16)	27.3 (17)	28.5 (15)	47.5 (32)	47.0 (32)	51.7 (36)
ln RMSSD	3.17 (0.69)	3.17 (0.58)	3.17 (0.58)	3.20 (0.66)	3.21 (0.65)	3.25 (0.59)	3.69 (0.78)	3.71 (0.73)	3.79 (0.78)
LF, ms²/Hz	872.1 (732)	861.8 (691)	883.8 (752)	746.8 (692)	730.8 (592)	737.5 (648)	926.3 (944)	822.0 (749)	991.9 (902)
ln LF	6.49 (1.06)	6.54 (0.92)	6.52 (1.02)	6.34 (1.12)	6.37 (0.98)	6.35 (1.05)	6.39 (1.48)	6.38 (1.20)	6.46 (1.30)
HF, ms²/Hz	231.8 (213)	218.4 (168)	232.5 (195)	261.9 (214)	260.1 (244)	278.8 (248)	933.9 (865)	870.9 (942)	1133.8 (1094)
ln HF	4.94 (1.42)	4.92 (1.20)	4.97 (1.25)	5.08 (1.27)	5.11 (1.36)	5.19 (1.22)	6.18 (1.50)	6.24 (1.51)	6.37 (1.66)
LF/HF	6.08 (4)	6.70 (4)	6.36 (4)	4.97 (3)	5.31 (3)	4.97 (3)	1.97 (2)	1.75 (1)	1.90 (2)
ln LF/HF	1.66 (0.68)	1.75 (0.69)	1.69 (0.80)	1.47 (0.72)	1.52 (0.76)	1.43 (0.81)	0.32 (1.05)	0.20 (1.01)	0.17 (1.29)

IBI Interbeat intervals, *SDNN* Standard deviation of RR intervals, *ln* Natural logarithm, *RMSSD* Square root of the mean squared differences of successive RR intervals, *LF* Low-frequency power, *HF* High-frequency power, *LF/HF* Sympathovagal balance

Table 3 Estimates, standard error and *P* value from the linear mixed models for heart rate variability indices showing the main effect of group, domain and the interaction (group × domain) in the crude and adjusted models in DPhacto (*n* = 568)

Variables	Crude model			Adjusted model*		
	Estimate	Standard error	*P*	Estimate	Standard error	*P*
IBI, ms						
Group			0.93			0.58
Pain-free	793.8	13.5		935.3	43.4	
Single-site pain	786.1	9.9		936.6	42.4	
Multisite pain	781.1	6.1		930.6	42.0	
Domain			< 0.01			< 0.01
Sleep	294.7	4.4		293.1	4.5	
Leisure	39.5	4.4		37.9	4.5	
Interaction			0.36			0.28
Pain-free at sleep	−21.8	10.7		−21.6	11.0	
Pain-free at leisure	−12.6	10.6		−11.4	10.9	
Single-site pain at sleep	−1.2	8.4		5.5	8.8	
Single-site pain at leisure	−1.5	8.3		1.2	8.7	
ln SDNN						
Group			0.55			0.61
Pain-free	3.92	0.03		4.92	0.11	
Single-site pain	3.95	0.02		4.95	0.11	
Multisite pain	3.95	0.01		4.94	0.11	
Domain			0.20			0.07
Sleep	0.00	0.01		0.00	0.01	
Leisure	−0.01	0.01		−0.01	0.01	
Interaction			0.36			0.13
Pain-free at sleep	−0.04	0.03		−0.05	0.03	
Pain-free at leisure	0.00	0.03		0.00	0.03	
Single-site pain at sleep	−0.05	0.03		−0.07	0.03	
Single-site pain at leisure	−0.01	0.03		−0.01	0.03	
ln RMSSD						
Group			0.54			0.81
Pain-free	3.17	0.05		4.32	0.17	
Single-site pain	3.17	0.04		4.31	0.16	
Multisite pain	3.17	0.02		4.30	0.16	
Domain			< 0.01			< 0.01
Sleep	0.61	0.01		0.61	0.02	
Leisure	0.07	0.01		0.07	0.02	
Interaction			0.16			0.13
Pain-free at sleep	−0.10	0.04		−0.11	0.04	
Pain-free at leisure	−0.04	0.04		−0.04	0.04	
Single-site pain at sleep	−0.06	0.03		−0.07	0.03	
Single-site pain at leisure	−0.03	0.03		−0.02	0.03	
ln LF						
Group			0.89			0.86
Pain-free	6.49	0.09		8.96	0.25	

Table 3 Estimates, standard error and *P* value from the linear mixed models for heart rate variability indices showing the main effect of group, domain and the interaction (group × domain) in the crude and adjusted models in DPhacto (*n* = 568) *(Continued)*

Variables	Crude model			Adjusted model*		
	Estimate	Standard error	P	Estimate	Standard error	P
Single-site pain	6.54	0.06		8.99	0.24	
Multisite pain	6.52	0.04		8.98	0.24	
Domain			< 0.01			< 0.01
Sleep	−0.06	0.03		−0.06	0.03	
Leisure	−0.17	0.03		−0.17	0.03	
Interaction			0.64			0.41
Pain-free at sleep	−0.04	0.09		− 0.07	0.09	
Pain-free at leisure	0.01	0.09		0.01	0.09	
Single-site pain at sleep	−0.09	0.07		−0.12	0.07	
Single-site pain at leisure	0.00	0.07		0.00	0.07	
ln HF						
Group			0.50			0.79
Pain-free	4.94	0.12		7.47	0.35	
Single-site pain	4.92	0.08		7.39	0.34	
Multisite pain	4.96	0.05		7.41	0.34	
Domain			< 0.01			< 0.01
Sleep	1.40	0.04		1.39	0.04	
Leisure	0.22	0.04		0.22	0.04	
Interaction			0.53			0.37
Pain-free at sleep	−0.17	0.10		−0.20	0.10	
Pain-free at leisure	−0.08	0.10		−0.07	0.10	
Single-site pain at sleep	−0.07	0.08		−0.08	0.08	
Single-site pain at leisure	−0.03	0.07		−0.02	0.08	
ln LF/HF						
Group			0.51			0.82
Pain-free	1.66	0.08		1.46	0.22	
Single-site pain	1.75	0.06		1.60	0.22	
Multisite pain	1.69	0.03		1.57	0.21	
Domain			< 0.01			< 0.01
Sleep	−1.51	0.03		−1.51	0.03	
Leisure	−0.26	0.03		−0.26	0.03	
Interaction			0.22			0.18
Pain-free at sleep	0.17	0.08		0.18	0.08	
Pain-free at leisure	0.07	0.08		0.06	0.08	
Single-site pain at sleep	−0.02	0.06		−0.04	0.07	
Single-site pain at leisure	0.03	0.06		0.02	0.07	

IBI Interbeat intervals, *SDNN* Standard deviation of RR intervals, *ln* Natural logarithm, *RMSSD* Square root of the mean squared differences of successive RR intervals, *LF* Low-frequency power, *HF* High-frequency power, *LF/HF* Sympathovagal balance. *Adjusted for: sex, age, BMI, smoking, moderate to vigorous physical activity at work and leisure, sitting time at work and leisure. Work domain was regarded as the reference

on a 0 to 10 scale. This high prevalence may be specific to the study population consisting of blue-collar workers, i.e., it refers to a disadvantaged socioeconomic group. Other studies have also shown a high prevalence of multisite pain in different populations, ranging from 35 to 64% [17, 30]. Although our findings showed that the imbalance of the autonomic modulation was not associated with multisite pain, this issue still deserves attention, since the theoretical framework support this relationship [25, 42]. Future studies should have a longitudinal design to verify if the autonomic imbalance precedes the occurrence of multisite pain.

Strengths and limitations

A strength of our study is the large sample size, which allowed for stratified analyses. A further strength was the relatively homogenous group of blue-collar workers, which minimized potential socioeconomic confounding. The control for lifestyle factors such as smoking, physical activity, sitting time, and individual characteristics such as sex, age, and BMI is also highly relevant as these factors are closely related to HRV and pain. A potential limitation is the lack of control for the respiration rate, circadian variation, sleep quality and psychosocial aspects of work. Additionally, we have only looked at HRV during sleep, work and leisure, while there exist several other ways of evaluating autonomic function, such as assessing autonomic reactivity to functional tests (e.g. Valsalva, cold pressor and handgrip tests). Finally, the cross-sectional design of this study does not allow determining whether an autonomic imbalance may occur before the development of multisite pain.

Conclusion

This cross-sectional study showed that multisite musculoskeletal pain is not associated with imbalanced cardiac autonomic regulation during work, leisure and sleep time.

Additional file

> **Additional file 1: Table S1.** Estimates, standard error and *P* value from the linear mixed models for heart rate variability indices showing the main effect of group, domain and the interaction (group × domain) in the crude and adjusted models using a strict definition of pain-free workers in DPhacto (*n* = 568). **Table S2.** Stratified analysis for age (< 50 years; ≥50 years). Estimates, standard error and *P* values from the linear mixed models for heart rate variability indices showing the main effect of group, domain and the interaction (group × domain) in the crude and adjusted models in DPhacto. **Table S3.** Stratified analysis for sex (male; female). Estimates, standard error and *P* values from the linear mixed models for heart rate variability indices showing the main effect of group, domain and the interaction (group × domain) in the crude and adjusted models in DPhacto. **Figure S1.** Original distribution of the HRV indices during work. **Figure S2.** Original distribution of the HRV indices during leisure. **Figure S3.** Original distribution of the HRV indices during sleep. (DOCX 1424 kb)

Abbreviations

ANOVA: Analysis of variance; BMI: Body mass index; DPhacto: Danish Physical activity cohort with objective measurements; HF: High frequency; HRV: Heart rate variability; IBI: Inter beat intervals; LF: Low frequency; LF/ HF: Sympathovagal balance; ln: Natural logarithm; MD: Mean difference; MSP: Multisite pain; MVPA: Moderate and vigorous physical activity; REML: Restricted maximum likelihood; RMSSD: Root mean square of successive differences of R-R intervals; SDNN: Standard deviation of R-R intervals; SE: Standard error; SSP: Single-site pain

Acknowledgments

We would like to thank the entire DPhacto research team for the project planning, data collection, handling and management.

Funding

This study was conducted with the financial support from The Danish Work Environment Research Fund and São Paulo Research Foundation (FAPESP), São Paulo, Brazil (grant#2015/18310–1). The funding body had no participation in the design of the study, data collection, data analysis and interpretation and in writing the manuscript.

Authors' contributions

TOS, DMH, JK, AH: contribution to conception and design. AH: acquisition of data. TOS, DMH, AH: analysis and interpretation of data. TOS, DMH, JK, AH: drafting the article, revising it critically for important intellectual content, final approval of the version to be published.

Competing interests

The authors declare that they have no competing interests.

Author details

[1]Physical Therapy Department, Federal University of São Carlos (UFSCar), Rodovia Washington Luís, km 235, São Carlos, SP 13565-905, Brazil. [2]Centre for Musculoskeletal Research, Department of Occupational and Public Health Sciences, University of Gävle, 801-76 Gävle, SE, Sweden. [3]National Research Centre for the Working Environment (NRCWE), Lersø Parkallé 105, 2100 Copenhagen Ø, DK, Denmark. [4]Department of Sports Science and Clinical Biomechanics, University of Southern Denmark, Odense, Denmark.

References

1. Acharya UR, Paul JK, Kannathal N, Lim CM, Suri JS. Heart rate variability: a review. Med Biol Eng Comput. 2006;44(12):1031–51.
2. Bernardi L, Valle F, Coco M, Calciati A, Sleight P. Physical activity influences heart rate variability and very-low-frequency components in Holter electrocardiograms. Cardiovasc Res. 1996;32(2):234–7.
3. Brage S, Brage N, Franks PW, Ekelund U, Wareham NJ. Reliability and validity of the combined heart rate and movement sensor Actiheart. Eur J Clin Nutr. 2005;59(4):561–70. https://doi.org/10.1038/sj.ejcn.1602118.
4. Carnes D, Parsons S, Ashby D, Breen A, Foster NE, Pincus T, Vogel S, Underwood M. Chronic musculoskeletal pain rarely presents in a single body site: results from a UK population study. Rheumatology. 2007;46(7): 1168–70. https://doi.org/10.1093/rheumatology/kem118.
5. Chan H-L, Lin M-A, Chao P-K, Lin C-H. Correlates of the shift in heart rate variability with postures and walking by time-frequency analysis. Comp Meth Program Biomed. 2007;86(2):124–30. https://doi.org/10.1016/j.cmpb. 2007.02.003.
6. Coggon D, Ntani G. Trajectories of multisite musculoskeletal pain and implications for prevention. Occup Environ Med. 2017;74(7):465–6. https://doi.org/10.1136/oemed-2016-104196.
7. Coggon D, Ntani G, Palmer KT, Felli VE, Harari R, Barrero LH, Felknor SA, Gimeno D, Cattrell A, Vargas-Prada S, Bonzini M, Solidaki E, Merisalu E, Habib RR, Sadeghian F, Masood Kadir M, Warnakulasuriya SS, Matsudaira K, Nyantumbu B, Sim MR, Harcombe H, Cox K, Marziale MH, Sarquis LM, Harari F, Freire R, Harari N, Monroy MV, Quintana LA, Rojas M, Salazar Vega EJ, Harris EC, Serra C, Martinez JM, Delclos G, Benavides FG, Carugno M, Ferrario MM, Pesatori AC, Chatzi L, Bitsios P, Kogevinas M, Oha K, Sirk T, Sadeghian A, Peiris-John RJ, Sathiakumar N, Wickremasinghe AR, Yoshimura N, Kelsall HL, Hoe VC, Urquhart DM, Derrett S, McBride D, Herbison P, Gray A. Patterns of multisite pain and associations with risk factors. Pain. 2013;154(9):1769–77. https://doi.org/10.1016/j.pain.2013.05.039.

8. Croft P, Dunn KM, Von Korff M. Chronic pain syndromes: you can't have one without another. Pain. 2007;131(3):237–8. https://doi.org/10.1016/j.pain.2007.07.013.

9. de Vries HJ, Brouwer S, Groothoff JW, Geertzen JH, Reneman MF. Staying at work with chronic nonspecific musculoskeletal pain: a qualitative study of workers' experiences. BMC Musculoskelet Disord. 2011;12:126. https://doi.org/10.1186/1471-2474-12-126.

10. Dinas PC, Koutedakis Y, Flouris AD. Effects of active and passive tobacco cigarette smoking on heart rate variability. Int J Cardiol. 2013;163(2):109–15. https://doi.org/10.1016/j.ijcard.2011.10.140.

11. Eckhoff C, Straume B, Kvernmo S. Multisite musculoskeletal pain in adolescence as a predictor of medical and social welfare benefits in young adulthood: the Norwegian Arctic adolescent health cohort study. Eur J Pain. 2017;21:1697–706. https://doi.org/10.1002/ejp.1078.

12. Fayaz A, Croft P, Langford RM, Donaldson LJ, Jones GT. Prevalence of chronic pain in the UK: a systematic review and meta-analysis of population studies. BMJ Open. 2016;6(6):e010364. https://doi.org/10.1136/bmjopen-2015-010364.

13. Fernandes RCP, Burdorf A. Associations of multisite pain with healthcare utilization, sickness absence and restrictions at work. Int Arch Occup Environ Health. 2016;89(7):1039–46. https://doi.org/10.1007/s00420-016-1141-7.

14. Generaal E, Vogelzangs N, Macfarlane GJ, Geenen R, Smit JH, de Geus EJ, Penninx BW, Dekker J. Biological stress systems, adverse life events and the onset of chronic multisite musculoskeletal pain: a 6-year cohort study. Ann Rheum Dis. 2016;75(5):847–54. https://doi.org/10.1136/annrheumdis-2014-206741.

15. Generaal E, Vogelzangs N, Macfarlane GJ, Geenen R, Smit JH, de Geus EJ, Dekker J, Penninx BW. Biological stress systems, adverse life events, and the improvement of chronic multisite musculoskeletal pain across a 6-year follow-up. J Pain. 2017;18(2):155–65. https://doi.org/10.1016/j.jpain.2016.10.010.

16. Hallman DM, Birk Jørgensen M, Holtermann A. On the health paradox of occupational and leisure-time physical activity using objective measurements: effects on autonomic imbalance. PLoS One. 2017;12(5):e0177042. https://doi.org/10.1371/journal.pone.0177042.

17. Haukka E, Kaila-Kangas L, Ojajärvi A, Saastamoinen P, Holtermann A, Jørgensen MB, Karppinen J, Heliövaara M, Leino-Arjas P. Multisite musculoskeletal pain predicts medically certified disability retirement among Finns. Eur J Pain. 2015;19(8):1119–28. https://doi.org/10.1002/ejp.635.

18. Jørgensen MB, Korshøj M, Lagersted-Olsen J, Villumsen M, Mortensen OS, Skotte J, Søgaard K, Madeleine P, Thomsen BL, Holtermann A. Physical activities at work and risk of musculoskeletal pain and its consequences: protocol for a study with objective field measures among blue-collar workers. BMC Musculoskelet Disord. 2013;20(14):213. https://doi.org/10.1186/1471-2474-14-213.

19. Kamaleri Y, Natvig B, Ihlebaek CM, Benth JS, Bruusgaard D. Number of pain sites is associated with demographic, lifestyle, and health-related factors in the general population. Eur J Pain. 2008;12(6):742–8.

20. Koenig J, Falvay D, Clamor A, Wagner J, Jarczok MN, Ellis RJ, Weber C, Thayer JF. Pneumogastric (vagus) nerve activity indexed by heart rate variability in chronic pain patients compared to healthy controls: a systematic review and meta-analysis. Pain Physician. 2016;19(1):E55–78.

21. Koenig J, Jarczok MN, Warth M, Ellis RJ, Bach C, Hillecke TK, Thayer JF. Body mass index is related to autonomic nervous system activity as measured by heart rate variability – a replication using short term measurements. J Nutr Health Aging. 2014;18(3):300–2. https://doi.org/10.1007/s12603-014-0022-6.

22. Kristiansen J, Korshøj M, Skotte JH, Jespersen T, Søgaard K, Mortensen OS, Holtermann A. Comparison of two systems for long-term heart rate variability monitoring in free-living conditions—a pilot study. Biomed Eng Online. 2011. https://doi.org/10.1186/1475-925X-10-27.

23. Kuorinka I, Jonsson B, Kilbom Å, Vinterberg H, Biering-Sörensen F, Anderson G, Jörgensen K. Standardised Nordic questionnaires for the analysis of musculoskeletal symptoms. Appl Ergon. 1987;18:233–7.

24. Linton SJ, Buer N. Working despite pain: factors associated with work attendance versus dysfunction. Int J Behav Med. 1995;2(3):252–62.

25. Maletic V, Raison CL. Neurobiology of depression, fibromyalgia and neuropathic pain. Front Biosci. 2009;14:5291–338.

26. Malik M, Bigger JT, Camm AJ, Kleiger RE, Malliani A, Moss AJ, Schwartz PJ. Heart rate variability standards of measurement, physiological interpretation, and clinical use. Eur Heart J. 1996;17(3):354–81.

27. Martínez-Lavín M. Is fibromyalgia a generalized reflex sympathetic dystrophy? Clin Exp Rheumatol. 2001;19(1):1–3.

28. Michael S, Graham KS, Oam DGM. Cardiac autonomic responses during exercise and postexercise recovery using heart rate variability and systolic time intervals - a review. Front Physiol. 2017;29(8):301. https://doi.org/10.3389/fphys.2017.00301.

29. Molfino A, Fiorentini A, Tubani L, Martuscelli M, Rossi Fanelli F, Laviano A. Body mass index is related to autonomic nervous system activity as measured by heart rate variability. Eur J Clin Nutr. 2009;63(10):1263–5. https://doi.org/10.1038/ejcn.2009.35.

30. Neupane S, Leino-Arjas P, Nygård CH, Oakman J, Virtanen P. Developmental pathways of multisite musculoskeletal pain: what is the influence of physical and psychosocial working conditions? Occup Environ Med. 2017;74(7):468–75. https://doi.org/10.1136/oemed-2016-103892.

31. Neupane S, Virtanen P, Leino-Arjas P, Miranda H, Siukola A, Nygård CH. Multi-site pain and working conditions as predictors of work ability in a 4-year follow-up among food industry employees. Eur J Pain. 2013;17(3):444–51. https://doi.org/10.1002/j.1532-2149.2012.00198.x.

32. Pan F, Laslett L, Blizzard L, Cicuttini F, Winzenberg T, Ding C, Jones G. Associations between fat mass and multisite pain: a five-year longitudinal study. Arthritis Care Res. 2017;69(4):509–16. https://doi.org/10.1002/acr.22963.

33. Perini R, Veicsteinas A. Heart rate variability and autonomic activity at rest and during exercise in various physiological conditions. Eur J Appl Physiol. 2003;90(3–4):317–25. https://doi.org/10.1007/s00421-003-0953-9.

34. Phillips CJ. The cost and burden of chronic pain. Rev Pain. 2009;3(1):2–5. https://doi.org/10.1177/204946370900300102.

35. Sato TO, Hallman DM, Kristiansen J, Skotte JH, Holtermann A. Different autonomic responses to occupational and leisure time physical activities among blue-collar workers. Int Arch Occup Environ Health. 2017. https://doi.org/10.1007/s00420-017-1279-y.

36. Skotte J, Korshøj M, Kristiansen J, Hanisch C, Holtermann A. Detection of physical activity types using triaxial accelerometers. J Phys Act Health. 2014;11(1):76–84. https://doi.org/10.1123/jpah.2011-0347.

37. Skotte JH, Kristiansen J. Heart rate variability analysis using robust period detection. Biomed Eng Online. 2014. https://doi.org/10.1186/1475-925X-13-138.

38. Solidaki E, Chatzi L, Bitsios P, Markatzi I, Plana E, Castro F, Palmer K, Coggon D, Kogevinas M. Work-related and psychological determinants of multisite musculoskeletal pain. Scand J Work Environ Health. 2010;36(1):54–61.

39. Tak LM, Riese H, de Bock GH, Manoharan A, Kok IC, Rosmalen JG. As good as it gets? A meta-analysis and systematic review of methodological quality of heart rate variability studies in functional somatic disorders. Biol Psychol. 2009;82(2):101–10. https://doi.org/10.1016/j.biopsycho.2009.05.002.

40. Tracy LM, Ioannou L, Baker KS, Gibson SJ, Georgiou-Karistianis N, Giummarra MJ. Meta-analytic evidence for decreased heart rate variability in chronic pain implicating parasympathetic nervous system dysregulation. Pain. 2016;157(1):7–29. https://doi.org/10.1097/j.pain.0000000000000360.

41. Walker-Bone K, Reading I, Coggon D, Cooper C, Palmer KT. The anatomical pattern and determinants of pain in the neck and upper limbs: an epidemiologic study. Pain. 2004;109(1–2):45–51. https://doi.org/10.1016/j.pain.2004.01.008.

42. Woda A, Picard P, Dutheil F. Dysfunctional stress responses in chronic pain. Psychoneuroendocrinology. 2016;71:127–35. https://doi.org/10.1016/j.psyneuen.2016.05.017.

22

Distal biceps tendon rupture: advantages and drawbacks of the anatomical reinsertion with a modified double incision approach

L. Tarallo[*], M. Lombardi, F. Zambianchi, A. Giorgini and F. Catani

Abstract

Background: Distal biceps tendon rupture occurs more often in middle-aged male population, involving the dominant arm. In this retrospective study, it's been described the occurrence of the most frequent adverse events and the clinical outcomes of patients undergoing surgical repair of distal biceps tendon rupture with the modified Morrey's double-incision approach, to determine better indications for patients with acute tendon injury.

Methods: Sixty-three patients with acute distal biceps tendon rupture treated with a modified double-incision technique between 2003 and 2015 were retrospectively evaluated at a mean 24 months of follow-up. Clinical evaluation including range of motion (ROM) and isometric strength recovery compared to the healthy contralateral side assessment, together with documentation of nerve injury, was performed. Patients were asked to answer DASH, OES and MEPS scores.

Results: The ROM recovery showed excellent results compared to the healthy contralateral side.
The reported major complications included: one case of proximal radio-ulnar synostosis, 3 cases of posterior interosseous nerve (PIN) palsy and one case of a-traumatic tendon re-rupture. Concerning minor complications, intermittent pain, ROM deficiency < 30° in flexion/extension and pronation/supination, isometric flexion strength deficiency < 30% and isometric supination strength deficiency < 60%, lateral antebrachial cutaneous nerve (LACBN) injury, were observed. The average DASH score was 8.5; the average OES was 41.5 and the MEPS was 96.3.

Conclusion: The Morrey modified double-incision technique finds its indication in young and active patients if performed within 2 weeks from injury. If performed by experienced surgeons, the advantages can exceed the drawbacks of possible complications.

Keywords: Distal biceps lesion, Tendon rupture, Biceps reinsertion, Double incision

Background

Distal biceps tendon rupture is a relatively uncommon injury, representing the 3% of all tendon lesions. It is predominantly affecting middle-aged, active men [1, 2]. Typically, the injury mechanism is represented by an eccentric muscle contraction against a heavy load in a semi-flexed position [2, 3].

At clinical examination, patients report acute pain in the cubital fossa and present edema, ecchymosis and palpable tendon defect on the volar side of the elbow. The Hook sign is usually positive. False negative is possible if the lacertus fibrosus is intact. Reduced strength in forearm supination and elbow flexion is usually observed [4]. Non-operative management of these injuries has been described, but significant strength reduction in flexion and supination often occurs in these patients. Therefore, such option is not suitable in young and demanding patients. On the other hand, surgical management of distal biceps tendon ruptures can be complicated by heterotopic ossification, tendon re-rupture, superficial wound infection, synostosis and nerve injury to the lateral antebrachial

* Correspondence: tarallo.luigi@policlinico.mo.it
Orthopaedics and Traumatology Department, University of Modena and Reggio Emilia, Via del Pozzo 71, 41124 Modena, Italy

cutaneous (LABC) nerve, anterior interosseous nerve (AIN), posterior interosseous nerve (PIN), median, radial and ulnar nerves [5–10].

Several techniques have been described for distal biceps tendon repair, including single anterior incision [11], often complicated by a high incidence of radial nerve palsy [12], double incision techniques exposing the radial tuberosity and allowing a smaller anterior approach, often complicated by frequent post-operative proximal radio-ulnar synostosis [13]. Others have also described a modified double-incision technique, introducing a muscle-splitting approach through the digits common extensor. More recently, with the advent of improved techniques and implants such as suture anchors, intraosseous screws and suspensory cortical buttons, single-incision techniques have once again gained popularity [14, 15].

At today's date, there is still no consensus regarding which is the best surgical solution to approach distal biceps tendon rupture [16]. Some authors sustain that complication rate does not significantly differ between one and two-incision approaches (23,9% for one-incision procedures and 25,7% for two-incision procedures) [17]. Others claim that the double-incision has significantly lower complication rates than the single-incision-approach [18]. The objective of the present retrospective study was to describe the occurrence of the most frequent adverse events and clinical outcomes of patients undergoing surgical repair of distal biceps tendon with a modified double-incision technique. It was hypothesized that the double-incision approach represents a reliable surgical solution for distal biceps tendon rupture in well selected patients.

Materials and methods

All distal biceps tendon ruptures undergoing surgical treatment in our department from January 2003 to January 2015 were considered eligible for study assessment. The inclusion criteria were as follows: age 18 years or above, acute or sub-acute tendon rupture (within 2 weeks from injury) treated with a modified double-incision surgical technique [19] and a minimum follow-up of 12 months. Only acute and sub-acute injuries were considered eligible because of proximal muscle retraction occurring in chronic ruptures [3]. We searched the department's surgical electronic database using the following keywords: distal biceps tendon, distal biceps rupture. A total of 85 cases were found. Twenty-two patients were excluded, as they did not meet the inclusion criteria or refused to take part to study assessments.

All the operations were performed by two surgeons, both being highly experienced in elbow surgery. The cohort exclusively included male patients, with an average age of 44.8 years (min. 28 – max. 66 years). The dominant arm was involved in 39 cases (61.9%). At an average follow up of 24 months (min. 12 – max. 120 months) patients were clinically evaluated by measuring the degrees of pronation/supination, flexion/extension, documenting areas of hypoesthesia or neurological pain and asked to answer the Elbow Oxford Score (EOS), the Disabilities of Arm, Shoulder and Hand score (DASH) and the Mayo Elbow Performance score (MEPS). Patients' overall satisfaction was recorded in a scale from 0 to 10.

Adverse events following surgical procedures were assessed and divided into two groups according to their frequency and severity, as described in the literature. Major complications included: persistent cramping or neurological pain, range of motion (ROM) deficiency > 30° in flexion-extension and pronation-supination compared to the healthy contralateral, isometric flexion strength deficiency > 30% and isometric supination strength deficiency > 60%, PIN palsy and non-traumatic re-rupture. Minor complications included: intermittent pain, ROM deficiency < 30° in flexion/extension and pronation/supination, isometric flexion strength deficiency < 30% and isometric supination strength deficiency < 60%, LACBN injury.

A digital Sauter FL dynamometer was used to test isometric muscle functioning in pronation/supination and flexion/extension with the elbow flexed at 90° and in full supination, with the aim to evaluate the strength of the injured joint. Results were compared with those achieved by the contralateral side, being compromised by the same injury in only one case. Patients with severe motion limitation were asked to undergo elbow radiographs.

Surgical technique

With the patients lying in supine position, the tourniquet is applied to the injured arm. A minimally invasive, 3 cm transverse incision, over the antecubital fossa is made. After dissection of the subcutaneous tissue, particular care must be given to the lateral antebrachial cutaneous nerve (LABCN), discerning it from the biceps brachii muscle to avoid secondary traction. The muscle-tendon junction must be identified, and the stump tendon caught. The distal degenerated portion of the biceps tendon is resected, and two 3 cm-Krackow sutures are placed in the torn tendon. The radial tuberosity is palped with the index finger first and then using a blunt, curved hemostat that must be carefully inserted into the biceps channel. The instrument slips past the tuberosity and is advanced below, so its tip can be appreciated over the dorsal aspect of the proximal forearm placed in maximal pronation. The second incision is made over the tip of the instrument. The radial tuberosity is exposed by a lateral muscle-splitting technique by passing the instrument between extensor ulnaris carpi (EUC) and extensor digitorum communis (EDC), while the ulnar periosteum is never exposed. The radial tuberosity is then cleaned up from soft tissues and prepared with a high-speed burr, forming a 1.5 cm wide and 1 cm deep trench (Fig. 1). Three drill holes are placed approximately at 7–8 mm intervals through the dorsal cortical margin of the tuberosity. In this phase, accurate washing and sucking are mandatory to prevent heterotopic ossification caused by bone debris spreading. The tendon is passed through the second incision and carefully introduced into the trench prepared in the tuberosity.

With the forearm in the neutral position, the sutures are passed through the holes, pulled tight and tied. A suction drain is placed in both wounds (Fig. 2). The elbow is then splinted at 90° of flexion, with the forearm at 45° of supination.

Results

Sixty-three patients were considered eligible for assessment and were evaluated at an average of 24 months of follow-up (min. 12 – max. 120 months). Adverse events following the surgical procedure were divided into two groups: major and minor complications, according to their frequency and severity, as described in the methods section.

The recovery rate compared to the healthy contralateral was: 95% flexion (min: 110° - max: 135°; average 125°), 97% extension (min: – 2° - max: 15°, average: 2°), 88.5% supination (min: 0° - max: 90°; average 70°), and 92% pronation (min: 0° - max: 90°; average: 73°).

The reported major complications included: 1 (1.5%) case of proximal radio-ulnar synostosis with radiographic documentation (Fig. 3), 3 (4.5%) cases of PIN palsy and 1 (1.5%) case of non-traumatic tendon re-rupture. No cases of ROM deficiency > 30° were found.

The reported minor complications included: 6 (9.5%) cases of ROM defiency < 30°, 3 (4.7%) cases of LACBN injury, 3 (4.7%) cases of intermittent pain, 1 (1.6%) cases of flexion strength deficiency < 30% and 1 (1.6%) case of isometric supination strength deficiency < 60%, (Tab. 1).

The average DASH score was 8.5, OES resulted 41.5, MEPS overall score was 96.3 with a very good satisfaction (8.9/10) (Tab. 2).

Discussion

The rupture of the distal portion of the biceps tendon is not a very common tendon lesion. It occurs more often in a selected portion of middle-aged, male people, more frequently involving the dominant arm. Risk factors involved in this type of injury include smoke and use of drugs (antibiotics), but none of these has been identified as certain.

In the last decades, literature has shown the superiority of surgical treatment over non-operative management, demonstrating functional improvement in particular for supination strength recover [20]. Several surgical options have been described in literature: one incision-approach, using suture anchors, endobutton, biotenodesis screw for fixation, and a double-incision approach, using bone tunnels [8, 15, 19, 21, 22]. Standard and modified double incision approach differ one to each other in ulnar periosteum exposure, avoided by the Morrey's muscle-splitting technique that reduces risk of synostosis [23, 24]. However, the minimal anterior incision on the cubital fossa, with muscle splitting technique, has not demonstrated to be a completely safe procedure to prevent the occurrence of nerve palsy (LACBN or radial) and heterotopic ossification. A recent comparison between the double-incision

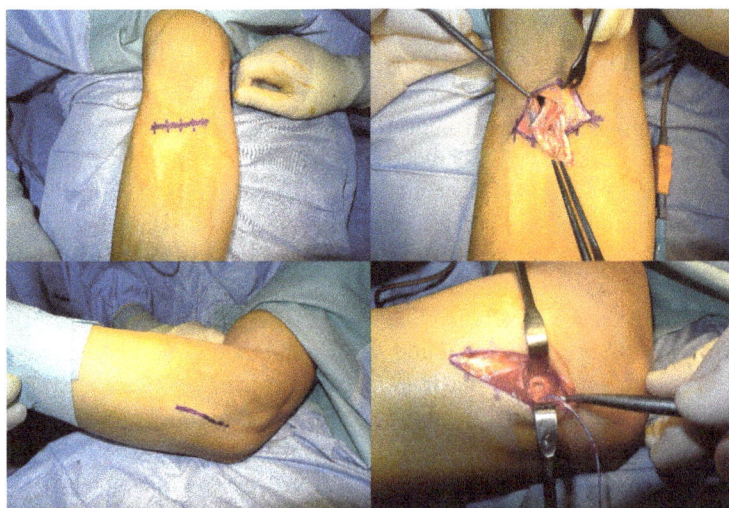

Fig. 1 Some surgical steps: fist the anterior incision, followed by the finding of the distal tendon, then the crucial passage of the curved blunt hemostat in the biceps channel that point the place of the posterior incision. The radial tuberosity is then cleaned up from soft tissues and prepared with a high-speed burr, forming a 1.5 cm wide and 1 cm deep trench

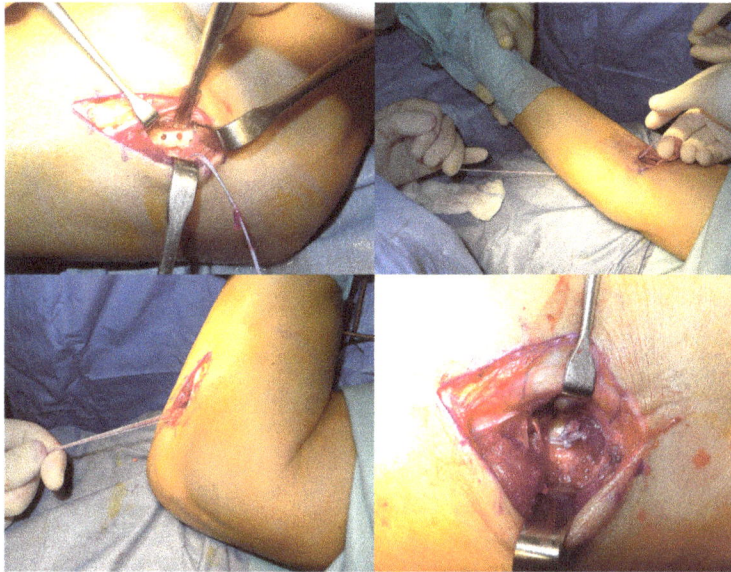

Fig. 2 Final surgical steps: three drill holes are placed through the dorsal cortical margin of the tuberosity, the tendon is passed through the second incision and carefully introduced into the trench prepared in the tuberosity. Finally, with the forearm in the neutral position, the sutures are passed through the holes, pulled tight and tied

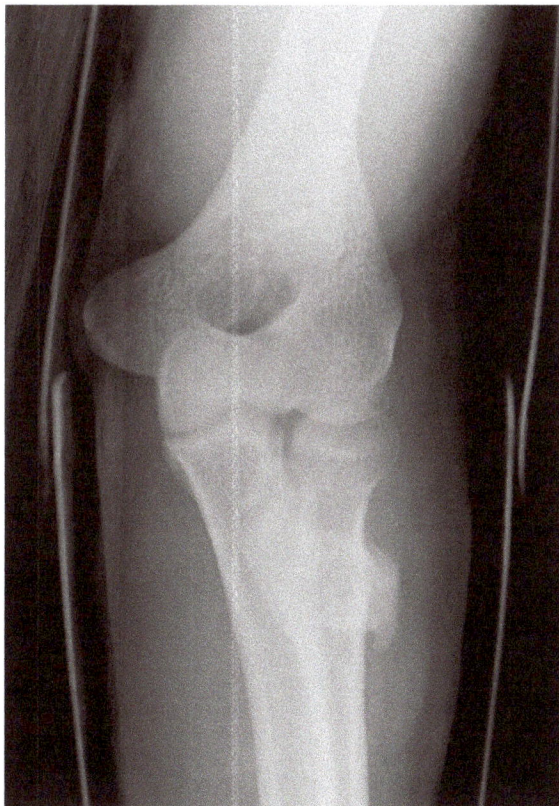

Fig. 3 A case of proximal radio-ulnar synostosis with radiographic documentation

approach and the single-incision using endo-buttons, has demonstrated no significant differences between the two techniques in mean DASH score (6.31 versus 5.91, $p = 0.697$), mean Work DASH score (10.49 versus 0.93, $p = 0.166$), mean Sports DASH score (10.54 versus 9.56, $p = 0.987$) and complication rates (39.39% versus 32.0%, respectively) [25].

In their systematic review of 22 papers describing the treatment of acute distal biceps tendon repair, among which 4 studies describing both single and double-incision techniques, 14 studies involving the single incision and 4 studies the double-incision approach exclusively, Watson et al. reported a 23.9% complication rate for the single-incision technique and 25.7% complication rate for the double-incision approach. LABCN neuroapraxia was the most common complication overall (11.6% for one-incision and 5.8% for two-incision techniques); heterotopic ossification, stiffness and synostosis were more frequently reported in the two-incision technique (7.0%, 5.7% and 2.3% respectively) [17]. Grewal et al., evaluating mid-term outcomes of single and double-incision techniques reported significantly higher overall complication rate inthesingle-incision technique. Regarding heterotopic ossification, a single case was reported both in the single and double-incision groups [13].

Citak et al. compared the clinical and functional outcomes after distal biceps tendon repair using a single-incision approach with suture anchors and with a double-incision exposure using transosseous sutures. No statistically significant differences among groups were observed relative to ROM recovery rate. While no

Table 1 Patients' case-series including dominant/non dominant forearm informations, follow-up visit, ROM and complication report. ROM values are expressed in degrees

N°	Age	Gender	Injured side	Follow up	ROM (ext-flex)	ROM (pron-sup)	Complications MAJOR	Complications MINOR
1	35	male	non dominant	12 months	0°-130°	90°-90°	no	no
2	42	male	dominant	15 months	0°-130°	90°-90°	no	intermittent pain
3	48	male	non dominant	2 years	0°-130°	90°-90°	no	no
4	62	male	non dominant	12 months	0°130°	90°-90°	no	no
5	43	male	non dominant	4 years	0°130°	90°-90°	no	no
6	28	male	dominant	19 months	0°-110°	80°-75°	no	ROM deficiency< 30°
7	37	male	non dominant	2 years	0°-130°	85°-90°	no	no
8	49	male	non dominant	5 years	0°-130°	90°-90°	no	no
9	66	male	dominant	1 years	0°-130°	75°-80°	no	ROM deficiency< 30°
10	30	male	dominant	8 years	0°-130°	90°90°	no	no
11	46	male	dominant	16 months	0°-130°	70°-50°	no	ROM deficiency< 30°
12	42	male	dominant	2 years	0°-130°	85°-90°	no	supination strength deficiency < 60%
13	62	male	non dominant	12 months	0°-130°	90°-90°	no	no
14	36	male	dominant	12 months	0°-130°	90°-90°	no	no
15	45	male	dominant	18 months	0°-130°	90°-85°	NIP transient palsy	no
16	59	male	dominant	15 months	0°-130°	90°-85°	no	no
17	48	male	dominant	18 months	0°-130°	65°-75°	no	ROM deficiency< 30°
18	39	male	dominant	2 years	0°-130°	85°-90°	no	no
19	37	male	non dominant	14 months	0°-130°	90°-90°	no	no
20	65	male	non dominant	4 years	15°-130°	90°-90°	no	no
21	52	male	dominant	2 years	0°-130°	90°-90°	no	no
22	59	male	non dominant	12 months	0°-130°	90°-90°	no	heterotopic ossifications
23	47	male	non dominant	16 months	0°-130°	90°-90°	no	no
24	42	male	non dominant	13 months	0°-130°	90°-90°	no	no
25	50	male	dominant	15 months	0°-130°	90°-90°	no	no
26	39	male	dominant	2 years	0°-130°	90°-90°	no	no
27	54	male	non dominant	12 months	0°-130°	90°-90°	no	no
28	47	male	non dominant	18 months	0°-130°	70°-80°	radio-ulnar synostosis	ROM deficiency< 30°
29	42	male	dominant	2 years	0°-130°	90°-90°	no	no
30	45	male	non dominant	19 months	0°-130°	90°-90°	no	intermittent pain
31	60	male	non dominant	16 months	0°-130°	90°-90°	no	no
32	36	male	non dominant	12 months	0°-130°	90°-85°	no	no
33	56	male	dominant	3 years	0°-130°	85°-90°	no	LACBN injury
34	47	male	dominant	12 months	0°-130°	90°-90°	no	no
35	40	male	dominant	14 months	0°-130°	90°-90°	no	no
36	54	male	non dominant	20 months	0°-130°	90°-90°	no	no
37	32	male	non dominant	4 years	0°-130°	90°-90°	no	no
38	42	male	dominant	2 years	0°-130°	90°-90°	no	no
39	36	male	dominant	13 months	0°-130°	90°-90°	no	no
40	40	male	dominant	12 months	0°-130°	75°-85°	atraumatic re-rupture	ROM deficiency< 30°
41	45	male	non dominant	2 years	0°-130°	90°-90°	no	no
42	57	male	dominant	17 months	0°-130°	90°-90°	no	no

Table 1 Patients' case-series including dominant/non dominant forearm informations, follow-up visit, ROM and complication report. ROM values are expressed in degrees *(Continued)*

N°	Age	Gender	Injured side	Follow up	ROM (ext-flex)	ROM (pron-sup)	Complications MAJOR	Complications MINOR
43	39	male	dominant	16 months	5°-125°	85°-90°	no	heterotopic ossifications
44	36	male	dominant	10 years	0°-130°	90°-90°	no	no
45	50	male	dominant	12 months	0°-130°	90°-90°	no	no
46	54	male	dominant	15 months	0°-130°	90°-90°	no	no
47	41	male	dominant	2 years	0°-130°	90°-90°	no	no
48	36	male	dominant	12 months	0°-130°	90°-90°	no	intermittent pain
49	29	male	non dominant	20 months	0°-130°	90°-90°	no	no
50	46	male	dominant	19 months	0°-100°	85°-90°	NIP transient palsy	no
51	51	male	dominant	4 years	0°-130°	90°-90°	no	no
52	56	male	dominant	18 months	20°-125°	90°-85°	no	no
53	47	male	dominant	2 years	0°-130°	85°-90°	NIP transient palsy	LACBN injury
54	39	male	dominant	15 months	0°-130°	90°-90°	no	no
55	35	male	non dominant	18 months	0°-130°	90°-90°	no	flexion strenght deficiency < 30%
56	41	male	dominant	1 years	5°-130°	90°-90°	no	no
57	28	male	dominant	13 months	0°-130°	90°-90°	no	no
58	40	male	dominant	17 months	0°-130°	90°-90°	no	no
59	41	male	dominant	3 years	0°-130°	90°-90°	no	no
60	46	male	dominant	14 months	0°-125°	90°-90°	no	LACBN injury
61	51	male	non dominant	12 months	0°-130°	90°-90°	no	no
62	37	male	dominant	6 years	0°-130°	90°-80°	no	no
63	42	male	non dominant	16 months	0°-120°	90°-90°	no	no

NIP: posterior interosseous nerve, LACBN: lateral antebrachial coutaneous nerve, ROM: range of motion

adverse events were described for the double-incision group, LACBN injury was reported in 5 cases in the single-incision cohort of patients [22].

Pairwise, Amin et al. conducted a meta-analysis of 87 articles, reporting higher frequencies of complications for the single-incision technique (performed with suture anchors, endobutton, biotenodesis screw), than for double-incision repair (performed with bone tunnels). Higher rates of nerve palsy (PIN, LACBN and radial

Table 2 Clinical scores. Values are reported as mean, min. and max

Categories	Scores
M.E.P.S.	96.3 (min:70; max 100)
O.E.S	41.5 (min:17; max:48)
DASH score	8.5 (min: 1; max: 37,5)
Lickert scale	8.9 (min: 0; max: 10)

MEPS Mayo Elbow Performance score
OES Elbow Oxford Score
DASH Disabilities of Arm, Shoulder and Hand score

nerve) and tendon re-rupture were reported in the single-incision group compared with the double-incision. On the other hand, heterotopic ossifications were described exclusively with the double-incision exposure.

As demonstrated by literature, advantages of the double-incision exposure include anatomic reinsertion on the radial tuberosity and consequent improved strength in supination and flexion [13], together with limited surgical costs. Limitations include higher rates of heterotopic ossifications.

In the present study including 63 subjects, the complications and clinical outcomes following the double-incision approach were examined and recorded in order to establish and determine appropriate indications for patients with acute ruptures of the distal biceps tendon. The obtained results were compared with those reported in literature relative to the surgical management of this injury.

Average ROM recovery showed excellent results compared to the healthy contralateral side, except from supination, which is the most impaired function in biceps tendon lesions [3, 22].

One case of radiographic radio-ulnar synostosis was observed in our series, determining complete block of

Table 3 Distal biceps tendon rupture surgical treatment as reported in literature, divided for single or double-incision approach. The rate of minor and major complications is reported

Study	Patients	Incision	Fixation method	ROM				Major complications	Minor complications
				Flexion	Extension	Pronation	Supination		
Tarallo et al. (present series)	63	2	Bone tunnels	125° (min:110°-max: 135°)	2° (min:-2-max:15°)	73° (min:0°-max:90°)	70° (min:0°-max:90°)	3(4.5%) PIN transient palsy 1 (1.5%) Radio-ulnar synostosis 1(1.5%) Atraumatic re-rupture	3 (4.7%) Intermittent pain 6 (9.5%) ROM deficiency < 30% 1 (1.5%) Isometric flexion strength defiency< 30° 1 (1.5%) Isometric supination strength defiency< 60° 3(4.47%) LACBN injury
				97%	92%	88.50%			
Grewal et al. [13]	43	2	Suture anchors	131.8°±9.1	1.9°±4.6	72.4°±12.6	59.5°±11.5	1(2.32%) Atraumatic re-rupture	3(6.9%)LACBN injury 1(2.32%) HO
	47	1	Bone tunnel	134.5°±6.9	3.0°±4.3	76.7°±8.2	63.9°±12.5	3(6.38%) Atraumatic re-rupture	19 (40.42%) LACBN injury 1 (2.12%) HO
Gupta at al. [24]	9	1	Endobutton	143°	0°	77° (min:70°-max:82°)	81° (min:78°-max:85°)	None	None
Citak et al. [25]	15	1	Intraosseous screw	147° (min:142.4°-max:150.7°)	1.3° (max:-0.6°-min:3.3°)	88° (min:85.7°-ma:90.3°)	89.3° (min:87.9°-max:90.8°)	None	2(13.3%) LACBN injury
	24	1	Suture anchors	134° (min:122.6°-max:145.3°)	1.3° (min:-0.2-max:2.7°)	82.5° (min:76.2°-max:88.8°)	81.7° (min:74.9°-max:88.5°)	3(12.5%) re-rupture	3(12.5%) LACBN injury 2(8.33%) ROM deficiency < 30%
	25	2	Bone tunnel	135° (min:118.9°-max:151.1°)	1° (min:-0.6°-max:2.6°)	85.7° (min:78.6°-max:92.5°)	84.7° (min:77.9°-max:91.5°)	None	None
Eardley et al. [26]	14	1	Intraosseous screw	130° (min:110°-145°)	0° (min:-10°-max:5°)	66° (min:50°-max:80°)	74° (min:50°-max:90°)	none	8(54%) LACBN injury 1(7.14%) HO
Johnson et al. [27]	12	1	Suture anchors	142°	-2°	83°	85°	None	1(8.33%) LACBN injury 1(8.33%) HO
Oke A. Anakwenze et al. [28]	14	2	Bone tunnel	145°	0°	80°	83°	None	3(21.42%)HO
	12	2	Bone tunnel	153°±12.0°	0°±0°	78.5°±9.6°	78.9°±10.0°	None	none
Amin et al. [29]	785	1	Suture anchors					17(2.1%) re-rupture	77(9.9%) LACBN injury

Table 3 Distal biceps tendon rupture surgical treatment as reported in literature, divided for single or double-incision approach. The rate of minor and major complications is reported (Continued)

Study	Patients	Incision	Fixation method	ROM				Major complications	Minor complications
				Flexion	Extension	Pronation	Supination		
			Endobutton					13(1.7%)PIN palsy	25(3.2%) HO
			Biotenodesis screw						49(6.24%) intermittent pain
	498	2	Bone tunnel					3(0.6%) re-rupture	11(2.2%) LACBN injury
								11(2.2%) synostosis	36(7.2%) HO
								13(1.7%) PIN palsy	
David M. Weinstein et al. [30]	32	1	Suture anchors	145° ± 8	0° ± 3	88° ± 10	73° ± 10	None	2(6.25%) LACBN injury
									1(3.12%) intermittent pain
Olsen JR et al. [31]	20	1	Cortical button + interference screw	140° ± 6.2	7° ± 5.1	79° ± 6.8	72° ± 9.5	4(20%) PIN palsy	3(18%) LACBN injury
	17	1	Suture anchors	139° ± 5.6	5° ± 3.9	75° ± 9.2	76° ± 5.3	1(6%) PIN palsy	None

PIN posterior interosseous nerve
ROM range of motion
HO heterotopic ossification
LACBN lateral ante brachial cutaneous nerve

prono-supination. The patient underwent surgical elbow arthrolysis with partial recovery of the limited movement. Three cases of transient PIN palsy, with complete recovery after 6 months, and 3 cases of transient LABC nerve palsy were reported in the examined cohort.

Relative to return at pre-injury activities, patients with high functional demand (sport professionals and manual workers) were found less satisfied than the majority of patients. Activities of daily living were possible for all the cohort, with an average DASH score of 8.5 and OES of 41.5. Complication rate and ROM recovery resulted comparable to available literature on surgical treatment of the same lesion (Tab. 3).

This study is not without limitations. The retrospective nature of the study design may have introduced selection bias and variations in treatment over time. In addition, being a single institution study may limit the generalizability of the results. Moreover, the mean follow-up was 24 months which, although adequate to determine results regarding pain relief, function and activity, may not be sufficient to draw conclusions regarding long term outcomes. No quantification of strength recovery in terms of Newton was reported and lastly, although post-operative MRI is described as a useful tool for tendon healing evaluation [23], no imaging examination was routinely performed in the study cohort.

On the other hand, strengths of the study include the large number of patients included, with the present series being the largest cohort in which clinical outcomes and complications of the double-incision technique in last decade's literature have been described. Moreover, all patients were operated with a unique surgical technique, determining a large sample size to analyze its advantages and drawbacks.

Conclusion

Although rate of complications and ROM recovery are similar among different surgical techniques, the Morrey-modified approach for distal biceps tendon repair represents a valid option to the single-incision techniques and finds its indication in young and active patients aiming to restore the pre-injury condition. Advantages of this approach include low costs and anatomical reinsertion, restoring flexion and supination strength. Surgery should be better performed within 2 weeks from injury to prevent proximal tendon retraction. To avoid frequent complications, including nerve palsy and severe ROM impairment, it's recommended that only well-trained elbow surgeons approach this technique.

Funding
We received no external funding for this study.

Authors' contributions
LT, FZ, AG and FC made substantial contributions to the design of the study. ML made contribution to acquisition of data, analysis and the interpretation of data. LT and ML have drafting the manuscript. All authors read and approved the final manuscript.

Competing interests
LT is a member of the Editorial Board of BMC Musculoskeletal Disorders. The other authors declare that they have no competing interests.

References

1. Anakwenze OA, Baldwin K, Abboud JA. Distal biceps tendon repair: an analysis of timing of surgery on outcomes. J Athl Train. 2013;48(1):9–11.
2. James P, Ward J, et al. Rupture of the distal biceps tendon. Bulletin of the Hospital for joint disease. 2014;72(1):110–9.
3. Dillon MT, King JC. Treatment of chronic biceps tendon ruptures. J Hand Surg. 2013;8(4):401–9.
4. Pascarelli L, et al. Technique and results after distal brachial biceps tendon reparation, through two anterior mini-incision. Acta Ortop Bras. 2013;21(2):76–9.
5. Bernstein AD, Breslow MJ, et al. Distal biceps tendon ruptures: a historical perspective and current concepts. Am J Orthop. 2001;30(3):193–200.
6. Bisson L, Moyer M et al. Complications associated with repair of a distal biceps rupture using the modified two-incision technique. J Shoulder Elbow Surg. 2008; 67(3):418–421.
7. Chavan PR, Duquin TR, et al. Repair of the ruptured distal biceps tendon: a systematic review. Am J Sports Med. 2008;36(8).
8. Balabaud L, Ruiz C, et al. Repair of distal biceps tendon ruptures using a suture anchor and an anterior approach. Journal of Hand Surgery. 2004;29(2):178–82.
9. Baratz M, King GJ, et al. Repair of distal biceps ruptures. J Hand Surg. 2012; 37(7):1462–6.
10. Blackmore SM, Jander RM, et al. Management of distal biceps and triceps ruptures. J Hand Ther. 2006;19(2):154–69.
11. Dobbie RP, et al. avulsion of the lower biceps brachii tendon: analysis of fifty-one previously unreported cases. Am J Surg. 1941;51(3):662–83.
12. Minton J, Meherin MD, Kilgore ES Jr. The treatment of ruptures of the distal biceps brachii tendon. Am J Surg. 1960;99(5):636–40.
13. Grewal R, Athwal GS, et al. Single versus double-incision technique for the repair of acute distal biceps tendon ruptures: a randomized clinical trial. J Bone Joint Surg (Am Vol). 2012;94(13):1166–74.
14. Boyd HB, Anderson LD, et al. A method for reinsertion of the distal biceps Brachii tendon. J Bone Joint Surg (Am Vol). 1961;43(7).
15. Christopher L Camp MD, et al. Single-incision technique for repair of distal biceps tendon avulsions with intramedullary cortical button. Arthroscopy Techniques. 2016;5(2):303–7.
16. Morrey F, Askew LJ, An KN, Dobyns JH. Rupture of the distal tendon of the biceps brachii. A biomechanical study. The Journal of Bone & Joint Surgery. 1985;67(3):418–21.
17. Watson JN, Moretti VM, et al. Repair techniques for acute distal biceps tendon ruptures: a systematic review. J Bone Joint Surg Am. 2014; 96A(24) 2086–2090.
18. Kodde F, et al. Refixation techniques and approaches for the distal biceps tendon ruptures: a systematic review of clinical studies. J Shoulder Elbow Surgery. 2016;25(2):29–37.
19. Tarallo L, Zambianchi F, Mugnai R, Costanzini CA, Catani F. Distal biceps tendon rupture reconstruction using muscle-splitting double-incision approach. World J Clin Cases. 2014;2(8):357–61.
20. Baker BE, et al. Rupture of the distal tendon of the biceps brachii. Operative versus non-operative treatment. The Journal of Bone & Joint Surgery. 1985;67(3):414–7.
21. Gupta RK, Bither N, et al. Repair of the torn distal biceps tendon by endobutton fixation. Indian J Orthop. 2012;46(1):71–6.
22. Citak M, et al. Surgical repair of the distal biceps brachii tendon: a comparative study of three surgical fixation techniques. Knee Surg Sports TraumatolArthrosc. 2011;19(11):1936–41.
23. Eardley WG, et al. Bioabsorbable interference screw fixation of distal biceps ruptures through a single anterior incision: a single-surgeon case series and review of the literature. Arch Orthop Trauma Surg. 2010;130(7):875–81.

23

A novel patient-specific three-dimensional-printed external template to guide iliosacral screw insertion: a retrospective study

Fan Yang[†], Sheng Yao[†], Kai-fang Chen, Feng-zhao Zhu, Ze-kang Xiong, Yan-hui Ji, Ting-fang Sun and Xiao-dong Guo[*] 🆔

Abstract

Background: Iliosacral screw fixation is a popular method for the management of posterior pelvic ring fractures or dislocations, providing adequate biomechanical stability. Our aim in this study was to describe the use of a new patient-specific external template to guide the insertion of iliosacral screws and to evaluate the efficacy and safety of this technique compared with the conventional fluoroscopy-guided technique.

Methods: This was a retrospective study of patients with incomplete or complete posterior pelvic ring disruptions who required iliosacral screw fixation. For analysis, patients were divided into two groups: the external template group (37 screws in 22 patients) and the conventional group (28 screws in 18 patients). The operative time per screw, radiation exposure time and the rate of screw perforation (accuracy) were compared between groups. In the external template group, the difference between the actual and planned iliosacral screw position was also compared.

Results: In the conventional group, the average operative time per screw was 39.7 ± 10.6 min, with an average radiation exposure dose of 1904.0 ± 844.5 cGy/cm^2, with 4 cases of screw perforation. In the external template group, the average operative time per screw was 17.9 ± 4.7 min, with an average radiation exposure dose of 742.8 ± 230.6 cGy/cm^2 and 1 case of screw perforation. In the template group, the mean deviation distance between the actual and planned screw position was 2.75 ± 1.0 mm at the tip, 1.83 ± 0.67 mm in the nerve root tunnel zone and 1.52 ± 0.48 mm at the entry point, with a mean deviation angle of $1.73 \pm 0.80°$.

Conclusions: The external template provides an accurate and safe navigation tool for percutaneous iliosacral screw insertion that could decrease the operative time and radiation exposure.

Keywords: External template, Iliosacral screw, Novel navigation tool, Pelvic fracture, Minimal invasive

Background

Iliosacral (IS) screw fixation is a popular method for the management of posterior pelvic ring fractures or dislocations, providing adequate biomechanical stability [1]. The classic percutaneous technique, as described by Matta and Saucedo [2], uses fluoroscopic guidance to reduce the extent of soft tissue disruption, decrease the volume of blood loss and shorten the overall operative time. However, fluoroscopic guidance is a significant source of radiation exposure to both the patient and medical staff. Additionally, patient-specific factors, such as obesity, intestinal gas and a dysmorphic sacrum, have been associated with a screw malposition rate of 2–15%, which may lead to catastrophic neurovascular injury [3, 4].

The use of computer-assisted navigation systems has been advocated to lower the risk of screw malposition, and of associated neurovascular injury, as well as to decrease exposure to radiation during IS screw insertion [5–7]. Although these systems do provide greater

---

* Correspondence: xiaodongguo@hust.edu.cn
[†]Fan Yang and Sheng Yao contributed equally to this work.
Department of Orthopaedics, Union Hospital, Tongji Medical College,
Huazhong University of Science and Technology, Wuhan 430022, China

accuracy and less radiation exposure, their high cost and the complexity of the setup have limited the widespread application of these systems in intermediate- and primary-care hospitals.

Individualized internal templates, based on three-dimensional (3D) image reconstruction and reverse engineering, provide an alternative to computer-guidance for the placement of a K-wire to guide the accurate insertion of the IS screw (Fig. 1a). Although use of an internal template provides an accuracy in screw placement that is similar to that of computer-assisted navigation, it does require an incision of approximately 5 cm and soft tissue dissection to provide a clear bone surface to match the template [8, 9]. Moreover, in our experience, we have found that the geometry of the posterior iliac crest is inadequate to restrain the internal plate, leading to slippage and malposition of the IS screw. As well, soft tissue residues on the bone may also contribute to a mismatch between the template and bone surface, again resulting in malposition of the IS screw.

Emergent external fixation is widely used for the primary management of pelvic fractures. The external fixator pins, which are inserted deep into the iliac crest, could provide a simple geometric surface and solid cornerstone for mounting an external template. Therefore, we developed a low-profile 3-dimensional (3D) printed external template that can be firmly attached to the external fixator pins, overcoming the abovementioned disadvantages of internal templates, to guide IS screw insertion (Fig. 1b and Fig. 2). The aim of our study was to describe the use of our new patient-specific external template to guide the insertion of iliosacral screws and to evaluate the efficacy and safety of this technique compared to the conventional fluoroscopy-guided technique. We hypothesized that use of the 3D-printed external template would lead to a superior outcome, in terms of the accuracy of screw insertion, a shorter operative time and lower radiation exposure, to the conventional technique.

Methods

Patients

The study group consisted of 40 patients who were treated at Wuhan Union Hospital, between January 2016 and September 2017, for traumatic incomplete or complete disruptions of the posterior pelvic ring (fractures of types B and C, per the AO/OTA classification) using IS screws [10]. The radiographs and medical records of these patients were retrospectively analyzed (Table 1).

IS screw placement, using an external template, was performed in 22 patients (template group), including 11 men and 11 women, 51.7 ± 15.2 years of age (range, 18–74 years). All 22 of these patients had undergone external fixation of the pelvic fracture in the emergency department at the time of admission. The conventional fluoroscopy-guided technique of IS screw insertion was used in 18 patients (conventional group), including 10 men and 8 women, 50.1 ± 13.7 years of age (range, 26–75 years). The distribution of the cause and classification of injuries for both groups is summarized in Table 1. All patients had experienced a high-energy trauma, with the distribution for the template and conventional group, respectively, as follows: motor vehicle accident, 9 (40.9%) versus 8 (44.4%); high-energy fall, 6 (27.3%) versus 7 (38.9%); motorcycle accident, 5 (22.7%) versus 3 (16.7%); and machinery injury, 2 (9.1%) versus 0. Using the Denis classification of sacral fractures [11], the distribution of the type of posterior pelvic fractures for the template and conventional group, respectively, was as follows; zone I fractures, 8 (36.4%) versus 7 (38.9%); zone II fractures, 11 (50.0%) versus 9 (50.0%); and sacroiliac joint fractures, 3 (13.6%) versus 3 (11.1%). None of the patients sustained a sacral fracture involving the spinal canal (Denis zone III).

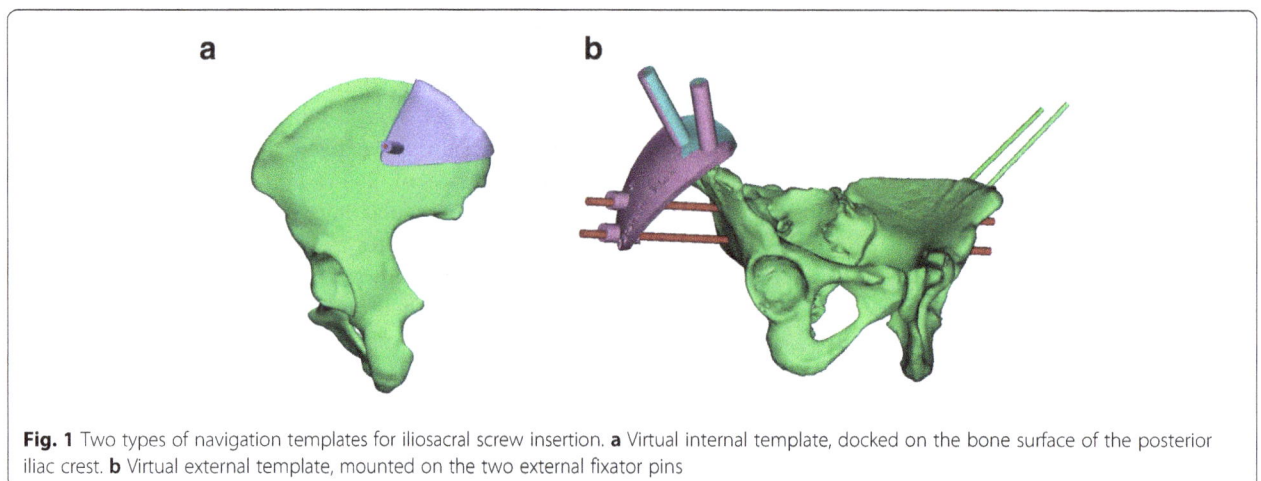

Fig. 1 Two types of navigation templates for iliosacral screw insertion. **a** Virtual internal template, docked on the bone surface of the posterior iliac crest. **b** Virtual external template, mounted on the two external fixator pins

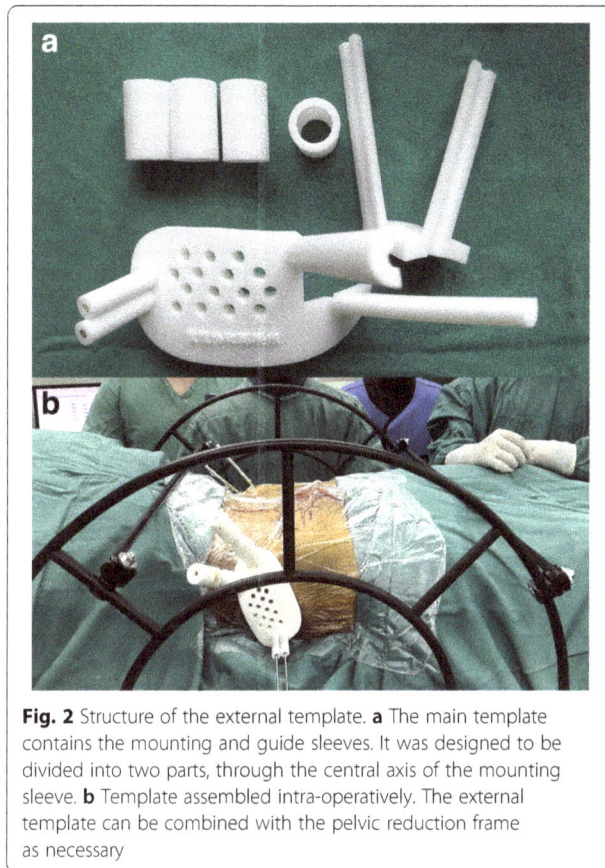

Fig. 2 Structure of the external template. **a** The main template contains the mounting and guide sleeves. It was designed to be divided into two parts, through the central axis of the mounting sleeve. **b** Template assembled intra-operatively. The external template can be combined with the pelvic reduction frame as necessary

Marker pin insertion and data collection

Two partially threaded Schanz 5 mm pins (inserted into the iliac crest for emergent fixation at the time of admission) were used as marker pins, as well as provided a stable mounting base for the external template. Consistent with the conventional technique of external fixation of the pelvis, the tips of the two pins were directed in convergent fashion toward the thick bony area above the acetabulum to obtain a firm insertion. Of note, a supra-acetabular pin, which is more commonly used for external fixation of the pelvis than iliac crest screws, was inappropriate for our purpose as it provides inadequate rotational stability to the mounted external template. Moreover, the supra-acetabular pin occupies the supra-acetabular corridor, which is needed to mount one of the pins of the pelvic reduction frame [12, 13] during definitive surgery. In our experience, we found that there was low deformation of the external template itself when it hung perpendicularly from the iliac crest pins (Fig. 2b) in short distance.

Thereafter, all patients in the template group underwent computed tomography (CT) imaging of the pelvis for both trauma assessment and template planning, with additional CT imaging avoided to minimize

patients' radiation exposure. CT data were saved in the Digital Imaging and Communications in Medicine (DICOM) format and used subsequently for design of the template.

The Schanz pins inserted as part of the external fixation of the pelvis were retained in situ until definitive surgery.

Template design and printing

The raw images of the pelvis and skin (DICOM format) were imported into Mimics 10.01 (Materialise, Leuven, Belgium) software for 3D reconstruction. In the 3D model of the pelvis, the trajectory was planned for placement of a virtual screw (7.0 mm diameter) into the S1 or S2 vertebra along the midline of the osseous corridor, with absence of penetration of the cortex confirmed on CT imaging along the three anatomical planes (sagittal, coronal and axial). The placement of another virtual screw into either the injured hemipelvis or contralateral hemipelvis, depending on the type of posterior pelvic ring injury, was also planned. The 3D model (including the bony pelvis, skin and virtual screws) was then exported into an STL format for use with the Geomagic Studio image-processing software (version 12.0; Geomagic, Cary, NC, USA). A virtual template, using the skin model as a substrate, was then designed using the *trim and curve* software, to connect the marker pins and the IS screws. The template design was also exported into the STL format for use with the 3-matic software (Materialise, Leuven, Belgium) to complete the virtual template through Boolean calculation (Fig. 3). The virtual template was then cut into two pieces, through the centric axis of the mounting sleeves so that it could easily be assembled on the marker pins intra-operatively (Fig. 2a). The data from the 3-matic software were imported into the 3D equipment software (UnionTech, SLA-Lite 450 HD, China) to print the external template (accuracy, 0.1 mm; material, photosensitive resin). The components of the template were sterilized, using a low-temperature plasma method, for use intra-operatively.

For patients who did not require fracture reduction, the template was designed to mount on the pins inserted in the iliac crest of the injured hemipelvis, as per the usual method (Fig. 3). For patients with an iliosacral dislocation or sacral fracture (Denis zone I and II fractures), requiring reduction as a component of the definitive surgery, the template was designed to mount on the pins inserted in the contralateral hemipelvis. As the spinal nerves are always contained in the contralateral sacral fragment in Denis zone I and II sacral fractures [14], the template mounted on the contralateral hemipelvis was used for the safe insertion of K-wires,

Table 1 Demographic and surgery details

	Template group (n = 22)	Conventional group (n = 18)	P value
Sex	Male 11, Female 11	Male 10, Female 8	0.726*
Age (years)	51.7 ± 15.2	50.1 ± 13.7	0.728#
Time from injury-to-surgery (days)	5.4 ± 2.0	4.1 ± 2.0	0.049#
AO/OTA classification of sacrum			0.723**
54B	7	4	
54C	15	14	
Posterior pelvic ring disruption, n (%)			1.000**
SI dislocation	3 (13.6%)	2 (11.1%)	
Denis zone I fracture	8 (36.4%)	7 (38.9%)	
Denis zone II fracture	11 (50.0%)	9 (50.0%)	
Number of screws			0.954*
S1	20	16	
S2	18	14	
Operation time (min)			< 0.001#
S1	18.7 ± 4.3	39.8 ± 10.6	
S2	17.1 ± 4.7	39.6 ± 11.1	
Average	17.9 ± 4.5	39.7 ± 10.7	
Radiation exposure (cGy/cm^2)			< 0.001#
S1	755.2 ± 239.5	1852.1 ± 844.5	
S2	729.1 ± 226.5	1963.3 ± 872.3	
Average	742.8 ± 230.6	1904.0 ± 844.5	

P value < 0.05 considered statistically significant
*Pearson chi-squared test
**Fisher's exact test
Two independent samples Student's t-test
SI sacroiliac joint
Values are presented as the mean ± standard deviation, unless otherwise indicated

even in cases with poor fracture reduction. However, for external template technique, no ideal solution has been obtained yet for Denis zone III or bilateral sacral fracture needing further reduction.

In our clinical setting, the cost for the design and printing of the template is approximately 250 dollars, requiring about 2 h for the design and more than 10 h for the printing. We cooperate with our affiliated 3D digital orthopaedic center, with a delay between CT imaging and definite surgery of 48–72 h, which takes into account the sterilization process and transportation. This cooperation obviates the need for the hospital to purchase this equipment.

Surgical technique

Patients were placed in the supine position on a radiolucent operation table, and surgery was performed under general anesthesia. A fluoroscopic C-arm was placed on the side opposite to the surgeon. The external pelvic fixation frame was removed, retaining the two marker pins to mount the template. The sacral fracture or dislocation was reduced using the pelvic

reduction frame described by Lefaivre et al. [12] (Fig. 2b). Then, the external template was mounted on the marker pins and a 2.5-mm K-wire was inserted into the planned corridor using the external template as a reference. Inlet and outlet fluoroscopy views were obtained to confirm the position of the K-wire (with minimum radiation exposure). A 6.5-mm cannulated screw was then inserted, following the K-wire (Fig. 4).

The same procedure was followed for the conventional group, up to the insertion of the K-wire. Specifically, once the sacral fracture or dislocation was reduced, a K-wire was inserted under C-arm fluoroscopy guidance, using lateral, inlet and outlet views. Adjustments in the position of the K-wire under fluoroscopy were made until the correct position was confirmed. A 6.5-mm cannulated screw was then inserted, following the K-wire.

Measurement and analysis

Postoperative pelvic radiographs and CT images were reviewed. Two observers independently evaluated the position of the screw from postoperative CT images, using

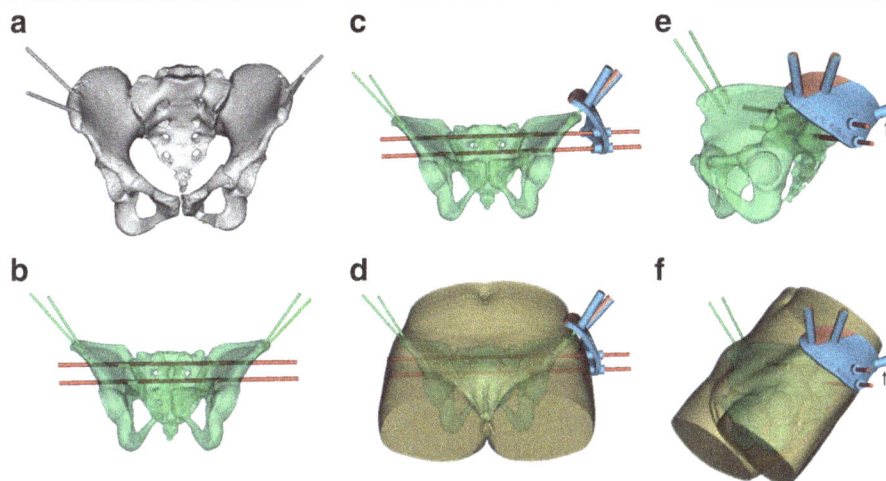

Fig. 3 External template designed using Mimics software. **a** A 3D model of the pelvis was reconstructed including the marker pins. **b** S1 and S2 virtual screws were placed into the sacrum and adjusted to the midway of the osseous corridor without any penetration. **c-f** The template was designed to connect the marker pins and virtual screws, providing sleeves to attach the template on the marker pins and guide the K-wire to the target corridor. Black arrow indicates the guide sleeve for the anterior column screw. (**d/f**) The plate is low-profile, minimizing the distance between both template and skin, and marker pins and virtual screws

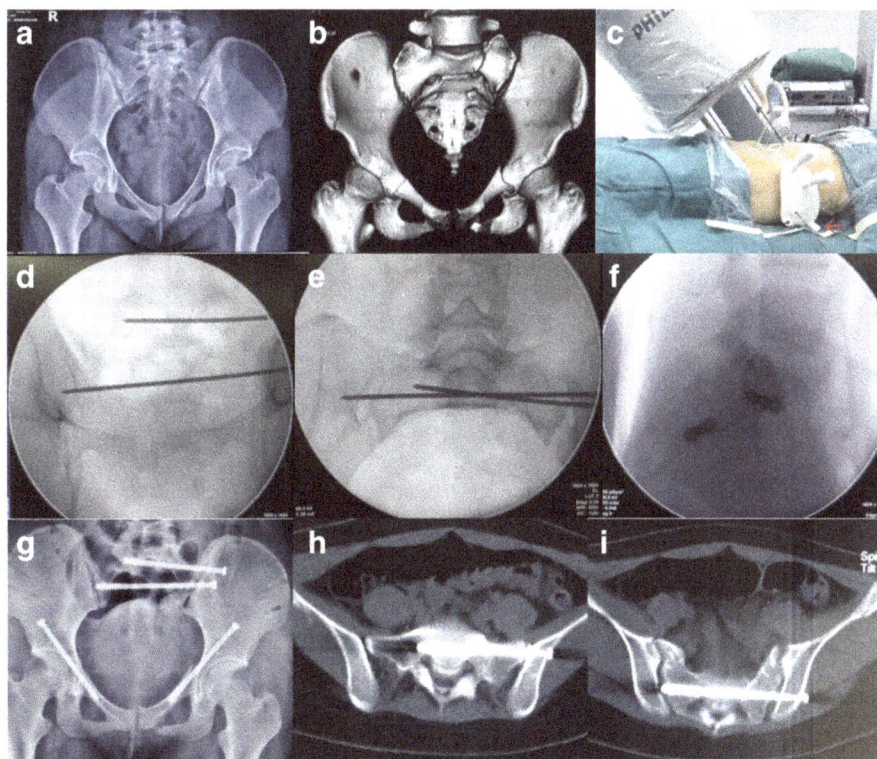

Fig. 4 Intraoperative application of the external template. **a-b** Preoperative AP radiographs/3D reconstruction of computed tomography images for a patient with a Denis zone II sacral fracture and bilateral pubic ramus fractures. **c-f** Intraoperative fluoroscopy (**d/e/f** outlet/inlet/lateral view) was used, minimally, to confirm the guide wire and screw in the target corridor. The red arrow in (**c**) indicates the guide sleeve for the anterior column screw. **g-i** Postoperative AP radiograph/computed tomography axial image confirmed the placement of the IS screws

the following grading criteria, as previously described [15]: grade 0, no violation; grade 1, < 2 mm; grade 2, 2–4 mm; and grade 3, > 4 mm. The amount of time required for screw insertion and radiation were also extracted from the surgical records for analysis. The quality of the reduction was graded using the criteria defined by Tornetta and Matta [16]: excellent, ≤4 mm; good, 4–10 mm; and fair, 10–20 mm. By matching pre- and postoperative CT images, the difference between the actual and planned screw positions was quantified by measuring the distance between the two screws at the point of entrance, nerve root tunnel zone and tip, measured in the sagittal plane of reconstructed CT images [17]. The offset angle was also measured (Fig. 5). Quantitative data are presented as the mean ± standard deviation. Between-group differences were evaluated using independent samples Student's t-test, the chi-squared test, and Fisher's exact test, as appropriate for the data type and distribution. All analyses were performed using SPSS (version 17.0; Chicago, IL, USA).

Results

A total of 65 screws were implanted in 40 patients: 37 screws (19 S1, 18 S2) in the template group (22 patients) and 28 screws (14 S1, 12 S2) in the conventional group (18 patients). The quality of the reduction was not significantly different between the two groups (Table 2). The average operative time per screw was 17.9 ± 4.5 min (range, 17–52 min) for the template group, which was significantly less than the 39.7 ± 10.7 min (range, 63–115 min) required for the conventional group ($p < 0.001$). The radiation exposure dose was lower for the template (742.8 ± 230.6 cGy/cm^2) than conventional (1904.0 ± 844.5 cGy/cm^2) group ($p < 0.001$; Table 1). The rate of screw perforation was also lower in the template (1 of 37 screws, 1 at grade 1) than conventional (4 of 28 screws, 2 at grade 1, 2 at grade 2) group ($P < 0.001$). No incidence of neurovascular injury was identified among cases of screw perforation (Table 3). No incidence of pin site infection was noted among patients treated with emergent external fixation.

In the template group, the mean distance between the actual and virtual screws was 2.7 ± 0.8 mm (tip), 1.8 ± 0.6 mm (nerve root zone) and 1.5 ± 0.5 mm (entrance point), with a mean deviation angle of 1.8 ± 0.8°.

Discussion

Use of our novel external template to guide K-wire insertion, and subsequent IS screw placement, provided high accuracy, with a shorter operative time and lower radiation exposure than the conventional fluoroscopy-guided technique. Moreover, despite the conventional use of inlet, outlet and lateral fluoroscopy views to guide percutaneous IS insertion, violation of the cortex remains an inherent problem of IS screw implantation [18–20], with additional fluoroscopic views often required intra-operatively to further improve accuracy. Ozmeric et al. [19] advised that two different inlet views should be used to evaluate the anterior and posterior borders of the sacral body, separately. Kim et

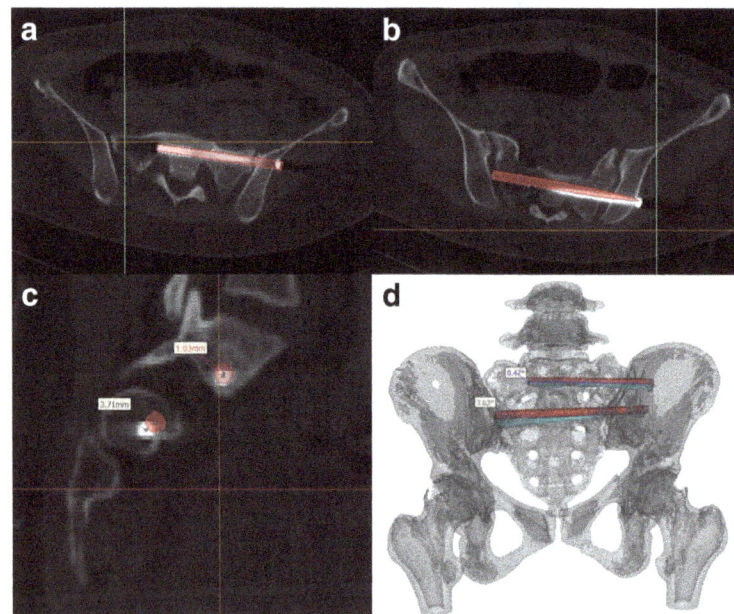

Fig. 5 The procedure for postoperative measurements. **a-b** The S1 and S2 axial views obtained after insertion of the partially threaded screws were merged with the pre-operative images used for planning (red bar). **c** The deviation distance between the inserted and planned virtual screw was measured on the sagittal plane at the nerve root tunnel zone. **d** The deviation angle was measured on the superimposed image of the pre- and postoperative 3D reconstructions

Table 2 Quality of the reduction

	Excellent (≤4 mm)	Good (4–10 mm)	Fair (10–20 mm)	P value
Template group	7	12	3	1.000*
Conventional group	5	11	2	

*Fisher's exact test; $p < 0.05$ considered statistically significant

al. [18] even suggested using two inlet views (at 25° and 55° from the vertical) and three outlet views (at 25°, 35° and 55° from the vertical) to avoid misperception of the local anatomy. However, any adjustment in the position of the guide wire required in one view should necessarily be reconfirmed on all fluoroscopic views. As such, improving the accuracy of placement of the guide wires using the conventional method increases both intra-operative time and radiation exposure, which limits the use of this iterative approach for accurate guide wire placement in clinical practice. Different assistive tools have been used to improve the accuracy and efficiency in placing guide wires, including the use of multidimensional fluoroscopy [20], an internal template [8, 9], thermoplastic membrane navigation [21], and computer-assisted navigation [5, 6, 17, 22]. Our external template is distinctive from these assistive approaches, with greater pre-operative time taken to design and print the navigation template, which avoids the need for repeated fluoroscopy during the surgery and reduces the overall operative time.

Radiation exposure is a significant concern for percutaneous IS screw insertion. Excessive amounts of radiation can cause muscle weakness, hair loss, cataracts, and even cancer [23]. Computer-assisted navigation does allow a surgeon to exit the operative theatre during image capture, reducing radiation exposure for the surgeon (and medical team). A distinct advantage of our external template is the shorter intra-operative time required to insert the guide wire within the target corridor. As such, the dose of radiation exposure was significantly lower (at 742.8 ± 230.6 cGy/cm^2), for both patients and the medical staff, compared to the conventional technique (at 1904.0 ± 844.5 cGy/cm^2).

The accuracy of IS screw insertion has traditionally been evaluated using the penetration grades [15]. In our

Table 3 The rate of screw perforation

	Grade 0	Grade 1	Grade 2	Perforation	P value
Template group	97.4%	2.6%	0%	5.3%	< 0.001*
S1 (n)	19	1	0		
S2 (n)	18	0	0		
Conventional group	86.7%	6.7%	6.7%	13.7%	
S1 (n)	14	1	1		
S2 (n)	12	1	1		

*Fisher's exact test; $p < 0.05$ considered statistically significant

study, the penetration grade was significantly lower for the external template than conventional group (Table 3). However, due to the ceiling effect, this grading system cannot be used to assess the accuracy of the large number of screws that did not penetrating the bone cortex. Takao et al. [17] described a method to evaluate the deviation distance between the planned and actual IS screw, measured at the tip of the screw, the nerve root tunnel zone and entry point, on sagittal view CT images. Using 3D CT fluoroscopy matching navigation, they reported mean deviations of 2.2 ± 0.8 mm (tip), 1.8 ± 0.7 mm (nerve root tunnel) and 2.5 ± 1.8 mm (entry point). A similar method was adopted by Takeba et al. [22], using the O-arm navigation system, with a mean deviation in the position of the tip of the screw of 1.3 ± 0.6 mm. In our study, we used the Takao et al.'s method, with deviation measures comparable to those of the above studies, in which computer navigation was used to guide IS screw insertion. The satisfactory results we obtained with regard to deviation between the planned and actual screw placement and low rate of penetration into the cortex reflect the precise planning of the IS screw trajectory, which was strictly along the midline of the osseous corridor and was confirmed on axial, coronal and sagittal planes in software. Moreover, the special strategy wherein the template was designed such that it could be mounted on the contralateral hemipelvis helped avoid screw penetration in cases with poor fracture reduction. Furthermore, with experience, we have developed the following tips for designing the template to decrease the extent of deformity of template system. First, the template should have a low profile, which minimizes the distance between the template and the skin and, thus, between the marker pins and the virtual screws (Fig. 3d-e). Second, the distance between the two pins inserted in the iliac crest needs to be sufficiently wide to provide good anti-rotation ability for the external template. Third, the guide sleeve in the external template should closely match the guide wire and be sufficiently long to adequately guide K-wire insertion. Fourth, the template system should be constructed using a high-strength material, such as stainless steel or photosensitive resin, providing a strong restraint to bending.

The delay in definitive surgery because of the time required for the design and printing of the template is a limitation of our technique. The mean time from injury to surgery for the template group in our study was 5.4 days, compared to 4.1 days for the conventional group ($p = 0.049$). This longer delay for the template group, however, did not negatively influence the quality of the fracture reduction, which was comparable between the two groups. Of note, all definitive surgeries of both groups were performed within 14 days of the trauma, and the use of the pelvic reduction frame for closed reduction [13] partly offset any adverse effects of a longer delay to surgery.

Pin site infection, which is a common complication of external fixation [24, 25], is also a potential weakness of our external template technique due to the need to insert pin into the iliac crest. However, there was no incidence of pin site infection in our study group. Use of a strict cleaning protocol for the pin sites [26] and effort to shorten the duration of pin fixation [27] can be important factors in preventing pin site infection. Furthermore, the marker pin insertion is an extra process for patients who did not need emergent external fixation. The decision to use this technique needs careful consideration and informed consent from these patients. The indications for the use of our external template technique among patients who did not require emergent external fixation, include, but are not limited to, the need for insertion of multiple percutaneous screws, dysmorphic sacrum and osteoporotic pelvic fractures.

Conclusions

In summary, the external template is an effective tool for percutaneous IS screw insertion, decreasing radiation exposure for both surgeon and patients and avoiding neurovascular injury caused by screw malposition. Considering the high accuracy in IS screw placement that we achieved using an external template, we propose that this technique could potentially be used for other percutaneous insertions of screws in pelvic or acetabular surgery (Fig. 3e-f and Fig. 4c). Further applications and studies are still required to confirm this hypothesis.

Abbreviations
3D: Three-dimensional; CT: Computed tomography; DICOM: Digital imaging and communications in medicine; IS: Iliosacral

Acknowledgements
The authors thank Minjie Gao and Hualun Sun, engineers of 3D digital orthopaedic center for their assistance in external template design, and Editage Corporation for the professional help in English language editing.

Funding
This work was financially supported by the National Natural Science Foundation of China (grant No. 81672158 and 81371939) and National Key R&D Program of China (2016YFC1100100).

Authors' contributions
XDG made substantial contributions to the design of template, performed the surgery, revised the manuscript. FY made substantial contributions to design and manuscript, assisted to perform surgery. SY made contributions to the manuscript, performed the statistical analysis, and assisted to perform surgery. KFC, FZZ, ZKX, YHJ and TFS assisted to perform surgery, collected the data and assessed the outcomes. All authors read and approved the final manuscript.

Competing interests
There are no competing interests to declare.

References

1. Lee CH, Hsu CC, Huang PY. Biomechanical study of different fixation techniques for the treatment of sacroiliac joint injuries using finite element analyses and biomechanical tests. Comput Biol Med. 2017;87:250–7.
2. Matta JM, Saucedo T. Internal fixation of pelvic ring fractures. Clin Orthop Relat Res. 1989;242:83–97.
3. Hinsche AF, Giannoudis PV, Smith RM. Fluoroscopy-based multiplanar image guidance for insertion of sacroiliac screws. Clin Orthop Relat Res. 2002;395:135–44.
4. Templeman D, Schmidt A, Freese J, Weisman I. Proximity of iliosacral screws to neurovascular structures after internal fixation. Clin Orthop Relat Res. 1996;329:194–8.
5. Theologis AA, Burch S, Pekmezci M. Placement of iliosacral screws using 3D image-guided (O-arm) technology and stealth navigation: comparison with traditional fluoroscopy. Bone Joint J. 2016;98-B(5):696–702.
6. Pishnamaz M, Wilkmann C, Na HS, Pfeffer J, Hänisch C, Janssen M, et al. Electromagnetic real time navigation in the region of the posterior pelvic ring: an experimental in-vitro feasibility study and comparison of image guided techniques. PLoS One. 2016;11(2):e0148199.
7. Gras F, Marintschev I, Wilharm A, Klos K, Mückley T, Hofmann GO. 2D-fluoroscopic navigated percutaneous screw fixation of pelvic ring injuries--a case series. BMC Musculoskelet Disord. 2010;11:153.
8. Zhang YZ, Lu S, Xu YQ, Shi JH, Li YB, Feng ZL. Application of navigation template to fixation of sacral fracture using three-dimensional reconstruction and reverse engineering technique. Chin J Traumatol. 2009;12(4):214–7.
9. Chen B, Zhang Y, Xiao S, Gu P, Lin X. Personalized image-based templates for iliosacral screw insertions: a pilot study. Int J Med Robot. 2012;8(4):476–82.
10. Kellam JF, Meinberg EG, Agel J, Karam MD, Roberts CS. Introduction: fracture and dislocation classification compendium-2018: international comprehensive classification of fractures and dislocations committee. J Orthop Trauma. 2018;32:S1–10.
11. Denis F, Davis S, Comfort T. Sacral fractures: an important problem. Retrospective analysis of 236 cases Clin Orthop Relat Res. 1988;227:67–81.
12. Lefaivre KA, Starr AJ, Reinert CM. Reduction of displaced pelvic ring disruptions using a pelvic reduction frame. J Orthop Trauma. 2009;23(4): 299–308.
13. Lefaivre KA, Starr AJ, Barker BP, Overturf S, Reinert CM. Early experience with reduction of displaced disruption of the pelvic ring using a pelvic reduction frame. J Bone Joint Surg Br. 2009;91(9):1201–7.
14. Takao M, Nishii T, Sakai T, Sugano N. CT-3D-fluoroscopy matching navigation can reduce the malposition rate of iliosacral screw insertion for less-experienced surgeons. J Orthop Trauma. 2013;27(12):716–21.
15. Smith HE, Yuan PS, Sasso R, Papadopolous S, Vaccaro AR. An evaluation of image-guided technologies in the placement of percutaneous iliosacral screws. Spine. 2006;31(2):234–8.
16. Tornetta P, Matta JM. Outcome of operatively treated unstable posterior pelvic ring disruptions. Clin Orthop Relat Res. 1996;329:186–93.
17. Takao M, Nishii T, Sakai T, Yoshikawa H, Sugano N. Iliosacral screw insertion using CT-3D-fluoroscopy matching navigation. Injury. 2014;45(6):988–94.
18. Kim JW, Quispe JC, Hao J, Herbert B, Hake M, Mauffrey C. Fluoroscopic views for a more accurate placement of iliosacral screws: an experimental study. J Orthop Trauma. 2016;30(1):34–40.
19. Ozmeric A, Yucens M, Gultaç E, Açar HI, Aydogan NH, Gül D, et al. Are two different projections of the inlet view necessary for the percutaneous placement of iliosacral screws. Bone Joint J. 2015;97-B(5):705–710.
20. Shaw JC, MLC R, Gary JL. Intra-operative multi-dimensional fluoroscopy of guidepin placement prior to iliosacral screw fixation for posterior pelvic ring injuries and sacroiliac dislocation: an early case series. Int Orthop. 2017; 41(10):2171–7.
21. Zheng Z, Zhang Y, Hou Z, Hao J, Zhai F, Su Y, et al. The application of a computer-assisted thermoplastic membrane navigation system in screw fixation of the sacroiliac joint--a clinical study. Injury. 2012;43(4):495–9.
22. Takeba J, Umakoshi K, Kikuchi S, Matsumoto H, Annen S, Moriyama N, et al. Accuracy of screw fixation using the O-arm® and StealthStation® navigation system for unstable pelvic ring fractures. Eur J Orthop Surg Traumatol. 2018; 28(3):431–8.
23. Mastrangelo G, Fedeli U, Fadda E, Giovanazzi A, Scoizzato L, Saia B. Increased cancer risk among surgeons in an orthopaedic hospital. Occup Med. 2005;55(6):498–500.
24. Jennison T, McNally M, Pandit H. Prevention of infection in external fixator pin sites. Acta Biomater. 2014;10(2):595–603.
25. Kazmers NH, Fragomen AT, Rozbruch SR. Prevention of pin site infection in external fixation: a review of the literature. Strategies Trauma Limb Reconstr. 2016;11(2):75–85.

24

Intensive therapy and remissions in rheumatoid arthritis

Catherine D. Hughes[*] [iD], David L. Scott, Fowzia Ibrahim and on behalf of TITRATE Programme Investigators

Abstract

Background: We systematically reviewed the effectiveness of intensive treatment strategies in achieving remission in patients with both early and established Rheumatoid Arthritis (RA).

Methods: A systematic literature review and meta-analysis evaluated trials and comparative studies reporting remission in RA patients treated intensively with disease modifying anti-rheumatic drugs (DMARDs), biologics and Janus Kinase (JAK) inhibitors. Analysis used RevMan 5.3 to report relative risks (RR) in random effects models with 95% confidence intervals (CI).

Results: We identified 928 publications: 53 studies were included (48 superiority studies; 6 head-to-head trials). In the superiority studies 3013/11259 patients achieved remission with intensive treatment compared with 1211/8493 of controls. Analysis of the 53 comparisons showed a significant benefit for intensive treatment (RR 2.23; 95% CI 1.90, 2.61). Intensive treatment increased remissions in both early RA (23 comparisons; RR 1.56; 1.38, 1.76) and established RA (29 comparisons RR 4.21, 2.92, 6.07). All intensive strategies (combination DMARDs, biologics, JAK inhibitors) increased remissions. In the 6 head-to-head trials 317/787 patients achieved remission with biologics compared with 229/671 of patients receiving combination DMARD therapies and there was no difference between treatment strategies (RR 1.06; 0.93. 1.21). There were differences in the frequency of remissions between early and established RA. In early RA the frequency of remissions with active treatment was 49% compared with 34% in controls. In established RA the frequency of remissions with active treatment was 19% compared with 6% in controls.

Conclusions: Intensive treatment with combination DMARDs, biologics or JAK inhibitors increases the frequency of remission compared to control non-intensive strategies. The benefits are seen in both early and established RA.

Keywords: Outcome, Early or established rheumatoid arthritis, Treatment response, Remission

Background

Remission has become a key treatment goal in rheumatoid arthritis (RA). Achieving remission with drug treatment is recommended in many clinical management guidelines [1–6]. It is also a central feature of the "treat-to-target" initiative [7, 8]. Patients who achieve remission have less disability and better quality of life than those with persisting inflammatory disease [9]. In early RA remission is particularly important due to the 'window of opportunity' during which early intensive treatment can halt or substantially reduce subsequent disease progression [10].

There are several definitions of remission in RA. The 2010 European League Against Rheumatism (EULAR) and American College of Rheumatology (ACR) criteria provided a framework for considering these different definitions [11]. A variety of composite measures are used to determine the presence of remission. These include the Disease Activity Score (DAS) and the Disease Activity Score for 28 joints (DAS28), the Simple Disease Activity Score (SDAI) and the Clinical Disease Activity Score (CDAI) [12–14]. DAS28 remission criteria have been used most frequently in trials of intensive treatments in RA, though there has been debate whether it is ideal [15].

Several systematic reviews have reported on treatment remissions in RA [16–20], patients likely to achieve remission [21, 22] and the strength of the rationale for treatment to target approaches in RA [23, 24]. The balance of evidence from these reviews is that intensive treatment increases remission. However, several uncertainties need

* Correspondence: chughes20@nhs.net
Department of Rheumatology, King's College London School of Medicine, Weston Education Centre, King's College London, Cutcombe Road, London SE5 9RJ, UK

to be resolved. Firstly, the relative merits of intensive treatment in early RA compared to established disease need to be considered. Secondly, it is important to know whether treatment with one type of therapy, such as biologics like tumour necrosis factor (TNF) inhibitors, will lead to more remissions than treatment with combinations of conventional disease modifying anti-rheumatic drugs (DMARDs) Finally it is important to know if one or other treatment strategy is preferable in early or established disease.

We have systematically reviewed RA clinical trials that report remissions. We evaluated both trials that compare an intensive treatment strategy with standard care and also head-to-head trials of different intensive treatment strategies. We analysed trials in early and established RA separately, taking the division between these groups as usually being 12 months since diagnosis.

Methods

Inclusion and exclusion criteria

The inclusion criteria were: randomized controlled trials or open label non-randomised comparative studies with at least one intensive treatment arm and one control arm; adult patients with RA; studies of at least 6 months duration; studies enrolling at least 50 patients; studies reporting remissions; studies using treatments in their licensed indication for RA. The intensive treatment arms used drugs considered more intensive than DMARD monotherapy. These included combination DMARDs (which could involve using short-term regular doses of steroids to control synovitis), TNF inhibitors, non-TNF biologics (tocilizumab, abatacept and rituximab), and Janus Kinase (JAK) inhibitors. We also noted whether studies used a treat-to-target approach with intensive treatments. Studies either compared one intensive treatment strategy against standard care or two different intensive treatment strategies (such as combination DMARDs and TNF inhibitors with DMARDs). Foreign language papers and published conference abstracts were excluded. Trials comparing similar types of treatment, such as two intensive DMARD regimens, were also excluded. The search identified publications from 1st January 2000 to 30th April 2017.

Search strategy

A systematic literature search was carried out using EMBASE, OVID Medline as well as hand searching the systematic reviews relevant to this topic found in the Cochrane library database. The key word search terms used were 'arthritis, rheumatoid' (MeSH), 'clinical trial' [Publication Type] (MeSH), randomised controlled trial [Publication Type] (MeSH), open label (free text) and 'remission' (free text). These were searched separately and in combination. The EMBASE search terms included 'arthritis, rheumatoid' (MeSH) all subheadings and FOCUS function, clinical trial (MeSH) Explode function.

Data collection

Two researchers (CH, DLS) independently assessed studies for eligibility and extracted data. This included year of publication, disease duration, number of treatment groups, study design, control and intensive treatment regimens, study size, remissions and study end-points. The numbers of patients achieving disease remission at the trial end-point was defined by Disease Activity Scores (DAS) < 1.6, DAS28 < 2.6 or equivalent criteria. The trials were classified as early (generally with disease durations < 1 year) or established (generally with disease durations > 1 year) reflecting the trial investigators assessments. When there were differences between assessors, they reviewed the reports together and came to a joint conclusion.

Assessing Bias

A quality assessment was completed for each paper using the Cochrane Collaboration tool for assessing risk of bias [25]. The types of bias assessed were: random sequence generation, selection bias, performance bias, detection bias, attrition bias, reporting bias and other bias (such as pharmaceutical funding). The risk was defined as low or high. We also used funnel plots to assess publication bias and associated issues [26].

Statistical analysis

Results were analysed using Review Manager 5.3 (Cochrane Collaboration, Oxford, UK). The random effects model based on DerSimonian and Laird's method [27] was used to estimate the pooled effect sizes; this gives more equal weighting to studies of different precision in comparison with a simple inverse variance weighted approach, so accommodating between study heterogeneity. For all meta-analyses, we performed Cochrane's chi-squared test to assess between study heterogeneity and quantified I^2 statistics [25]. P-values < 0.05 were considered significant.

Some of the randomised controlled trials had more than two treatment arms: when there were two control groups the results were combined; when there were two or more intensive treatment groups only those reporting licensed dosage regimens were included.

Results

Study selection

We identified 928 publications: 440 were duplicated studies and 414 were excluded after reviewing abstracts. Seventy four full text papers were reviewed in detail; 21 were excluded and 53 selected for inclusion (Fig. 1). These papers comprised 48 superiority trials, in which an intensive treatment strategy was compared with a less intensive strategy, and 6 head-to-head trials comparing combination DMARDs with biologic treatments. The BeST paper is included in both of these groups.

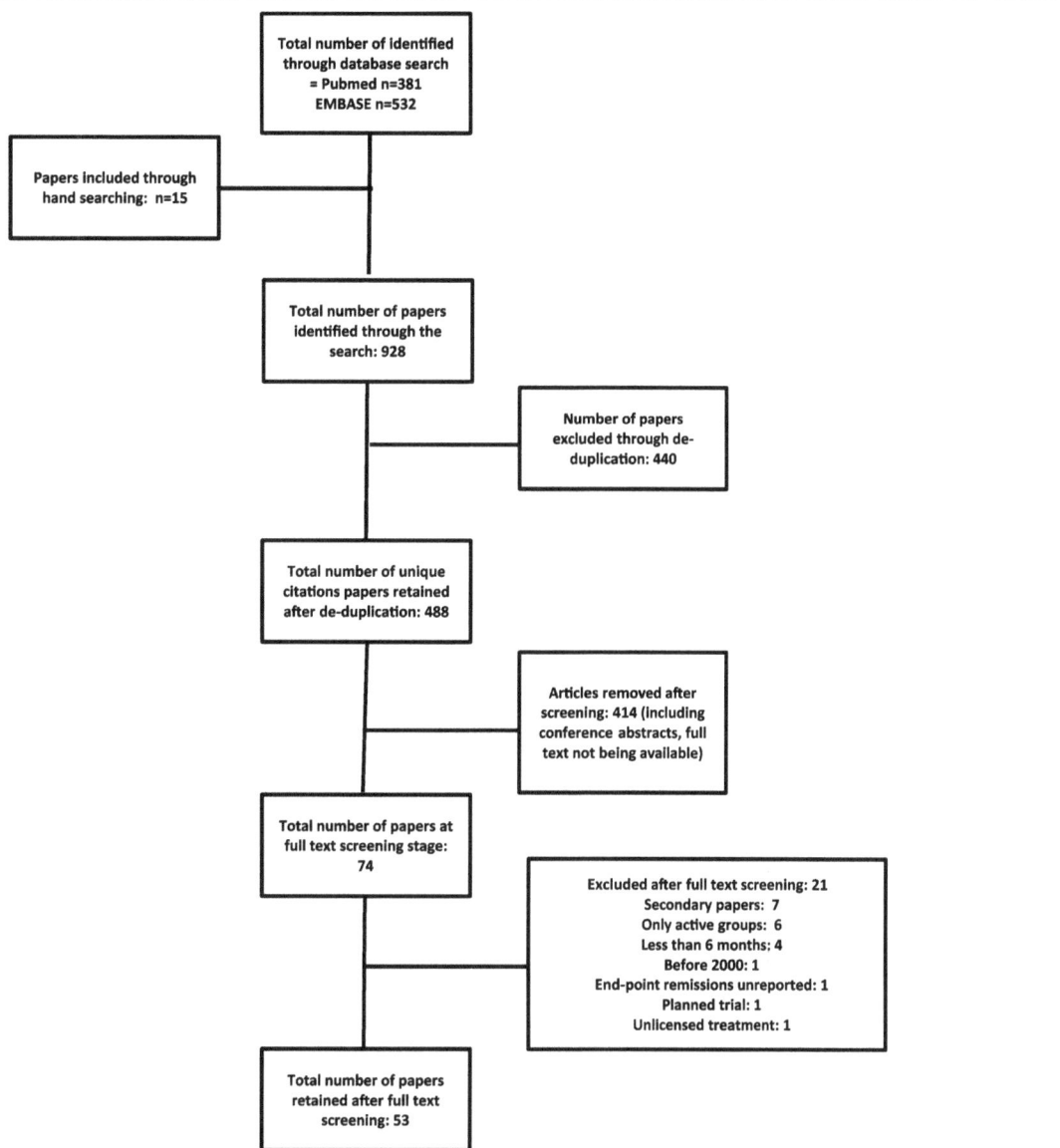

Fig. 1 PRISMA Diagram Outlining Search Strategy

Characteristics of included studies

Twenty two superiority trials evaluated patients reported as having early RA. Their maximum disease durations ranged from 3 months to 3 years. Mean or median disease durations, reported in 20 of these trials, ranged from 1 to 11 months (mean 6 months). Four of these trials studied patients with very early disease, less than 6 months from diagnosis. One trial had two different intensive treatment arms (combination DMARDs and biologics) which were both included. Six trials had two or three intensive treatment arms: in three trials biologic monotherapy treatment arms were omitted; in another three trials only licensed combination regimens were included.

Twenty six superiority trials evaluated patients with established RA. Six of these trials specified maximum

disease durations (from 5 to 20 years). Mean or median disease durations, reported in all of these trials, ranged from 1 to 12 years (mean 8 years). One trial had two control groups (methotrexate or sulfasalazine monotherapy) and these were combined. Sixteen trials had two or more intensive treatment arms: three had two different licensed intensive treatments (biologics and JAK inhibitors) which were both included; in one trial the biologic monotherapy treatment arm was omitted; in a further 12 trials only licensed combination regimens were included.

Overall 19,752 RA patients were studied: 7300 in early RA and 12,452 with established RA (Table 1). There were 46 conventional RCTs, one was open label and one quasi-experimental. Twenty four trials had 2-arms, 17 had 3-arms and 7 had over three arms. The trials often reported

Table 1 Details of Studies with Control Groups

First Author	Study	Year	Design	Groups	RA Duration	Quality Assessments			Months Follow-up	Treatments	
						Allocation	Blinding	Bias Analysis		Control	Intensive
Atsumi [28]	C-Opera	2016	RCT	2	Early	Low risk	Low risk	Low risk	12	MTX	Certolizumab/MTX
Bakker [29]	Camera II	2012	RCT	2	Early	Low risk	Low risk	Low risk	24	MTX	Prednisolone/MTX
Bijlsma [30]	U-Act-Early	2016	RCT	3	Early	Low risk	Low risk	Low risk	24	MTX	Tocilizumab/MTX
Breedveld [31]	Premier	2005	RCT	3	Early	Low risk	Low risk	Low risk	24	MTX	Adalimumab/MTX
Burmester [32]	Function	2015	RCT	4	Early	Unclear	Unclear	Low risk	12	MTX	Tocilizumab/MTX
Capell [33]	Mascot	2007	RCT	3	Est'lishd	Low risk	Low risk	Low risk	12	MTX or SZP	MTZ/SZP
Cohen [34]	Reflex	2006	RCT	2	Est'lishd	Low risk	Low risk	Low risk	6	MTX	Rituximab/MTX
Detert [35]	Hit Hard	2012	RCT	2	Early	Low risk	Low risk	Low risk	6	MTX	Adalimumab/MTX
Dougadas [36]	Act-Ray	2013	RCT	2	Est'lishd	Low risk	Low risk	Low risk	6	Tocilizumab	Tocilizumab/MTX
Emery [37]	Avert	2014	RCT	3	Early	Low risk	Low risk	Low risk	12	MTX	Abatacept/MTX
Emery [38]	Comet	2008	RCT	2	Early	Low risk	Low risk	Low risk	12	MTX	Etanercept/MTX
Emery [39]	Go Before	2009	RCT	4	Est'lishd	Low risk	Low risk	Low risk	6	MTX	Golimumab/MTX
Emery [40]	Radiate	2008	RCT	3	Est'lishd	Low risk	Low risk	Low risk	6	MTX	Tocilizumab/MTX
Emery [41]	Serene	2010	RCT	3	Est'lishd	Low risk	Low risk	Low risk	12	MTX	Rituximab/MTX
Emery [42]	C-Early	2017	RCT	2	Early	Low risk	Low risk	Low risk	12	MTX	Certolizumab/MTX
Genovese [43]	RA Beacon	2016	RCT	3	Est'lishd	Low risk	Low risk	Low risk	6	DMARD	Baracitinib/DMARDs
Genovese [44]	Toward	2008	RCT	2	Est'lishd	Low risk	Low risk	Low risk	6	DMARD	Tocilizumab/DMARD
Goekoop Ruitermann [45]	BeSt	2005	RCT	4	Early	Low risk	Low risk	Low risk	12	DMARDs	Infliximab/DMARDs or Combination DMARDs
Grigor [46]	Ticora	2004	RCT	2	Est'lishd	Low risk	Low risk	Low risk	18	Usual Care	Combination DMARDs
Hetland [47]	Cimestra	2006	RCT	2	Early[a]	Unclear	Low risk	Low risk	12	MTX	MTX/Ciclosporin
Horslev Petersen [48]	Opera	2014	RCT	2	Early[a]	Low risk	Low risk	Low risk	12	MTX	Adalimumab/MTX
Kavanaugh [49]	Optima	2013	RCT	2	Est'lishd	Low risk	Low risk	Low risk	6	MTX	Adalimumab/MTX
Kivitz [50]	Brevacta	2014	RCT	2	Est'lishd	Low risk	Low risk	Low risk	6	DMARD	Tocilizumab/DMARD
Klareskog [51]	Tempo	2004	RCT	3	Est'lishd	Low risk	Low risk	Low risk	6	MTX	Etanercept/MTX
Kremer [52]	–	2005	RCT	3	Est'lishd	Low risk	Low risk	Low risk	6	MTX	Abatacept/MTX
Kremer [53]	Lithe	2011	RCT	3	Est'lishd	Low risk	Low risk	Low risk	12	MTX	Tocilizumab/MTX
Kremer [54]	–	2012	RCT	7	Est'lishd	Low risk	unclear	Low risk	24	MTX	Tofacitinib/MTX
Kremer [55]	–	2013	RCT	4	Est'lishd	Low risk	Low risk	Low risk	6	DMARD	Tofacitinib/DMARD
Nam [56]	Empire	2014	RCT	2	Early[a]	Low risk	Low risk	Low risk	12	MTX	Etanercept/MTX
Nam [57]	Idea	2014	RCT	2	Early	Low risk	Low risk	Low risk	18	MTX	MTX/Infliximab
Schiff [58]	Attest	2007	RCT	3	Est'lishd	Low risk	Low risk	Low risk	12	MTX	Abatacept/MTX or

Table 1 Details of Studies with Control Groups *(Continued)*

First Author	Study	Year	Design	Groups	RA Duration	Quality Assessments			Months Follow-up	Treatments	
Schipper [59]	–	2012	Quasi-Exp	2	Early	High risk	High risk	Indeterminate	12	Usual care	Infliximab/MTX
Smolen [60]	Certain	2014	RCT	2	Est'lishd	Low risk	Low risk	Low risk	12	DMARD	Tight control[b]
Smolen [61]	Go After	2009	RCT	3	Est'lishd	Low risk	Low risk	Low risk	6	DMARD	Certolizumab/DMARD
Smolen [62]	Option	2008	RCT	3	Est'lishd	Low risk	Low risk	Low risk	6	MTX	Golimumab/DMARD
Smolen [63]	Rapid2	2008	RCT	4	Est'lishd	Low risk	Low risk	Low risk	6	MTX	Tocilizumab/MTX
Soubrier [64]	Guepard	2009	RCT	2	Early[a]	Low risk	Low risk	Unclear	12	MTX	Certolizumab/MTX
St. Clair [65]	–	2004	RCT	3	Early	Low risk	High risk	Low risk	12	MTX	Adalimumab/MTX
Symmons [66]	Brosg	2006	RCT	2	Est'lishd	High risk	Low risk	Low risk	36	Symptomatic	Infliximab/MTX
Tak [67]	Image	2010	RCT	3	Early	Low risk	Low risk	Low risk	12	MTX	Combination DMARDs
Takeuchi [68]	Hopeful-1	2014	RCT	2	Early	Low risk	Low risk	Low risk	6	MTX	Rituximab/MTX
Taylor [69]	RA Beam	2017	RCT	3	Est'lishd	Low risk	Low risk	Low risk	6	MTX	Adalimumab/MTX
van der Heijde [70]	Oral Scan	2013	RCT	3	Est'lishd	Low risk	Low risk	Low risk	6	MTX	Baracitinib/MTX or Adalimumab/MTX
Van Ejik [71]	Stream	2012	RCT	2	Early	Uncertain	Low risk	Low risk	24	Usual care	MTX/Tofacitinib
van Vollenhoven [72]	Oral Standard	2012	RCT	4	Est'lishd	Low risk	Low risk	Low risk	6	MTX	Intensive treatment
Verstappen [73]	Camera	2007	Open label	2	Early	High risk	High risk	Indeterminate	24	Usual care	Tofacitinib/MTX or Adalimumab/MTX
Weinblatt [74]	Go Further	2013	RCT	2	Est'lishd	Low risk	Low risk	Low risk	6	MTX	Combination DMARDs
Westhovens [75]	–	2009	RCT	2	Early	Low risk	Low risk	Low risk	12	MTX	Golimumab/MTX
											Abatacept/MTX

a. These trials enrolled patients with disease durations no more than 6 months. b. In Schipper et al. study by 12 months 16% controls had combination DMARDs and 6% had TNF inhibitors; with intensive treatment 30% had combination DMARDs and 12% TNF inhibitors. The trial was classified as comparing combination DMARDs

Abbreviations: *RCT* Randomised controlled trial, *Est'lishd* Established, *MTX* Methotrexate, *SZP* Sulfasalazine, *DMARD* Disease modifying anti-rheumatic drugs

outcomes at several different time-points, but their primary outcomes were reported at 6 months in 21 trials, at 12 months in 19 trials and at longer intervals in 8 trials (2 at 18 months, 5 at 24 months and 1 at 36 months).

DAS28 remissions (DAS28 < 2.6) were reported in 38/48 superiority trials and 4/6 head-to-head trials. DAS remissions (DAS < 1.6) were reported in 5/48 superiority trials and 2/6 head-to-head trials. Five superiority trials reported other remissions (using SDAI in 3 and unique study-specific criteria in 2). In addition, 12 superiority trials reported some or all of the new EULAR/ACR remission criteria.

Treat-to-target strategies were included within 8/48 superiority trials and 3/6 head-to-head trials, though there were substantial differences in how these strategies were delivered.

Remission in superiority trials

Overall in the 48 trials 3013/11,259 patients achieved remission with intensive treatment compared with 1211/8493 patients receiving non-intensive therapy (Table 2). Analysis of the 53 comparisons in these trials using the random effects relative risk model showed there was a highly significant benefit for intensive treatment (RR 2.23; 95% CI

1.90, 2.61). There was marked heterogeneity between studies; I2 was 84%.

In the 38 trials (40 comparisons) reporting DAS28 remissions the random risk ratio was 2.26 (95% CI 1.89, 2.71); in the 10 trials (12 comparisons) reporting other remission criteria the random risk ratio was 2.13 (95% CI 1.53, 2.98). The random risk ratios showed significant effects with trials of 6 months, 12 months and longer durations. Although the random ratio was somewhat higher in trials of 6 months duration, 17/21 trials (20/24 comparisons) were in established RA and in these the random risk ratio was 4.82 (95% CI 2.85, 8.13); in the 4 trials (4 comparisons) lasting 6 months in early RA the random risk ratio was 1.94 (95% CI 1.21, 3.11). In the 8 trials (9 comparisons) involving TTT strategies as part of intensive treatment the random risk ratio was 1.62 (95% CI 1.30, 2.03).

In the 22 trials in early RA with intensive treatments trials with 1756/3993 patients achieved remission with intensive treatment compared with 903/3307 patients receiving monotherapy. One trial evaluated two intensive treatment regimens and there were consequently 23 comparisons; 13 evaluated TNF inhibitors, 5 evaluated other biologics and 5 evaluated combination DMARDs. Analysis of the 23 comparisons in these trials showed a significant overall benefit for intensive treatment (RR

Table 2 Effectiveness In Superiority Trials Assessed By Random Risk Ratio and Heterogeneity

	Treatments	Trials	Comparisons	Random Risk Ratio (95% CI)	Heterogeneity
All	All	48	52	2.23 (1.90, 2.61)	$I^2 = 84\%$
	DAS28 Remissions	38	40	2.26 (1.89, 2.71)	$I^2 = 85\%$
	Other Remission Criteria	10	12	2.13 (1.53, 2.98)	$I^2 = 81\%$
	6 Month Duration	21	24	3.78 (2.60, 5.51)	$I^2 = 86\%$
	12 Month Duration	19	20	1.73 (1.44, 2.09)	$I^2 = 82\%$
	18–36 Month Duration	8	8	1.84 (1.39, 2.42)	$I^2 = 79\%$
	Used TTT Strategy	8	9	1.62 (1.30, 2.03)	$I^2 = 75\%$
Early	All[a]	22	23	1.56 (1.38, 1.76)	$I^2 = 74\%$
	TNF Inhibitors	13	13	1.44 (1.26, 1.66)	$I^2 = 62\%$
	Other Biologics	5	5	2.00 (1.53, 2.63)	$I^2 = 79\%$
	Combination DMARDS[b]	5	5	1.46 (1.11, 1.93)	$I^2 = 73\%$
	Used TTT Strategy	6	7	1.51 (1.22, 1.88)	$I^2 = 72\%$
Established	All	26	29	4.21 (2.92, 6.07)	$I^2 = 86\%$
	TNF Inhibitors	10	10	3.59 (2.14, 6.03)	$I^2 = 70\%$
	Other Biologics	10	10	6.81 (2.62, 17.7)	$I^2 = 95\%$
	Combination DMARDS	3	3	2.41 (1.14, 5.10)	$I^2 = 67\%$
	JAK Inhibitors	6	6	3.39 (2.14, 5.36)	$I^2 = 0\%$
	Used TTT Strategy	2	2	2.39 (0.90, 6.32)	$I^2 = 83\%$

[a]The 4 very early trials which enrolled patients with disease durations no more than 6 months involved 4 comparisons with a random risk ratio (95% CI) of 1.47 (1.03, 2.10) and I^2 72%
[b]Excluding the Schipper et al. study in which some patients in both groups had DMARD monotherapy, DMARD combination therapy and TNF inhibitors leaves 4 trials with 4 comparisons with a random risk ratio (95% CI) of 1.38 (1.01, 1.88) and I^2 71%
Abbreviations: *DAS28* Disease Activity Score for 28 joints, *TNF* Tumour necrosis factor, *DMARDs* Disease modifying anti-rheumatic drugs, *JAK* Janus kinase, *TTT* Treat To Target

1.56; 95% CI 1.38, 1.76). There was marked heterogeneity in these studies; I^2 was 74% (Table 2). A funnel plot showed a symmetrical pattern in these trials (result not shown). Four trials enrolled patients with disease durations no more than 6 months and these showed a similar benefit for intensive treatment (RR 1.47; 95%CI 1.03, 2.10) Comparison of the different intensive treatment regimens in early RA patients showed similar impacts of different intensive treatments; these ranged from a random risk ratio of 1.43 with TNF inhibitors to 2.00 with other biologics. TTT strategies also increased remissions with a random risk ratio of 1.51.

In the 26 established RA trials 1257/7266 patients achieved remission with intensive treatment compared with 308/5186 patients receiving monotherapy. Three trials evaluated two intensive treatment regimens and consequently there were 29 comparisons: 10 evaluated TNF inhibitors, 10 evaluated other biologics, 3 evaluated combination DMARDs and 6 evaluated JAK inhibitors. Analysis of these 29 comparisons trials showed a significant overall benefit for intensive treatment (RR 4.21; 95% CI 2.92, 6.07). There was marked heterogeneity in these studies; I^2 was 86% (Table 2). A funnel plot showed an asymmetrical pattern in these trials (result not shown). Comparison of the different intensive treatment regimens in established RA patients showed some differences in the magnitude of effects; random risk ratios ranged from 2.41 with combination DMARDs to 6.81 with other biologics (tocilizumab, adalimumab and rituximab); however, as the confidence intervals overlapped there was no evidence these differences were significant. Only two trials used TTT strategies and although these increase remissions the 95% confidence intervals showed the finding may not have been significant (random risk ratio 2.39; 95% CI 0.90, 6.32).

Using a fixed effects model gave similar findings. In all trials the risk ratio was 2.06 (95%CI 1.94, 2.18), in early RA trials it was 1.64 (95% CI 1.54, 1.74) and in established RA the risk ratio was 3.32 (95% CI 2.94, 3.74). Interestingly the fixed model indicated TTT strategies in established RA in two trials may have been significant (risk ratio 2.19, 95% CI 1.50, 3.19.

Remission in head to head trials

Overall in the 6 trials 317/787 patients achieved remission with TNF inhibitors compared with 229/671 of patients receiving combination DMARD therapies. Analysis of these 6 trials using the random effects relative risk model (Table 3) showed there was a no different between treatment strategies (RR 1.06; 95% CI 0.93. 1.21). There was little heterogeneity between studies; I^2 was 21%. Comparing 4 early RA and 2 established RA trials separately also showed no evidence of a significant difference between groups (Table 3). However, comparisons of the first 6 months results in the two established

Table 3 Effectiveness In Head To Head Trials Comparing Biologic with Combination DMARD Strategies Assessed By Random Risk Ratio and Heterogeneity

	Trials	Random Risk Ratio (95% CI)	Heterogeneity
All	6	1.06 (0.93, 1.21)	$I^2 = 21\%$
Early	4	1.05 (0.88, 1.24)	$I^2 = 40\%$
Established	2	1.21 (0.88, 1.68)	$I^2 = 0\%$
Established First 6 Months	2	1.74 (1.14, 2.64)	$I^2 = 0\%$

RA trials showed more remissions with TNF inhibitors using the random effects relative risk model (RR 1.74, 95% CI 1.14, 2.64). The fixed effects model gave similar findings (RR 1.90; 95% CI 1.17, 3.10).

Frequency of remissions

There were marked differences in the frequency of remissions in active and control groups in both early and established RA (Fig. 2). In early RA the average frequency of remissions with active treatment was 49%: in 10 early RA trials 50% or more active patients achieved remissions; the highest rate was 86% in the U-Act-Early (tocilizumab) trial and the lowest rate was 18% in the St Clair (Infliximab) trial. In early RA controls the average frequency of remission was 34%: in four trials 50% or more controls achieved remissions; and the lowest rate in controls was 18% in the Image (rituximab) trial. The average difference in remission rates between active and control group in early RA trials was 15%.

In established RA the average frequency of remissions with active treatment was 19%: in only one trial did 50% or more active patients achieved remission (65% in the Ticora trial of combination DMARDs); in 14 trials 10% or less active patients achieved remission and, in the Reflex, (rituximab) and RA Beam (baricitinib and adalimumab) trials only 3% of patients achieved remissions. In established RA controls the average frequency of remission was 6%: in 22 trials less than 5% of controls achieved remissions; and in the Reflex (rituximab) trial no control patient achieved an end-point remission. The average difference in remission rates between active and control group in early RA trials was 13%.

Quality and risk of Bias

Quality assessment, using the Cochrane Collaboration tool for assessing risk of bias, showed overall quality was high with low risks of bias (Table 1).

Discussion

TNF Inhibitors, other biologics and combination DMARDS were all effective in increasing remission in early and established RA. Treat to target strategies, which usually involved intensive DMARDs, were also

Early RA

Established RA

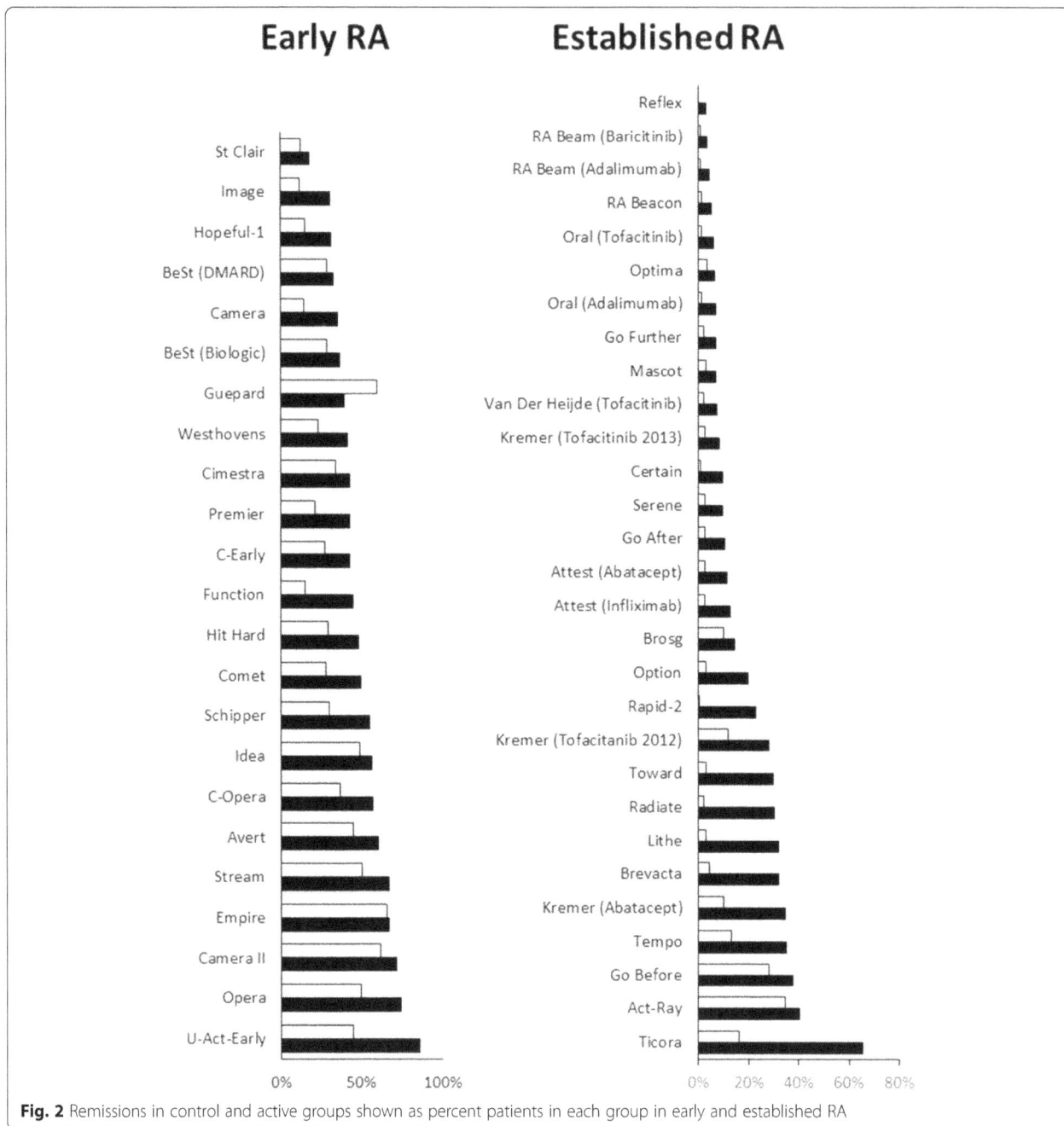

Fig. 2 Remissions in control and active groups shown as percent patients in each group in early and established RA

effective. JAK inhibitors were similarly effective in established RA; there was no data about their impact in early disease. Although other biologics achieved numerically higher risk ratios in both early and established RA the overlapping confidence intervals gave no support to the view that these differences are clinically significant. The benefits of different types of intensive treatment were therefore broadly similar. Trials of varying durations, from 6 months to more than 12 months, all showed intensive treatments increased remissions. There was no evidence that patients with very early RA of no more

than 6 months disease duration benefited more from intensive treatments. We excluded trials with durations of less than 6 months to ensure we did not disadvantage the assessment of intensive treatment strategies using slower acting DMARDs. The head-to-head trials supported the similarities between treatments with combination DMARD strategies and TNF inhibitor strategies, which achieved similar end-point remission rates. There was however, some evidence that TNF inhibitors increased the early remission rates, in keeping with their relatively rapid onset of action compared to conventional DMARD combinations.

TNF Inhibitors, other biologics and combination DMARDS were all effective in increasing remission in early and established RA. There was no evidence that patients with very early RA of no more than 6 months disease duration benefited more from intensive treatments. JAK inhibitors were similarly effective in established RA; there was no data about their impact in early disease. Although other biologics achieved numerically higher risk ratios in both early and established RA the overlapping confidence intervals gave no support to the view that these differences are clinically significant. The head-to-head trials supported the similarities between treatments with combination DMARD strategies and TNF inhibitor strategies, which achieved similar end-point remission rates. There was however, some evidence that TNF inhibitors increased the early remission rates, in keeping with their relatively rapid onset of action compared to conventional DMARD combinations.

The overall quality of the studies was relatively high. However, there was evidence of marked heterogeneity in their findings with most comparisons having high I^2 values. This heterogeneity meant that in some intensive treatment arms in early RA over 70% patients achieved remission while in other intensive treatment arms in established RA under 10% patients achieved remission. These differences are likely to reflect patient selection more than treatment efficacy, with very early RA patients having no previous DMARDs are highly likely to achieve remission with intensive treatment while established RA patients who have failed multiple prior treatments are unlikely to do so.

The most likely explanation for the asymmetrical funnel plot in trials in established RA relates to specifically including studies using treatments in their licensed indication which were published between 2000 and 2017. A consequence is that potential intensive treatments which were evaluated in RA patients but were not found to be effective, were not included. Firstly, small initial studies with new drugs which would have shown negative results for remissions were not included as the treatments were never licensed for RA. An example is the spleen tyrosine kinase inhibitors [81]. Secondly, some TNF inhibitors were not effective in RA and were therefore not licensed; an example is Lenercept, which failed to show sustained benefit in clinical trials [82]. Finally, combinations with DMARDs were tried in the 1980's, before remission was measured or reported; these trials were mainly negative [83]; subsequent trials of intensive DMARD combinations reporting remission which were published after 2000 studied treatments which were known to be effective in combination. These factors mean the funnel plot of remissions in established RA

would not include small trials with negative findings because of the selection criteria used. As this report focuses on the benefits of different intensive treatment strategies using licensed treatments given at their approved dosages we do not think an asymmetric funnel plot changes our conclusions.

Our systematic review has a number of limitations. Firstly, studies not reporting remission data were excluded, though they often show clinically important improvements with intensive treatment. Secondly, studies reported remissions differently; for example, DAS and DAS28 remissions are similar but not identical. Thirdly, studies were of variable duration and comparing remission rates over 6 and 12 months or more is not ideal; however, variations in treatments and patient selection meant there was no evidence for one particular time point being best. Fourthly, studies differed in the way they handled non-responders, with some trials stopping treatment if patients had not responded within 3 months or so and applying non-responder imputations. This approach may alter the remission rates in the non-intensive treatment by making it appear smaller than it might have been if treatment was continued. Fifthly, as mentioned previously, studies enrolled different patient groups in whom the likelihood of achieving remissions was very different. Sixthly, the intensive combination DMARD regimens used in the trials have been combined together, even though they represent a wide range of different strategies, not all of which appeared highly effective. In one study by Schipper et al. [58] some patients in active and control groups had monotherapy and others had biologics, so the trial is not just a comparison of one treatment strategy; however, excluding it made no difference to the conclusions. Finally, there is debate about the benefits of combining the results of different trials in a meta-analysis, considering their potential degrees of clinical heterogeneity. As we have also undertaken extensive sub-group analyses we consider the approach we have taken is justified in this particular clinical context.

Our results have several implications for clinical practice. Firstly, they show that intensive treatment strategies lead to more remissions than conventional care in both early and established RA. This finding is generally supportive of the treat-to-target approach currently recommended [7, 8], although we have not attempted to dissociate the impact of giving intensive treatment from the impact of the target. Secondly, they show that initial treatment with conventional DMARD combinations has similar effectiveness to early biologics. This finding is supportive of the current recommendations about biologic treatments from the National Institute for Health and Care Excellence (NICE), which recommend trying combination DMARDs before biologic treatment [84]. Thirdly, they question whether remission is necessarily

Table 4 Details Of Head-To-Head Studies

| First Author | Study | Year | Design | Groups | RA Duration | Quality Assessments | | | Months Follow-up | Treatments | |
						Allocation	Blinding	Bias Analysis		Non-Biologic	Biologic
Goekoop Ruitermann [45]	BeSt	2005	RCT	4	Early	Low risk	Low risk	Low risk	12	Combination DMARDs	Infliximab/DMARDs
Heimans [76]	Improved	2014	RCT	2	Early	Low risk	High risk	Unclear	12	Triple DMARDs	Adalimumab/MTX
Leirisalo-Repo [77]	Neo-Fin RA Co	2013	RCT	2	Early	Low risk	Low risk	Low risk	24	Triple DMARDs	Infliximab/Triple DMARDs
O'Dell [78]	Racat	2013	RCT	2	Est'lishd	Low risk	Low risk	Low risk	12	Triple DMARDs	Etanercept/MTX
Scott [79]	Tacit	2015	RCT	2	Est'lishd	Low risk	High risk	Indeterminate	12	Combination DMARDs	TNF inhibitors/DMARDs
Moreland [80]	Tear	2012	RCT	4	Early	Low risk	Low risk	Low risk	24	Triple DMARDs	Etanercept/MTX

Abbreviations: *RCT* Randomised controlled trial, *Est'lishd* Established, *MTX* Methotrexate, *DMARD* Disease modifying anti-rheumatic drugs, *TNF* Tumour necrosis factor

the ideal target for treatment in established RA, as it is only achieved by a minority of patients in most trials of intensive treatment. There may be greater value of aiming for low disease activity states, in which case these need to be measured in future trials. The EULAR good response criteria can be used to assess the frequency of achieving low disease activity states measures using DAS28. Current guidance on treat to target includes aiming for low disease activity in some patients.

One issue this review cannot address is treatment sequencing. Some experts believe most early RA patients should receive methotrexate monotherapy initially for a few months and only have intensive treatments if they fail to respond. Other experts recommend early intensive treatment followed by treatment tapering. It is possible to find individual trials within our systematic review, which support both options, but there is no systematic evidence to support or refute either approach. One final pair of inter-related uncertainties is the optimal time to assess remission and the most suitable assessment to evaluate its presence. Combining superiority and head-to-head trials (Tables 1 and 4) shows 23 (43%) lasted 12 months, 20 (38%) lasted 6 months and 10 (19%) lasted over 12 months, with the longest (BROSG trial evaluating combination DMARDs) lasting 3 years. This finding suggests trials of 12 months or longer seem preferable. Although most trials reported DAS28 remissions, this represents an historical target and there is now greater emphasis on stricter remission criteria.

Conclusions

Intensive treatment with combination DMARDs, biologics or JAK inhibitors increases the frequency of remission compared to control non-intensive strategies. The benefits are seen in both early and established RA. The relative merits of different remission criteria in trials is a complex question but changing criteria has the disadvantage of making it difficult to compare trials with newer criteria and those using more historic methods.

Abbreviations

ACR: American College of Rheumatology; BROSG: British rheumatoid outcome study group; CDAI: Clinical disease activity score; CI: Confidence intervals; DAS: Disease activity score; DAS28: Disease activity score for 28 joints; DMARDs: Disease modifying anti rheumatic drugs; EULAR: European league against rheumatism; JAK inhibitors: Janus kinase inhibitors; NICE: National Institute for Health and Care Excellence; RA: Rheumatoid arthritis; RR: Relative risks; SDAI: Simple diseasee activity score; TNF inhibitors: Tumour necrosis factor inhibitors; TTT: Treat to target

Acknowledgements

On behalf of TITRATE Programme Investigators.
Work Stream A: Heidi Lempp, Jackie Sturt and Louise Prothero;
Work Stream B: Isabel Neatrour, Rhiannon Baggott, Fowzia Ibrahim, Brian Tom, Allan Wailoo, James Galloway, Gabrielle Kingsley and David Scott.
Work Stream C: Brian Tom, Fowzia Ibrahim & David L Scott.

Funding

CH is a South Thames Rheumatology Specialist Registrar working in Kings College Hospital. FI is supported by the Academic department of Rheumatology. DLS is supported by TITRATE study programme. The TITRATE study is funded by the National Institute for Health Research (NIHR) as one of its Programme Grants For Applied Research (Grant Reference Number: RP-PG-0610-10066; Programme Title: Treatment Intensities and Targets in Rheumatoid Arthritis Therapy: Integrating Patients' And Clinicians' Views – The TITRATE Programme. The views expressed are those of the authors and not necessarily those of the NHS, the NIHR or the Department of Health and Social care.

Authors' contributions

CH reviewed the articles, extracted data and drafted the manuscript. FI & DS participated in data extraction and commented on draft manuscript. All authors read and approved the final manuscript.

Competing interests

The authors declare that they have no competing interests.

References

1. Smolen JS, Landewe R, Bijlsma J, Burmester G, Chatzidionysiou K, Dougados M, et al. EULAR recommendations for the management of rheumatoid arthritis with synthetic and biological disease-modifying antirheumatic drugs: 2016 update. Ann Rheum Dis. 2017;76:960–77.
2. Singh JA, Saag KG, Bridges SL Jr, Akl EA, Bannuru RR, Sullivan MC, et al. 2015 American College of Rheumatology Guideline for the treatment of rheumatoid arthritis. Arthritis Rheumatol. 2016;68:1–26.
3. Gaujoux-Viala C, Gossec L, Cantagrel A, Dougados M, Fautrel B, Mariette X, et al. Recommendations of the French Society for Rheumatology for managing rheumatoid arthritis. Joint Bone Spine. 2014;81:287–97.
4. Albrecht K, Kruger K, Wollenhaupt J, Alten R, Backhaus M, Baerwald C, et al. German guidelines for the sequential medical treatment of rheumatoid arthritis with traditional and biologic disease-modifying antirheumatic drugs. Rheumatol Int. 2014;34:1–9.
5. Bykerk VP, Akhavan P, Hazlewood GS, Schieir O, Dooley A, Haraoui B, et al. Canadian rheumatology association recommendations for pharmacological management of rheumatoid arthritis with traditional and biologic disease-modifying antirheumatic drugs. J Rheumatol. 2012;39:1559–82.
6. (UK) NCCfCC. Rheumatoid arthritis: national clinical guideline for management and treatment in adults: National institute for health and clinical excellence: guidance. National collaborating centre for chronic conditions (UK). London: Royal College of Physicians (UK); 2009.
7. Smolen JS, Breedveld FC, Burmester GR, Bykerk V, Dougados M, Emery P, et al. Treating rheumatoid arthritis to target: 2014 update of the recommendations of an international task force. Ann Rheum Dis. 2016;75:3–15.
8. Huizinga T, Knevel R. Rheumatoid arthritis: 2014 treat-to-target RA recommendations--strategy is key. Nat Rev Rheumatol. 2015;11:509–11.
9. Alemao E, Joo S, Kawabata H, Al MJ, Allison PD, Rutten-van Molken MP, et al. Effects of achieving target measures in rheumatoid arthritis on functional status, quality of life, and resource utilization: analysis of clinical practice data. Arthritis Care Res. 2016;68:308–17.
10. van Nies JA, Tsonaka R, Gaujoux-Viala C, Fautrel B, van der Helm-van Mil AH. Evaluating relationships between symptom duration and persistence of

rheumatoid arthritis: does a window of opportunity exist? Results on the Leiden early arthritis clinic and ESPOIR cohorts. Ann Rheum Dis. 2015;74:806–12.

11. Felson DT, Smolen JS, Wells G, Zhang B, van Tuyl LH, Funovits J, et al. American College of Rheumatology/European league against rheumatism provisional definition of remission in rheumatoid arthritis for clinical trials. Ann Rheum Dis. 2011;70:404–13.

12. Prevoo ML, van Gestel AM, van THMA, van Rijswijk MH, van de Putte LB, van Riel PL. Remission in a prospective study of patients with rheumatoid arthritis. American rheumatism association preliminary remission criteria in relation to the disease activity score. Br J Rheumatol. 1996;35:1101–5.

13. Smolen JS, Breedveld FC, Schiff MH, Kalden JR, Emery P, Eberl G, et al. A simplified disease activity index for rheumatoid arthritis for use in clinical practice. Rheumatology. 2003;42:244–57.

14. Aletaha D, Ward MM, Machold KP, Nell VP, Stamm T, Smolen JS. Remission and active disease in rheumatoid arthritis: defining criteria for disease activity states. Arthritis Rheum. 2005;52:2625–36.

15. Sheehy C, Evans V, Hasthorpe H, Mukhtyar C. Revising DAS28 scores for remission in rheumatoid arthritis. Clin Rheumatol. 2014;33:269–72.

16. Schipper LG, van Hulst LT, Grol R, van Riel PL, Hulscher ME, Fransen J. Meta-analysis of tight control strategies in rheumatoid arthritis: protocolized treatment has additional value with respect to the clinical outcome. Rheumatology. 2010;49:2154–64.

17. Knevel R, Schoels M, Huizinga TW, Aletaha D, Burmester GR, Combe B, et al. Current evidence for a strategic approach to the management of rheumatoid arthritis with disease-modifying antirheumatic drugs: a systematic literature review informing the EULAR recommendations for the management of rheumatoid arthritis. Ann Rheum Dis. 2010;69:987–94.

18. Jurgens MS, Welsing PM, Jacobs JW. Overview and analysis of treat-to-target trials in rheumatoid arthritis reporting on remission. Clin Exp Rheumatol. 2012;30(4 Suppl 73):S56–63.

19. Bykerk VP, Keystone EC, Kuriya B, Larche M, Thorne JC, Haraoui B. Achieving remission in clinical practice: lessons from clinical trial data. Clin Exp Rheumatol. 2013;31:621–32.

20. Stoffer MA, Schoels MM, Smolen JS, Aletaha D, Breedveld FC, Burmester G, et al. Evidence for treating rheumatoid arthritis to target: results of a systematic literature search update. Ann Rheum Dis. 2016;75:16–22.

21. Hamann P, Holland R, Hyrich K, Pauling JD, Shaddick G, Nightingale A, et al. Factors associated with sustained remission in rheumatoid arthritis in patients treated with anti-tumor necrosis factor. Arthritis Care Res. 2017;69:783–93.

22. Katchamart W, Johnson S, Lin HJ, Phumethum V, Salliot C, Bombardier C. Predictors for remission in rheumatoid arthritis patients: a systematic review. Arthritis Care Res. 2010;62:1128–43.

23. Pincus T, Castrejon I, Bergman MJ, Yazici Y. Treat-to-target: not as simple as it appears. Clin Exp Rheumatol. 2012;30(4 Suppl 73):S10–20.

24. Solomon DHBA, Katz JN, Radner H, Brown EM, Fraenkel L. Review: treat to target in rheumatoid arthritis: fact, fiction, or hypothesis? Arthritis Rheumatol. 2014;66:775–82.

25. Higgins JPT, Green S (editors). Cochrane Handbook for Systematic Reviews of Interventions Version 5.1.0 [updated March 2011]. The Cochrane Collaboration, 2011. Available from http://handbook.cochrane.org.

26. Sterne JA, Sutton AJ, Ioannidis JP, Terrin N, Jones DR, Lau J, et al. Recommendations for examining and interpreting funnel plot asymmetry in meta-analyses of randomised controlled trials. BMJ. 2011;343:d4002.

27. DerSimonian R, Laird N. Meta-analysis in clinical trials. Control Clin Trials. 1986;7:177–88.

28. Atsumi T, Yamamoto K, Takeuchi T, Yamanaka H, Ishiguro N, Tanaka Y, et al. The first double-blind, randomised, parallel-group certolizumab pegol study in methotrexate-naive early rheumatoid arthritis patients with poor prognostic factors, C-OPERA, shows inhibition of radiographic progression. Ann Rheum Dis. 2016;75:75–83.

29. Bakker MF, Jacobs JW, Welsing PM, Verstappen SM, Tekstra J, Ton E, et al. Low-dose prednisone inclusion in a methotrexate-based, tight control strategy for early rheumatoid arthritis: a randomized trial. Ann Intern Med. 2012;156:329–39.

30. Bijlsma JWJ, Welsing PMJ, Woodworth TG, Middelink LM, Petho-Schramm A, Bernasconi C, et al. Early rheumatoid arthritis treated with tocilizumab, methotrexate, or their combination (U-act-early): a multicentre, randomised, double-blind, double-dummy, strategy trial. Lancet. 2016;388:343–55.

31. Breedveld FC, Weisman MH, Kavanaugh AF, Cohen SB, Pavelka K, van Vollenhoven R, et al. The PREMIER study: a multicenter, randomized, double-blind clinical trial of combination therapy with adalimumab plus methotrexate versus methotrexate alone or adalimumab alone in patients

with early, aggressive rheumatoid arthritis who had not had previous methotrexate treatment. Arthritis Rheum. 2006;54:26–37.

32. Burmester GR, Rigby WF, van Vollenhoven RF, Kay J, Rubbert-Roth A, Kelman A, et al. Tocilizumab in early progressive rheumatoid arthritis: FUNCTION, a randomised controlled trial. Ann Rheum Dis. 2016;75:1081–91.

33. Capell HA, Madhok R, Porter DR, Munro RA, McInnes IB, Hunter JA, et al. Combination therapy with sulfasalazine and methotrexate is more effective than either drug alone in patients with rheumatoid arthritis with a suboptimal response to sulfasalazine: results from the double-blind placebo-controlled MASCOT study. Ann Rheum Dis. 2007;66:235–41.

34. Cohen SB, Emery P, Greenwald MW, Dougados M, Furie RA, Genovese MC, et al. Rituximab for rheumatoid arthritis refractory to anti-tumor necrosis factor therapy: results of a multicenter, randomized, double-blind, placebo-controlled, phase III trial evaluating primary efficacy and safety at twenty-four weeks. Arthritis Rheum. 2006;54:2793–806.

35. Detert J, Bastian H, Listing J, Weiss A, Wassenberg S, Liebhaber A, et al. Induction therapy with adalimumab plus methotrexate for 24 weeks followed by methotrexate monotherapy up to week 48 versus methotrexate therapy alone for DMARD-naive patients with early rheumatoid arthritis: HIT HARD, an investigator-initiated study. Ann Rheum Dis. 2013;72:844–50.

36. Dougados M, Kissel K, Sheeran T, Tak PP, Conaghan PG, Mola EM, et al. Adding tocilizumab or switching to tocilizumab monotherapy in methotrexate inadequate responders: 24-week symptomatic and structural results of a 2-year randomised controlled strategy trial in rheumatoid arthritis (ACT-RAY). Ann Rheum Dis. 2013;72:43–50.

37. Emery PBG, Bykerk VP, Combe BG, Furst DE, Barre E, Karyekar CS, et al. Evaluating drug-free remission with abatacept in early rheumatoid arthritis: results from the phase 3b, multicentre, randomised, active-controlled AVERT study of 24 months, with a 12-month double-blind treatment period. Ann Rheum Dis. 2015;74:19–26.

38. Emery P, Breedveld FC, Hall S, Durez P, Chang DJ, Robertson D, et al. Comparison of methotrexate monotherapy with a combination of methotrexate and etanercept in active, early, moderate to severe rheumatoid arthritis (COMET): a randomised, double-blind, parallel treatment trial. Lancet. 2008;372:375–82.

39. Emery P, Fleischmann RM, Moreland LW, Hsia EC, Strusberg I, Durez P, et al. Golimumab, a human anti-tumor necrosis factor alpha monoclonal antibody, injected subcutaneously every four weeks in methotrexate-naive patients with active rheumatoid arthritis: twenty-four-week results of a phase III, multicenter, randomized, double-blind, placebo-controlled study of golimumab before methotrexate as first-line therapy for early-onset rheumatoid arthritis. Arthritis Rheum. 2009;60:2272–83.

40. Emery P, Keystone E, Tony HP, Cantagrel A, van Vollenhoven R, Sanchez A, et al. IL-6 receptor inhibition with tocilizumab improves treatment outcomes in patients with rheumatoid arthritis refractory to anti-tumour necrosis factor biologicals: results from a 24-week multicentre randomised placebo-controlled trial. Ann Rheum Dis. 2008;67:1516–23.

41. Emery P, Deodhar A, Rigby WF, Isaacs JD, Combe B, Racewicz AJ, et al. Efficacy and safety of different doses and retreatment of rituximab: a randomised, placebo-controlled trial in patients who are biological naive with active rheumatoid arthritis and an inadequate response to methotrexate (study evaluating Rituximab's efficacy in MTX iNadequate rEsponders (SERENE)). Ann Rheum Dis. 2010;69:1629–35.

42. Emery P, Bingham CO 3rd, Burmester GR, Bykerk VP, Furst DE, Mariette X, et al. Certolizumab pegol in combination with dose-optimised methotrexate in DMARD-naive patients with early, active rheumatoid arthritis with poor prognostic factors: 1-year results from C-EARLY, a randomised, double-blind, placebo-controlled phase III study. Ann Rheum Dis. 2017;76:96–104.

43. Genovese MC, Kremer J, Zamani O, Ludivico C, Krogulec M, al XL. Baricitinib in patients with refractory rheumatoid arthritis. N Engl J Med. 2016;374:1243–52.

44. Genovese MC, McKay JD, Nasonov EL, Mysler EF, da Silva NA, Alecock E, et al. Interleukin-6 receptor inhibition with tocilizumab reduces disease activity in rheumatoid arthritis with inadequate response to disease-modifying antirheumatic drugs: the tocilizumab in combination with traditional disease-modifying antirheumatic drug therapy study. Arthritis Rheum. 2008;58:2968–80.

45. Goekoop-Ruiterman YP, de Vries-Bouwstra JK, Allaart CF, van Zeben D, Kerstens PJ, Hazes JM, et al. Clinical and radiographic outcomes of four different treatment strategies in patients with early rheumatoid arthritis (the BeSt study): a randomized, controlled trial. Arthritis Rheum. 2005;52:3381–90.

46. Grigor C, Capell H, Stirling A, McMahon AD, Lock P, Vallance R, et al. Effect of a treatment strategy of tight control for rheumatoid arthritis (the TICORA study): a single-blind randomised controlled trial. Lancet. 2004;364:263–9.

47. Hetland ML, Stengaard-Pedersen K, Junker P, Lottenburger T, Ellingsen T, Andersen LS, et al. Combination treatment with methotrexate, cyclosporine, and intraarticular betamethasone compared with methotrexate and intraarticular betamethasone in early active rheumatoid arthritis: an investigator-initiated, multicenter, randomized, double-blind, parallel-group, placebo-controlled study. Arthritis Rheum. 2006;54:1401–9.

48. Horslev-Petersen K, Hetland ML, Junker P, Podenphant J, Ellingsen T, Ahlquist P, et al. Adalimumab added to a treat-to-target strategy with methotrexate and intra-articular triamcinolone in early rheumatoid arthritis increased remission rates, function and quality of life. The OPERA study: an investigator-initiated, randomised, double-blind, parallel-group, placebo-controlled trial. Ann Rheum Dis. 2014;73:654–61.

49. Kavanaugh A, Fleischmann RM, Emery P, Kupper H, Redden L, Guerette B, et al. Clinical, functional and radiographic consequences of achieving stable low disease activity and remission with adalimumab plus methotrexate or methotrexate alone in early rheumatoid arthritis: 26-week results from the randomised, controlled OPTIMA study. Ann Rheum Dis. 2013;72:64–71.

50. Kivitz A, Olech E, Borofsky M, Zazueta BM, Navarro-Sarabia F, Radominski SC Bao M, et al. Subcutaneous tocilizumab versus placebo in combination with disease-modifying antirheumatic drugs in patients with rheumatoid arthritis. Arthritis Care Res. 2014;66:1653–61.

51. Klareskog L, van der Heijde D, de Jager JP, Gough A, Kalden J, Malaise M, et al. Therapeutic effect of the combination of etanercept and methotrexate compared with each treatment alone in patients with rheumatoid arthritis: double-blind randomised controlled trial. Lancet. 2004;363:675–81.

52. Kremer JM, Dougados M, Emery P, Durez P, Sibilia J, Shergy W, et al. Treatment of rheumatoid arthritis with the selective costimulation modulator abatacept: twelve-month results of a phase iib, double-blind, randomized, placebo-controlled trial. Arthritis Rheum. 2005;52:2263–71.

53. Kremer JM, Blanco R, Brzosko M, Burgos-Vargas R, Halland AM, Vernon E, et al. Tocilizumab inhibits structural joint damage in rheumatoid arthritis patients with inadequate responses to methotrexate: results from the double-blind treatment phase of a randomized placebo-controlled trial of tocilizumab safety and prevention of structural joint damage at one year. Arthritis Rheum. 2011;63:609–21.

54. Kremer JM, Cohen S, Wilkinson BE, Connell CA, French JL, Gomez-Reino J, et al. A phase IIb dose-ranging study of the oral JAK inhibitor tofacitinib (CP-690,550) versus placebo in combination with background methotrexate in patients with active rheumatoid arthritis and an inadequate response to methotrexate alone. Arthritis Rheum. 2012;64:970–81.

55. Kremer J, Li ZG, Hall S, Fleischmann R, Genovese M, Martin-Mola E, et al. Tofacitinib in combination with nonbiologic disease-modifying antirheumatic drugs in patients with active rheumatoid arthritis: a randomized trial. Ann Intern Med. 2013;159:253–61.

56. Nam JL, Villeneuve E, Hensor EM, Wakefield RJ, Conaghan PG, Green MJ, et al. A randomised controlled trial of etanercept and methotrexate to induce remission in early inflammatory arthritis: the EMPIRE trial. Ann Rheum Dis. 2014;73:1027–36.

57. Nam JL Villeneuve EHE, Hensor EM, Conaghan PG, Keen HI, Buch MH, Gough AK, Green MJ, et al. Remission induction comparing infliximab and high-dose intravenous steroid, followed by treat-to-target: a double-blind, randomised, controlled trial in new-onset, treatment-naive, rheumatoid arthritis (the IDEA study). Ann Rheum Dis. 2014;73:75–85.

58. Schiff M, Keiserman M, Codding C, Songcharoen S, Berman A, Nayiager S, et al. Efficacy and safety of abatacept or infliximab vs placebo in ATTEST: a phase III, multi-Centre, randomised, double-blind, placebo-controlled study in patients with rheumatoid arthritis and an inadequate response to methotrexate. Ann Rheum Dis. 2008;67:1096–103.

59. Schipper LG, Vermeer M, Kuper HH, Hoekstra MO, Haagsma CJ, Den Broeder AA, et al. A tight control treatment strategy aiming for remission in early rheumatoid arthritis is more effective than usual care treatment in daily clinical practice: a study of two cohorts in the Dutch rheumatoid arthritis monitoring registry. Ann Rheum Dis. 2012;71:845–50.

60. Smolen JS, Emery P, Ferraccioli GF, Samborski W, Berenbaum F, Davies OR, et al. Certolizumab pegol in rheumatoid arthritis patients with low to moderate activity: the CERTAIN double-blind, randomised, placebo-controlled trial. Ann Rheum Dis. 2015;74:843–50.

61. Smolen JS, Kay J, Doyle MK, Landewe R, Matteson EL, Wollenhaupt J, et al. Golimumab in patients with active rheumatoid arthritis after treatment with tumour necrosis factor alpha inhibitors (GO-AFTER study): a multicentre, randomised, double-blind, placebo-controlled, phase III trial. Lancet. 2009; 374:210–21.

62. Smolen JS, Beaulieu A, Rubbert-Roth A, Ramos-Remus C, Rovensky J, Alecock E, et al. Effect of interleukin-6 receptor inhibition with tocilizumab in patients with rheumatoid arthritis (OPTION study): a double-blind, placebo-controlled, randomised trial. Lancet. 2008;371:987–97.

63. Smolen J, Landewe RB, Mease P, Brzezicki J, Mason D, Luijtens K, et al. Efficacy and safety of certolizumab pegol plus methotrexate in active rheumatoid arthritis: the RAPID 2 study. A randomised controlled trial. Ann Rheum Dis. 2009;68:797–804.

64. Soubrier M, Puechal X, Sibilia J, Mariette X, Meyer O, Combe B, et al. Evaluation of two strategies (initial methotrexate monotherapy vs its combination with adalimumab) in management of early active rheumatoid arthritis: data from the GUEPARD trial. Rheumatology. 2009;48:1429–34.

65. St Clair EW, van der Heijde DM, Smolen JS, Maini RN, Bathon JM, Emery P, et al. Combination of infliximab and methotrexate therapy for early rheumatoid arthritis: a randomized, controlled trial. Arthritis Rheum. 2004;50:3432–43.

66. Symmons D, Tricker K, Harrison M, Roberts C, Davis M, Dawes P, et al. Patients with stable long-standing rheumatoid arthritis continue to deteriorate despite intensified treatment with traditional disease modifying anti-rheumatic drugs--results of the British rheumatoid outcome study group randomized controlled clinical trial. Rheumatology. 2006;45:558–65.

67. Tak PP, Rigby WF, Rubbert-Roth A, Peterfy CG, van Vollenhoven RF, Stohl W, et al. Inhibition of joint damage and improved clinical outcomes with rituximab plus methotrexate in early active rheumatoid arthritis: the IMAGE trial. Ann Rheum Dis. 2011;70:39–46.

68. Takeuchi T, Yamanaka H, Ishiguro N, Miyasaka N, Mukai M, Matsubara T, et al. Adalimumab, a human anti-TNF monoclonal antibody, outcome study for the prevention of joint damage in Japanese patients with early rheumatoid arthritis: the HOPEFUL 1 study. Ann Rheum Dis. 2014;73:536–43.

69. Taylor PC, Keystone EC, van der Heijde D, Weinblatt ME, Del Carmen Morales L, Reyes Gonzaga J, et al. Baricitinib versus placebo or adalimumab in rheumatoid arthritis. N Engl J Med. 2017;376:652–62.

70. van der Heijde D, Tanaka Y, Fleischmann R, Keystone E, Kremer J, Zerbini C, et al. Tofacitinib (CP-690,550) in patients with rheumatoid arthritis receiving methotrexate: twelve-month data from a twenty-four-month phase III randomized radiographic study. Arthritis Rheum. 2013;65:559–70.

71. van Eijk IC, Nielen MM, van der Horst-Bruinsma I, Tijhuis GJ, Boers M, Dijkmans BA, et al. Aggressive therapy in patients with early arthritis results in similar outcome compared with conventional care: the STREAM randomized trial. Rheumatology. 2012;51:686–94.

72. van Vollenhoven RF, Fleischmann R, Cohen S, Lee EB, Garcia Meijide JA, Wagner S, et al. Tofacitinib or adalimumab versus placebo in rheumatoid arthritis. N Engl J Med. 2012;367:508–19.

73. Verstappen SM, Jacobs JW, van der Veen MJ, Heurkens AH, Schenk Y, ter Borg EJ, et al. Intensive treatment with methotrexate in early rheumatoid arthritis: aiming for remission. Computer assisted Management in Early Rheumatoid Arthritis (CAMERA, an open-label strategy trial). Ann Rheum Dis. 2007;66:1443–9.

74. Weinblatt ME, Bingham CO 3rd, Mendelsohn AM, Kim L, Mack M, Lu J, Baker D, et al. Intravenous golimumab is effective in patients with active rheumatoid arthritis despite methotrexate therapy with responses as early as week 2: results of the phase 3, randomised, multicentre, double-blind, placebo-controlled GO-FURTHER trial. Ann Rheum Dis. 2013;72:381–9.

75. Westhovens R, Robles M, Ximenes AC, Nayiager S, Wollenhaupt J, Durez P, et al. Clinical efficacy and safety of abatacept in methotrexate-naive patients with early rheumatoid arthritis and poor prognostic factors. Ann Rheum Dis. 2009;68:1870–7.

76. Heimans L, Wevers-de Boer KV, Visser K, Goekoop RJ, van Oosterhout M, Harbers JB, et al. A two-step treatment strategy trial in patients with early arthritis aimed at achieving remission: the IMPROVED study. Ann Rheum Dis. 2014;73:1356–61.

77. Leirisalo-Repo M, Kautiainen H, Laasonen L, Korpela M, Kauppi MJ, Kaipiainen-Seppanen O, et al. Infliximab for 6 months added on combination therapy in early rheumatoid arthritis: 2-year results from an investigator-initiated, randomised, double-blind, placebo-controlled study (the NEO-RACo study). Ann Rheum Dis. 2013;72:851–7.

78. O'Dell JR, Mikuls TR, Taylor TH, Ahluwalia V, Brophy M, Warren SR, et al. Therapies for active rheumatoid arthritis after methotrexate failure. N Engl J Med. 2013;369:307–18.

79. Scott DL, Ibrahim F, Farewell V, O'Keeffe AG, Walker D, Kelly C, et al. Tumour necrosis factor inhibitors versus combination intensive therapy with conventional

disease modifying anti-rheumatic drugs in established rheumatoid arthritis: TACIT non-inferiority randomised controlled trial. BMJ. 2015;350:h1046.

80. Moreland LW, O'Dell JR, Paulus HE, Curtis JR, Bathon JM, St Clair EW, et al. A randomized comparative effectiveness study of oral triple therapy versus etanercept plus methotrexate in early aggressive rheumatoid arthritis: the treatment of early aggressive rheumatoid arthritis trial. Arthritis Rheum. 2012;64:2824–35.

81. Scott DL. Role of spleen tyrosine kinase inhibitors in the management of rheumatoid arthritis. Drugs. 2011;71:1121–32.

82. Rau R, Sander O, van Riel P, van de Putte L, Hasler F, Zaug M, et al. Intravenous human recombinant tumor necrosis factor receptor p55-fc IgG1 fusion protein Ro 45-2081 (lenercept): a double blind, placebo controlled dose finding study in rheumatoid arthritis. J Rheumatol. 2003;30:680–90.

83. Felson DT, Anderson JJ, Meenan RF. The efficacy and toxicity of combination therapy in rheumatoid arthritis. A meta-analysis. Arthritis Rheum. 1994;37:1487-91.

84. (NICE). NIfHaCE: Adalimumab, etanercept, infliximab, certolizumab pegol, golimumab, tocilizumab and abatacept for rheumatoid arthritis not previously treated with DMARDs or after conventional DMARDs only have failed. https://www.nice.org.uk/guidance/ta375

25

The impact of thigh and shank marker quantity on lower extremity kinematics using a constrained model

Annelise A. Slater, Todd J. Hullfish and Josh R. Baxter[*] (iD)

Abstract

Background: Musculoskeletal models are commonly used to quantify joint motions and loads during human motion. Constraining joint kinematics simplifies these models but the implications of the placement and quantity of markers used during data acquisition remains unclear. The purpose of this study was to establish the effects of marker placement and quantity on lower extremity kinematics calculated using a constrained-kinematic model. We hypothesized that a constrained-kinematic model would produce lower-extremity kinematics errors that correlated with the number of tracking markers removed from the thigh and shank.

Methods: Healthy-young adults ($N = 10$) walked on a treadmill at slow, moderate, and fast speeds while skin-mounted markers were tracked using motion capture. Lower extremity kinematics were calculated for 256 combinations of leg and shank markers to establish the implications of marker placement and quantity on joint kinematics. Marker combinations that yielded differences greater than 5 degrees were tested with paired t-tests and the relationship between number of markers and kinematic errors were modeled with polynomials to determine goodness of fit (R^2).

Results: Sagittal joint and hip coronal kinematics errors were smaller than documented errors caused by soft-tissue artifact, which tends to be approximately 5 degrees, when excluding thigh and shank markers. Joint angle and center kinematic errors negatively correlated with the number of markers included in the analyses ($R^2 > 0.97$) and typically showed the greatest error reductions when two markers were included on the thigh or shank segments. Further, we demonstrated that a simplified marker set that included markers on the pelvis, lateral knee condyle, lateral malleolus, and shoes produced kinematics that strongly agreed with the traditional marker set that included 3 tracking markers for each segment.

Conclusion: Constrained-kinematic models are resilient to marker placement and quantity, which has implications on study design and post-processing workflows.

Keywords: Motion capture, Musculoskeletal model, Constrained-kinematic model, Lower extremity

Background

Musculoskeletal modeling relies on accurate experimental data to calculate the motions and loads generated during human motion. Despite recent advances in motion capture technology that have improved marker tracking to sub-millimeter precision, soft-tissue artifact continues to be a major limiter of the clinical efficacy of motion capture data [1]. A recent special edition of the Journal of Biomechanics proposed new and innovative techniques to mitigate some of the effects of soft-tissue artifact [2]. While these techniques improve the overall fidelity of motion capture data, they introduce new challenges to both the collection and processing workflows [3–7]. This study takes a different approach to the problem. Instead, seeking to understand how currently implemented techniques can be streamlined to preserve kinematic accuracy while reducing the burdens placed on subjects and researchers.

Unconstrained-kinematic models – often referred to as 'six degree-of-freedom' – are commonly utilized to quantify joint motion using skin-based motion capture

* Correspondence: josh.baxter@uphs.upenn.edu
Human Motion Laboratory, Department of Orthopaedic Surgery, University of Pennsylvania, 3737 Market Street, Suite 702, Philadelphia, PA 19104, USA

[8, 9]; however, their accuracy has been challenged by fluoroscopy and bone-pin studies [10, 11]. For example, knee valgus and internal rotation errors of 117 and 192%, respectively, have been reported despite utilizing techniques that are aimed at minimizing soft tissue artifact [12]. In addition, unconstrained joints increase the complexities of musculoskeletal models, making simulation of human motion challenging.

Constrained-kinematic models leverage well-known characteristics of joint function [13, 14] to compensate for soft-tissue artifact while minimizing the number of markers needed to quantify motion [15]. These models also make possible advanced analyses of neuromuscular function and forward dynamic simulations [16] without the need of simulating joint contact, which is impractical to implement on large data sets. Despite these inherent strengths of constrained-kinematic models, experimental considerations of marker placement and quantity have not yet been associated with kinematic fidelity; specifically, whether marker placement and quantify alter lower extremity range of motion, root mean square errors, and cross-correlations when compared to a kinematic model that utilizes four markers on each segment.

The purpose of this study was to quantify the implications of marker placement and quantity on lower extremity kinematics using a constrained-kinematic model. To do this, we tested 256 combinations of marker number and placement and characterized their effects on lower extremity kinematics and joint centers – a surrogate measure of joint kinetics [17]. We hypothesized that (1) joint kinematics calculated using constrained and unconstrained models would not differ and (2) lower extremity kinematic errors (root mean square errors) would positively correlate with the number of markers excluded from the analyses. The secondary aim of this study was to identify a 'simplified' marker set that provides kinematic fidelity while minimizing the number of markers needed for model definition and kinematic tracking. Additionally, we tested the effects of marker sets on three different walking speeds (slow, medium, and fast) to determine if a 'simplified' marker set could detect subtle changes in joint kinematics. If successful, these findings will provide support to modify existing laboratory standards regarding marker placement and quantify in order to streamline subject setup and accommodate other experimental constraints – such as wearable devices, braces, and other measurement equipment.

Methods
Subjects and motion capture
Motion capture was performed on 10 healthy-young adults (24 ± 4 years, 6 females, BMI 24.2 ± 3.4) who provided written consent in this IRB approved study. Subjects were excluded if they had a recent lower-extremity

injury that limited their activity levels. Retro-reflective markers (9.5 mm, B&L Engineering, Santa Ana, CA) were placed on the lower-extremities of each subject and tracked using a 12-camera motion capture system (Raptor Series, Motion Analysis Corp, Santa Rosa, CA) while subjects walked on a treadmill (TMX428, Trackmaster, Newton, KS). Markers were placed over anatomic landmarks (Fig. 1) of the pelvis: anterior and posterior superior iliac spines; legs: lateral knee condyle and lateral ankle malleolus; and feet: calcaneus, first and fifth metatarsal heads, and the great toe that were placed on the shoes. Additional tracking markers were placed on the proximal-lateral (#1), distal-lateral (#2), and middle-anterior (#3) regions of the thigh and shank [18]. Marker positions were acquired while subjects stood in a neutrally-aligned position, which were used to scale a generic musculoskeletal model. Next, subjects walked on a treadmill at a slow (0.9 m/s), moderate (1.2 m/s), and

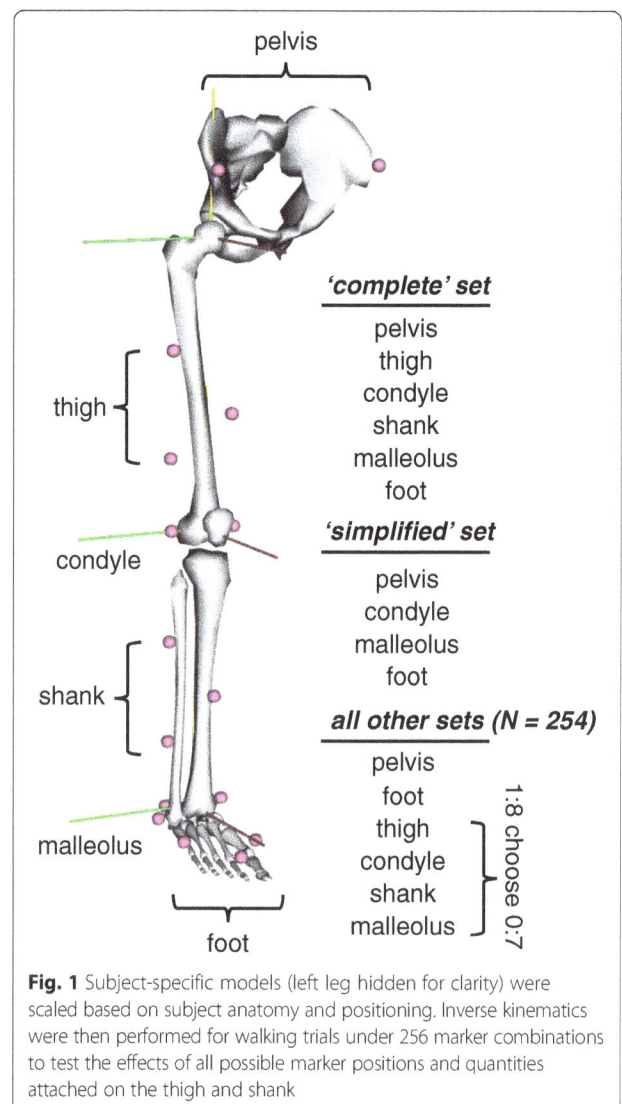

Fig. 1 Subject-specific models (left leg hidden for clarity) were scaled based on subject anatomy and positioning. Inverse kinematics were then performed for walking trials under 256 marker combinations to test the effects of all possible marker positions and quantities attached on the thigh and shank

fast (1.5 m/s) pace. Each trial lasted 2 min and generated approximately 100 strides for each leg. Joint angles and centers during each of the 100 measured strides were averaged over each walking speed and marker combination then compared to the kinematics calculated from the complete marker set. Heel strike events were identified using a kinematic-based algorithm [19].

Constrained-kinematic model

Lower extremity kinematics were calculated for 256 different combinations of thigh and shank markers using a constrained-kinematic model implemented in opensource musculoskeletal modeling software (Opensim v3.3; [20]). This lower extremity model [18] – defined the hip as a ball joint, the knee as a mobile-hinge joint, the foot and ankle as an oblique universal joint, and the forefoot as a hinge joint – was scaled based on anatomic landmarks captured in the neutrally-aligned position. We used this single degree-of-freedom knee joint that proscribed non-sagittal motions [13] for two reasons: 1 – soft-tissue artifacts cause errors greater in magnitude than the actual joint motion in the coronal and transverse planes [10, 21, 22] and 2 – the muscles that cross the knee joint do have limited leverage outside of the sagittal plane. Marker trajectories were interpolated using a cubic-spline and low-pass filtered at 6 Hz [8]. Hip, knee, and ankle kinematics were calculated using inverse kinematics and all markers received equal weighting [20]. Markers on the thigh and shank segments were systematically excluded from the analysis (Fig. 1), so every combination of markers ranging from 0 to all 8 were tested (pseudocode. 1). This combinatory study tested 256 marker combinations tested to characterize the effects of marker location and inclusion on joint kinematics.

Pseudocode: for $i = 1$ to 8, for $j = 1$ to i-1, i choose j, endfor, endfor.

Subject-specific musculoskeletal models were scaled using a previously reported generic model [18] and marker positions captured while subjects stood in the anatomic position. The pelvis, thighs, shanks, and feet were scaled based on markers placed on anatomic landmarks: pelvis – right and left anterior superior iliac spines; thigh – anterior superior iliac spine and lateral condyle; shank – lateral condyle and lateral malleolus; and foot – lateral malleolus and toe. The scaled model was then moved to the anatomic position by fitting the model to the anatomic marker positions and recorded joint angles. The anterior superior iliac spines, lateral condyles and malleoli, heel, 1st and 5th metatarsal heads, and toe markers were all given equal weighting. Similarly, the hips, knees, ankles, and toe joints were all weighted towards neutral sagittal alignments. Since hip adduction and rotation varied amongst subjects during the anatomic pose, those coordinates received no

weighting. Finally, scaled models were confirmed by superimposing the marker positions over the model.

During the pilot testing for this study ($N = 3$), we calculated the functional hip joint centers [23] and compared these locations to the hip joint centers from the scaled models [18]. We found that the functional hip joint centers were 30% wider than the generic model, which agrees with prior reports of pelvic morphology [24]. Therefore, we increased the hip joint center width in the unscaled generic model and scaled this modified model for all research subjects based on pelvis anatomy. This had appreciable effects on the initialization of models during pilot testing, where the model positioning agreed more strongly with the marker positions when the wider hip joint center locations were implemented.

Unconstrained-kinematic model

Unconstrained joint kinematics were calculated to confirm if the unconstrained and constrained calculations yielded similar results. Anatomic coordinate systems were assigned to each segment using established definitions [25, 26] that mirrored the coordinate systems defined in the constrained-kinematic model (Fig. 1). Briefly, flexion axes were assigned to the proximal segment, internal rotation axes were assigned to the distal segment, and the shared axes of the two segments represented joint adduction. Four markers on each segment, which three 'tracking' markers and a distal-lateral joint marker, were used to track and define joint motions with a least squares approach to minimize the effects of soft-tissue artifact [27]. Euler rotations were calculated using a flexion-adduction-rotation sequence [26], and joint angles during the anatomic pose trial were matched with the joint angles calculated in the constrained-kinematic model in order to perform a true one-to-one comparison.

Accounting for uncertainty associated with soft-tissue artifact

Soft-tissue artifact is an inherent limitation of marker-based motion capture. Biplane fluoroscopy studies, which are considered to be a gold standard for quantifying skeletal kinematics, have demonstrated that lower extremity kinematics quantified using motion capture vary approximately 5 degrees from true skeletal motion [1, 21]. In order to establish an equivalence between different kinematic models and marker sets, we analyzed each condition in order to detect differences in peak joint rotations and range of motions that exceeded than this 5 degrees threshold of uncertainty. In order to approximate the soft-tissue artifact in the current study, we calculated the root mean square between the experimentally collected marker trajectories and the constrained-model marker trajectories that were output from the inverse kinematics algorithm.

Statistical analysis

Joint kinematics were first post-processed to calculate summary statistics and kinematic error data for further statistical analysis. Two primary analyses were performed: 1 – joint angles calculated using the unconstrained and constrained models that included all tracking markers and 2 – joint angles and centers for each marker combination using the constrained-kinematic model were compared to the constrained model that included all tracking markers. Joint center displacements in the anterior-posterior, superior-inferior, and medial-lateral directions were calculated with respect to joint center positions from the complete marker set. Maximal and minimal joint rotations as well as joint range of motion were calculated for hip flexion and adduction as well as knee flexion and ankle plantarflexion. Cross-correlation coefficients [28] and root mean square (RMS) errors were calculated for joint kinematics. Ninety-five percent bootstrap confidence intervals were calculated (bootci, MATLAB, The Mathworks, Natick, MA, USA) using a using the average kinematic curves from each subject [28] to demonstrate the amount of certainty in the joint kinematics and visualized in plots. Prior to data analysis, we defined a 'substantially different' cross correlation coefficient (r_{xy}) to be less than 0.9. Hip internal rotations were also calculated as part of a secondary analysis.

To test our first hypothesis that joint kinematics calculated using constrained and unconstrained models would not differ, we determined if these kinematic models produced kinematic curves that did not differ past the 5 degree threshold. To test our second hypothesis that lower extremity kinematic errors would be positively correlated with the number of markers excluded from the analyses, we calculated the root mean square error of the kinematic curves with respect to the full marker constrained model. We then fit polynomials to these root mean square error data as a function of the number of markers included in the analysis. Additionally, we tested each marker set for differences in lower extremity kinematics between different marker combinations using the constrained kinematic model that exceeded the 5 degree threshold. Paired t-tests were performed on instances in which this 5 degree thresholds were exceeded to test for statistically significant differences ($p < 0.05$) between the full and modified marker sets. These boot-strapped confidence intervals calculated from the complete marker set data were expanded by 5 degrees to demonstrate the uncertainty associated with skin mounted markers compared to more direct techniques [1, 21]. Marker sets that produced joint kinematics that fell within the 5 degree threshold and were strongly

correlated ($r_{xy} > 0.90$) compared to the full marker set were considered to be 'high fidelity'.

Joint kinematics calculated at three walking speeds were compared to determine if a 'simplified' marker set – consisting of markers on the pelvis, lateral condyles, lateral malleoli, and shoes – detects speed-dependent changes in joint excursions similarly to a traditional marker set. This simplified marker set was selected because it is easily implemented and the markers placed on the lateral knee and ankle joints are needed to initialize the musculoskeletal model. Group means were compared using paired t-tests and corrections of multiple comparisons were not performed to decrease the likelihood of type II errors, thus making these analyses less conservative and more likely to reject the null hypothesis (no difference between marker sets) when a difference exists.

Results

Constrained and unconstrained kinematic models

Constrained and unconstrained-kinematic models calculated sagittal plane and hip adduction kinematics that differed less than the a priori 5 degree threshold (RMS errors: 1.6–3.2°; Fig. 2). Hip and knee flexion patterns were strongly correlated ($r_{xy} \geq 0.90$), ankle sagittal motions fell just below the cutoff value for 'substantially different' ($0.85 < r_{xy} < 0.90$). Hip adduction patterns were moderately correlated ($0.65 < r_{xy} < 0.71$). Despite any detected differences in kinematic patterns, joint excursions varied by less than five degrees between unconstrained and constrained models. Estimated soft-tissue artifact of markers on the thigh segment were almost twice as large as markers on the shank segment (RMS error 12.6 and 6.7 mm, respectively, Table 1).

Effects of marker placement and quantity on kinematics

Lower extremity sagittal kinematics, calculated using the constrained kinematic model, were not strongly affected by removing thigh and shank markers from the kinematic analysis (Fig. 3). Specifically, including markers on the lateral knee condyles and malleoli generated high-fidelity sagittal kinematics compared to the constrained-kinematic model that utilized all tracking markers ($r_{xy} \geq 0.94$; RMS errors < 2.3°). Regardless of the number of markers included in the kinematic analyses, adduction patterns were similar ($0.85 < r_{xy} < 0.90$) and joint range of motion as well as flexion and extension peaks did not deviate beyond the 5° uncertainty threshold. Hip adduction was accurately measured by all but two marker sets – when all markers proximal to the lateral malleoli were removed.

Joint angle and center kinematic errors were negatively correlated with the number of markers included in the constrained-kinematic analysis (Fig. 4). Joint angle errors

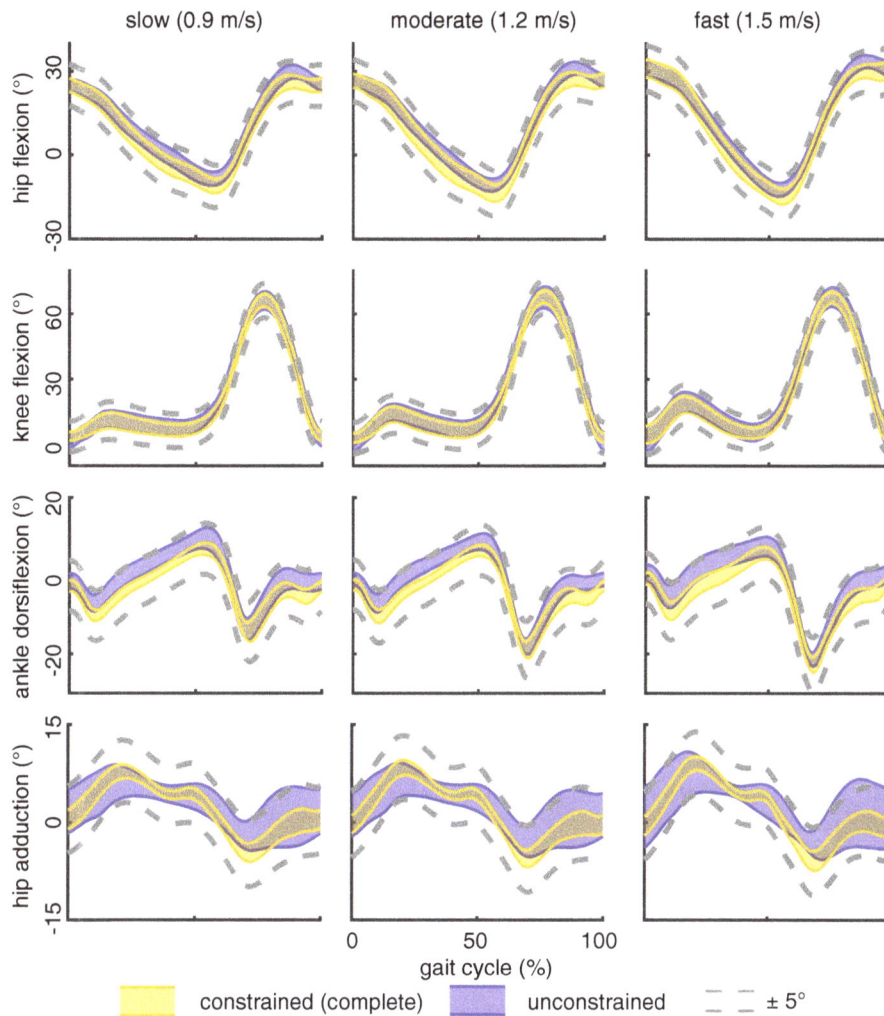

Fig. 2 Lower extremity kinematics calculated using the constrained (gold band) and unconstrained (purple band) models were similar to within 5°. Sagittal knee and hip kinematics had the strongest agreement ($r_{xy} \geq 0.90$), ankle sagittal kinematics fell just below our threshold for 'substantially different' ($0.85 < r_{xy} < 0.90$), and hip abduction was only moderately correlated between the two kinematic models ($0.65 < r_{xy} < 0.71$)

Table 1 Calculated root mean square errors (mm) between experimentally and model marker trajectories using the full markers set

	Slow (0.9 m/s)	Moderate (1.2 m/s)	Fast (1.5 m/s)
Thigh1	13.0	13.5	14.2
Thigh2	9.0	10.4	10.4
Thigh3	12.3	11.8	13.7
Lateral Knee	13.0	13.6	15.7
Shank1	9.5	9.6	9.2
Shank2	5.4	5.5	5.7
Shank3	6.1	6.7	7.1
Lateral Ankle	5.0	5.2	5.7

decayed at rates that were best fit by non-linear polynomials ($R^2 > 0.97$, Fig. 4), where most of the errors were reduced by including two markers placed on either the thigh or shank in the kinematic analyses. Knee joint center errors were 2–4 fold greater than hip and ankle joint center errors, respectively. Including additional markers in the kinematic analyses had a strong-linear effect ($R^2 > 0.97$, Fig. 4) on hip and ankle joint center errors, while knee joint center errors decayed at a cubic rate ($R^2 = 0.99$, Fig. 3b) with diminishing improvements after two markers were included. Hip and ankle joint center positions were less affected by reduced markers (RMS error < 6 mm) than the knee joint (RMS error < 19 mm).

Increased joint excursions with walking speed were identified with both the complete and simplified marker sets (Table 2; Fig. 2). The complete and simplified marker sets demonstrated similar sensitivities to

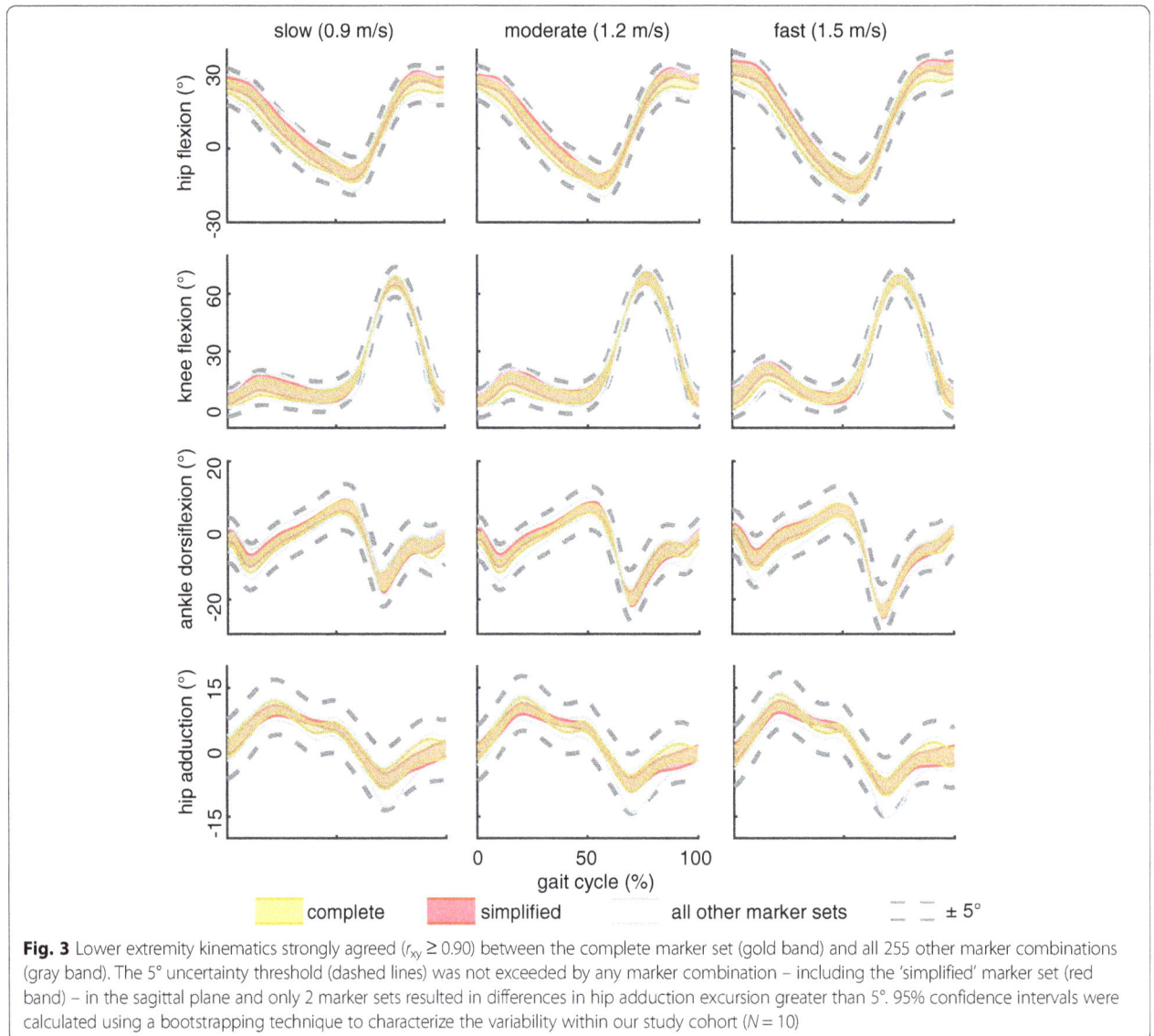

Fig. 3 Lower extremity kinematics strongly agreed ($r_{xy} \geq 0.90$) between the complete marker set (gold band) and all 255 other marker combinations (gray band). The 5° uncertainty threshold (dashed lines) was not exceeded by any marker combination – including the 'simplified' marker set (red band) – in the sagittal plane and only 2 marker sets resulted in differences in hip adduction excursion greater than 5°. 95% confidence intervals were calculated using a bootstrapping technique to characterize the variability within our study cohort ($N = 10$)

detecting increases in sagittal joint excursion. Similarly, hip adduction increased with walking speed; however, subtle increases of less than 2° between moderate and fast walking speeds were only detected with the complete marker set.

Hip internal rotation patterns were weakly correlated ($0.10 < r_{xy} < 0.21$) with calculations using an unconstrained-kinematic model and demonstrated differences that exceed five degrees (RMS errors: 3.9–5.4°). The effects of removing thigh and shank markers from the constrained-kinematic model had moderate effects ($0.55 < r_{xy} < 0.90$). However, hip internal rotation excursions were within five degrees of the complete marker set in 95% of the marker combinations.

Discussion

We demonstrated that constrained-kinematic models accurately reproduce lower extremity kinematics of walking as well as a complete marker set when numerous markers are excluded from the analyses. The effects of reducing markers on sagittal kinematics and hip adduction are smaller than kinematic uncertainty caused by soft tissue artifact [1, 21, 22]. Joint center trajectories, which govern the joint moment arm of the ground reaction force – and thus joint kinetics (Myers, 2015) – appear to also be resilient to decreased markers. Since marker placement minimally affects joint kinematics, researchers can tailor marker sets based on experimental constraints. For example, a 'simplified' marker set (Fig. 1), that excludes the traditional tracking markers adhered to the thigh and shank, can be utilized without compromising kinematic fidelity to increase motion capture workflow and provide more flexibility for the placement of other sensors and wearable devices.

Lower extremity kinematics quantified in this study compared favorably with prior reports. Similar to prior

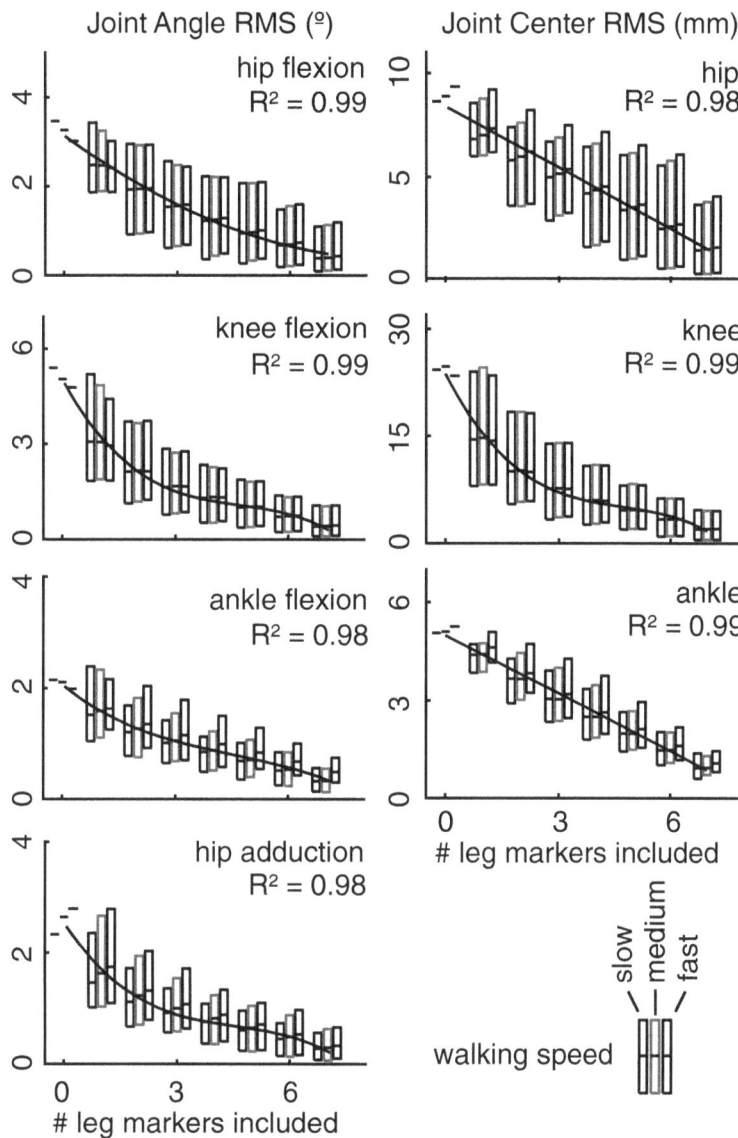

Fig. 4 Lower extremity RMS errors negatively correlated with the number of leg markers included in the kinematic analyses. Joint kinematics (angles; left column) errors were best described by a 3rd order polynomial ($R^2 > 0.98$). Knee center errors were also best characterized by a 3rd polynomial ($R^2 = 0.99$; right column), while hip and ankle center errors linearly correlated with the number of leg markers included in the analyses ($R^2 > 0.98$; right column). Boxes show the range of all RMS values and the dark bar indicates the average RMS value. Walking speed did not affect kinematic errors

Table 2 95% confidence intervals for lower extremity ranges of motion – calculated using the constrained-kinematic model with full and simplified marker sets – during walking at increasing speeds

	slow (0.9 m/s)	moderate (1.2 m/s)	fast (1.5 m/s)
hip flexion	(37.2–40.4) | (38.6–43.1)	(41.2–44.2)^s | (42.8–47.0)^s	(44.7–49.7)^{sm} | (46.7–53.2)^{sm}
knee flexion	(58.7–67.5) | (56.8–66.2)	(61.3–69.8)^s | (59.4–68.4)^s	(61.7–68.5) | (60.7–67.4)^s
ankle dorsiflexion	(20.3–24.5) | (20.9–25.5)	(23.3–28.8)^s | (24.2–29.5)^s	(26.3–32.0)^{sm} | (26.7–32.5)^{sm}
hip adduction	(15.2–18.7) | (14.6–18.2)	(16.5–21.0)^s | (15.6–20.0)^s	(18.0–22.7)^{sm} | (16.3–21.2)^s
hip rotation	(7.9–12.0) | (11.1–16.0)	(10.5–14.1)^s | (13.5–18.7)^s	(11.4–16.2)^{sm} | (14.9–20.1)^s

95% confidence intervals for joint range of motion for the full and simplified marker sets are reported for each joint coordinate and walking speed (full \| simplified).
^{s}increased range of motion compared to slow speed. ^{m} increased range of motion compared to medium speed. $p < 0.05$

work [29, 30], we found that sagittal hip, knee, and ankle excursion increased with walking speed (Table 2). Hip coronal kinematics measured in this study demonstrated stereotypical patterns that are well described in the literature [31, 32]. Since much of the literature implements six degree-of-freedom marker sets, we calculated the unconstrained motion of the lower extremity and implemented a least squares approach [27] to minimize the effects of soft tissue artifact on resulting joint kinematics. Sagittal joint and hip coronal motions were similar between the unconstrained and constrained-kinematic results (Fig. 2). Hip internal rotation differed between the unconstrained and constrained model, which may be explained by well documented soft tissue artifact of the thigh segment [33]. However, these differences were less pronounced between constrained marker sets, likely due to the lack of knee rotation in the musculoskeletal model.

Our findings demonstrate that constrained-kinematic models are resilient to marker placement and dropout. Although we did not directly track skeletal motion in this study, we approximated the uncertainty introduced by soft-tissue artifact by calculating the difference between experimentally-measured marker and model-fixed marker trajectories. We found that the markers placed on the thigh, lateral knee, and shank had average RMS values of 12.5, 14.1, and 7.1 mm, respectively (Table 1); compared to direct measurements of soft-tissue artifact in the literature of 13.8, 13.9, and 10.8 mm, respectively [21]. Despite the lateral knee being prone to soft-tissue artifact, its inclusion improved kinematic tracking when fewer than five leg markers were included in the kinematic analyses (Fig. 5). Increasing the number of markers used for gait analysis has diminishing returns with regard to lower extremity kinematics (Fig. 4).

Excluding all of the markers attached to the thigh and shank generated sagittal joint kinematics that were in strong agreement with the complete marker set but adversely affected knee joint center kinematics, which impacts joint loads [17]. Adding markers to the lateral condyles and malleoli – which were used to scale the musculoskeletal model – mitigated the majority of kinematic errors ($r_{xy} \geq 0.94$; RMS errors < 2.3°). To improve experimental consistency and workflow, markers can be permanently fixed to lab shoes, which reduces the number of markers applied to the subject to eight: four on the pelvis and two on each leg. Thus, a 'simplified' marker set accurately characterizes joint kinematics and joint center motions by providing essential inputs to constrained-kinematic models.

Changing the placement and quantity of tracking markers can reduce experimental setup time, allows for more comfortable attire to be worn during data collection, and provides fewer obstructions for other experimental equipment while being resistant to errors kinematic errors

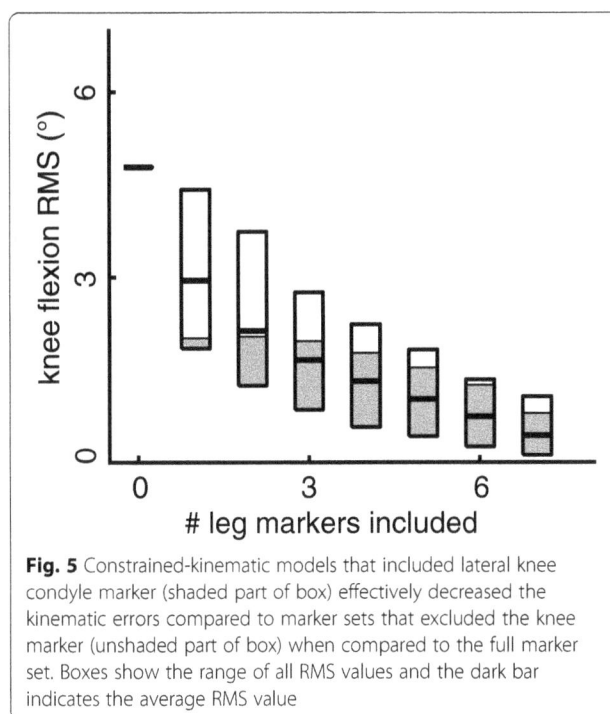

Fig. 5 Constrained-kinematic models that included lateral knee condyle marker (shaded part of box) effectively decreased the kinematic errors compared to marker sets that excluded the knee marker (unshaded part of box) when compared to the full marker set. Boxes show the range of all RMS values and the dark bar indicates the average RMS value

(Figs. 3, 4 and 5). While unconstrained-kinematic models require at least three markers on each segment at all times, our results demonstrate that constrained-kinematic models can perform well with no markers on certain segments; for example, the thigh and shank. Hierarchical marker sets track segment kinematics by assuming the location of a joint center based on a nearby segment [34]. However, this approach is susceptible to soft-tissue artifact [35] and does not provide the necessary joint constraints for advanced musculoskeletal analyses [36]. Our findings also benefit researchers utilizing wearable-assistive devices [37, 38], ultrasonography during human motion [39], and high-density electromyography sensors [40] – all techniques that require unobstructed access to the lower extremities.

Processing and analyzing motion capture data can be streamlined into a turn-key routine utilizing open-source musculoskeletal modeling software [20] and batched scripts. In addition to calculating joint kinematics, constrained-kinematic models are well-suited for performing both inverse and forward dynamic simulations. Integrating gait analysis into a single musculoskeletal modeling environment provides investigators with a standardized workflow while maintaining the flexibility needed to perform specific analyses [41, 42]. Further, many analyses are not possible to perform without imposing joint constraints or contact [43, 44]. Therefore, migrating kinematic analyses into a constrained-kinematic model may minimize workflow complexity without compromising kinematic fidelity (Fig. 2).

Several limitations should be considered when interpreting these findings. We did not directly measure skeletal motion but did show similarities in joint kinematics with prior studies that utilized intracortical bone pins and fluoroscopy [21, 45]. Instead, we demonstrated that both the constrained and unconstrained kinematic models produced equivalent lower extremity kinematics, based on the fact that these kinematics were within a previously determined 5 degree threshold [1, 21]. Subject walked at three different speeds but did not perform more dynamic tasks such as jump-cut that are associated with large errors due to soft-tissue artifact [46], which limits the study findings to lower impact activities like walking. Subjects in the present study were healthy-young adults that were generally fit with a healthy body mass index (BMI 24.2 ± 3.4), which may not be representative of clinical populations. Joint kinematics are sensitive to joint-axis location and orientation [47, 48], which may be affected when scaling generic musculoskeletal models to subject-specific anthropometry. To mitigate these potential errors, we visually confirmed that each subject-specific model closely matched the neutrally-aligned position. Further, we confirmed joint kinematics using unconstrained-kinematic models that shared the same joint axis definitions as the constrained-kinematic models (Fig. 2). Due to knee valgus and internal rotation errors as high as twice that of skeletal motion [12], we limited knee joint kinematics to a single degree-of-freedom and prescribed other rotations and translations based on flexion angle [13]. Accurately measuring frontal plane knee kinematics during gait requires advanced imaging or invasive techniques [21], which was outside of the scope of this study. Walking trials were acquired on a commercial treadmill that did not have an integrated force plate, so we were unable to calculate joint reaction moments. We instead decided to quantify the changes in the joint center trajectories, which governs the ground reaction force moment arm and thus joint moments. In order to show the robustness of the constrained-kinematic model, we chose not to modify the hip joint center locations based on subject-specific functional hip joint locations. However, hip kinetics are sensitive to joint center location and employing more rigorous scaling techniques should be considered when high-fidelity hip kinetics are required.

Conclusion

Constrained-kinematic models provide the flexibility to change the position and quantity of tracking markers used during gait analysis. Experiments can be designed to attain the lower-extremity kinematic fidelity necessary to answer specific research questions while adjusting marker placement and quantity to suit the constraints of the experimental setup. In addition, integrating constrained-kinematic models into a gait analysis workflow offers several advantages that can improve post-processing efficiency while providing access to unique analysis tools to test specific questions. However, investigators should weigh the strengths and weaknesses of both constrained and unconstrained-kinematic models to determine which approach is best suited for the specific research question.

Abbreviations
BMI: body mass index; RMS: root mean square; r_{xy}: cross correlation coefficient

Acknowledgements
The Authors have no acknowledgements.

Funding
No funding has been provided for this research.

Authors' contributions
AS, TH, and JB designed the experiment; AS and TH collected the data; AS and JB analyzed and interpreted the data; AS and JB drafted the manuscript; AS, TH, and JB revised the intellectual content of the manuscript; AS, TH, and JB approved the final version of the manuscript; and AS, TH, and JB agreed to be accountable for all aspects of the study.

Competing interests
One author (JB) is an associate editor for BMC Musculoskeletal Disorders. None of the other authors have any competing interests.

References
1. Leardini A, Chiari L, Della Croce U, Cappozzo A. Human movement analysis using stereophotogrammetry. Part 3. Soft tissue artifact assessment and compensation. Gait Posture. 2005;21:212–25.
2. Camomilla V, Dumas R, Cappozzo A. Human movement analysis: the soft tissue artefact issue. J Biomech. 2017;62:1–4.
3. Barré A. Assessment of the lower limb soft tissue artefact at marker-cluster level with a high-density marker set during walking; 2017.
4. Begon M, Bélaise C, Naaim A, Lundberg A, Chèze L. Multibody kinematics optimization with marker projection improves the accuracy of the humerus rotational kinematics. J Biomech. 2017;62:117–23.
5. Masum MA, Pickering MR, Lambert AJ, Scarvell JM, Smith PN. Multi-slice ultrasound image calibration of an intelligent skin-marker for soft tissue artefact compensation. J Biomech. 2017;62:165–71.
6. Richard V, Cappozzo A, Dumas R. Comparative assessment of knee joint models used in multi-body kinematics optimisation for soft tissue artefact compensation. J Biomech. 2017;62:95–101.
7. Sangeux M, Barré A, Aminian K. Evaluation of knee functional calibration with and without the effect of soft tissue artefact. J Biomech. 2016. https://doi.org/10.1016/j.jbiomech.2016.10.049.
8. Collins TD, Ghoussayni SN, Ewins DJ, Kent JA. A six degrees-of-freedom marker set for gait analysis: repeatability and comparison with a modified Helen Hayes set. Gait Posture. 2009;30:173–80.
9. Schmitz A, Buczek FL, Bruening D, Rainbow MJ, Cooney K, Thelen D. Comparison of hierarchical and six degrees-of-freedom marker sets in analyzing gait kinematics. Comput Methods Biomech Biomed Engin 2016;19:199–207.
10. Benoit DL, Ramsey DK, Lamontagne M, Xu L, Wretenberg P, Renström P. Effect of skin movement artifact on knee kinematics during gait and cutting motions measured in vivo. Gait Posture. 2006;24:152–64.
11. Fiorentino NM, Atkins PR, Kutschke MJ, Goebel JM, Foreman KB, Anderson AE. Soft tissue artifact causes significant errors in the calculation of joint angles and range of motion at the hip. Gait Posture. 2017;55:184–90.
12. Stagni R, Fantozzi S, Cappello A, Leardini A. Quantification of soft tissue artefact in motion analysis by combining 3D fluoroscopy and stereophotogrammetry: a study on two subjects. Clin Biomech. 2005;20:320–9.
13. Nisell R, Németh G, Ohlsén H. Joint forces in extension of the knee. Analysis of a mechanical model. Acta Orthop Scand. 1986;57:41–6.
14. Isman RE, Inman VT, Poor P. Anthropometric studies of the human foot and ankle. Bull Prosthet Res. 1969;11:97–108.
15. Lu TW, O'Connor JJ. Bone position estimation from skin marker co-ordinates using global optimisation with joint constraints. J Biomech. 1999;32:129–34.

16. Anderson FC, Pandy MG. Static and dynamic optimization solutions for gait are practically equivalent. J Biomech. 2001;34:153–61.

17. Schwartz MH, Rozumalski A. A new method for estimating joint parameters from motion data. J Biomech. 2005;38:107–16.

18. Rajagopal A, Dembia C, DeMers M, Delp D, Hicks J, Delp S. Full body musculoskeletal model for muscle-driven simulation of human gait. IEEE Trans Biomed Eng. 2016;9294(c):1–1.

19. Zeni J, Richards J, Higginson JS. Two simple methods for determining gait events during treadmill and overground walking using kinematic data. Gait Posture. 2008;27:710–4.

20. Delp SL, Anderson FC, Arnold AS, Loan P, Habib A, John CT, et al. OpenSim: open-source software to create and analyze dynamic simulations of movement. IEEE Trans Biomed Eng. 2007;54:1940–50.

21. Akbarshahi M, Schache AG, Fernandez JW, Baker R, Banks S, Pandy MG. Non-invasive assessment of soft-tissue artifact and its effect on knee joint kinematics during functional activity. J Biomech. 2010;43:1292–301.

22. Reinschmidt C, Van Den Bogert AJ, Lundberg A, Nigg BM, Murphy N, Stacoff A, et al. Tibiofemoral and tibiocalcaneal motion during walking: external vs. skeletal markers. Gait Posture. 1997;6:98–109.

23. Piazza SJ, Okita N, Cavanagh PR. Accuracy of the functional method of hip joint center location: effects of limited motion and varied implementation. J Biomech. 2001;34:967–73.

24. Daysal GA, Goker B, Gonen E, Demirag MD, Haznedaroglu S, Ozturk MA, et al. The relationship between hip joint space width, center edge angle and acetabular depth. Osteoarthr Cartil. 2007;15:1446–51.

25. Grood ES, Suntay WJ. A joint coordinate system for the clinical description of three-dimensional motions: application to the knee. J Biomech Eng. 1983;105:136–44.

26. Wu G, Siegler S, Allard P, Kirtley C, Leardini A, Rosenbaum D, et al. ISB recommendation on definitions of joint coordinate system of various joints for the reporting of human joint motion--part I: ankle, hip, and spine. International Society of Biomechanics. J Biomech. 2002;35:543–8.

27. Challis JH. A procedure for determining rigid body transformation parameters. J Biomech. 1995;28:733–7.

28. Baxter JR, Sturnick DR, Demetracopoulos CA, Ellis SJ, Deland JT. Cadaveric gait simulation reproduces foot and ankle kinematics from population-specific inputs. J Orthop Res. 2016;34:1663–8.

29. Murray MP, Mollinger LA, Gardner GM, Sepic SB. Kinematic and EMG patterns during slow, free, and fast walking. J Orthop Res. 1984;2:272–80.

30. Zeni JA Jr, Higginson JS. Differences in gait parameters between healthy subjects and persons with moderate and severe knee osteoarthritis: a result of altered walking speed? Clin Biomech. 2009;24:372–8.

31. Hurwitz DE, Foucher KC, Sumner DR, Andriacchi TP, Rosenberg AG, Galante JO. Hip motion and moments during gait relate directly to proximal femoral bone mineral density in patients with hip osteoarthritis. J Biomech. 1998;31:919–25.

32. Buczek FL, Rainbow MJ, Cooney KM, Walker MR, Sanders JO. Implications of using hierarchical and six degree-of-freedom models for normal gait analyses. Gait Posture. 2010;31:57–63.

33. Arampatzis A, De Monte G, Karamanidis K, Morey-Klapsing G, Stafilidis S, Brüggemann G-P. Influence of the muscle-tendon unit's mechanical and morphological properties on running economy. J Exp Biol. 2006;209 Pt 17:3345–57.

34. Kadaba MP, Ramakrishnan HK, Wootten ME. Measurement of lower extremity kinematics during level walking. J Orthop Res. 1990;8:383–92.

35. Lamberto G, Martelli S, Cappozzo A, Mazzà C. To what extent is joint and muscle mechanics predicted by musculoskeletal models sensitive to soft tissue artefacts? J Biomech. 2017;62:68–76.

36. Li J-D, Lu T-W, Lin C-C, Kuo M-Y, Hsu H-C, Shen W-C. Soft tissue artefacts of skin markers on the lower limb during cycling: effects of joint angles and pedal resistance. J Biomech. 2017;62:27–38.

37. Elliott G, Sawicki GS, Marecki A, Herr H. The biomechanics and energetics of human running using an elastic knee exoskeleton. In: 2013 IEEE 13th international conference on rehabilitation robotics (ICORR); 2013. p. 1–6.

38. Sawicki GS, Ferris DP. Powered ankle exoskeletons reveal the metabolic cost of plantar flexor mechanical work during walking with longer steps at constant step frequency. J Exp Biol. 2009;212(Pt 1):21–31.

39. Lichtwark GA, Wilson AM. In vivo mechanical properties of the human Achilles tendon during one-legged hopping. J Exp Biol. 2005;208(Pt 24):4715–25.

40. Huang C, Chen X, Cao S, Zhang X. Muscle-tendon units localization and activation level analysis based on high-density surface EMG array and NMF algorithm. J Neural Eng. 2016;13:066001.

41. Kainz H, Graham D, Edwards J, Walsh HPJ, Maine S, Boyd RN, et al. Reliability of four models for clinical gait analysis. Gait Posture. 2017;54:325–31.

42. Schmitz A, Piovesan D. Development of an Open-Source, Discrete Element Knee Model. IEEE Trans Biomed Eng. 2016;63:2056–67.

43. Kar J, Quesada PM. A numerical simulation approach to studying anterior cruciate ligament strains and internal forces among young recreational women performing valgus inducing stop-jump activities. Ann Biomed Eng. 2012;40:1679–91.

44. Marques F, Souto AP, Flores P. On the constraints violation in forward dynamics of multibody systems. Multibody Syst Dyn. 2017;39:385–419.

45. Nester C, Jones RK, Liu A, Howard D, Lundberg A, Arndt A, et al. Foot kinematics during walking measured using bone and surface mounted markers. J Biomech. 2007;40:3412–23.

46. Miranda DL, Rainbow MJ, Crisco JJ, Fleming BC. Kinematic differences between optical motion capture and biplanar videoradiography during a jump–cut maneuver. J Biomech. 2013;46:567–73.

47. Kainz H, Modenese L, Lloyd DG, Maine S, Walsh HPJ, Carty CP. Joint kinematic calculation based on clinical direct kinematic versus inverse kinematic gait models. J Biomech. 2016;49:1658–69.

48. Kainz H, Carty CP, Maine S, Walsh HPJ, Lloyd DG, Modenese L. Effects of hip joint Centre mislocation on gait kinematics of children with cerebral palsy calculated using patient-specific direct and inverse kinematic models. Gait Posture. 2017;57:154–60.

26

Association of *COL9A3* trp3 polymorphism with intervertebral disk degeneration

Donghua Huang[†], Xiangyu Deng[†], Kaige Ma, Fashuai Wu, Deyao Shi, Hang Liang, Sheng Chen and Zengwu Shao[*]

Abstract

Background: Intervertebral disk degeneration (IDD) is a common musculoskeletal disease associated with genetic factors. *COL9A3* gene encodes the α3 (IX) chain of type IX collagen that is part of the interior structure of the disc. Mutations in COL9A3 gene sequence, leading to an Arg103Trp substitution in its 3 chain (the Trp3 allele at rs61734651 site), respectively, have been found to be connected with IDD occurrence in several studies. However, those studies have showed conflict results. Thus, a meta-analysis has been performed to assess the associations between the *COL9A3* trp3 polymorphism and IDD.

Methods: Data were gathered from the following four electronic databases: PubMed, Web of Science (WOS), Embase and Cochrane library up to January 01, 2018. The pooled odds ratio (polled ORs) and 95% confidence interval (CI) were calculated to evaluate the strength of relationship between the *COL9A3* trp3 polymorphism and IDD.

Results: Eleven eligible studies with 1631 cases of IDD and 1366 controls were included in this meta-analysis. The results indicated that the *COL9A3* trp3 polymorphism was not associated with IDD (trp3 positive versus trp3 negative: OR = 1.31, 95%CI = 0.78–2.21, $P = 0.309$). Furthermore, the Egger's test and the Begg funnel plot did not show any evidence of publication bias.

Conclusions: Our results suggest that the *COL9A3* trp3 polymorphism might not be associated with IDD. Nor did we find any relationship in subgroup analyses stratified by gender and ethnicity. Future researches with larger samples are required to verify this outcome.

Keywords: *COL9A3*, Single nucleotide polymorphism, trp3, Intervertebral disk degeneration, Meta-analysis

Background

Low back pain (LBP), a common musculoskeletal disorder, involves the muscle, nerve, and bone tissues of back [1–3]. It has been reported that LBP ranked first in terms of disability and sixth in terms of total burden as part of the Global Burden of Disease 2010 Study [4]. Intervertebral disk degeneration (IDD), describing the natural destruction of intervertebral disk inside the spine, has been considered as one of the major causes to motor losses and LBP. The etiology and pathogenesis of IDD is so complicated that IDD is thought to be the results of co-effects of ageing and relevant environmental factors such as sporting activities, damage, occupation, and smoking [5–9]. However, there have been many articles establishing a close relationship between heredity and IDD recently [10–12].

For the last several years, many genes have been discovered to be associated with IDD, some of which are collagen genes, such as Collagen I, IX and XI genes [12–14]. Among these genes, the association of collagen type IX alpha 3 chain (*COL9A3)* gene polymorphism with IDD risk has been studied much frequently. *COL9A3* gene, located in the chromosome 20q13.3, encodes the α3 (IX) chain of type IX collagen which is part of the interior structure of the disc, nucleus pulposus [14–16]. Mutations in *COL9A3* gene leading to an Arg103Trp substitution in its 3 chain (the Trp3 allele at rs61734651 site), in other words, this change in collagen IX by substitution of

---

[*] Correspondence: szwpro@163.com
[†]Donghua Huang and Xiangyu Deng contributed equally to this work.
Department of Orthopaedics, Union Hospital, Tongji Medical College, Huazhong University of Science and Technology, Wuhan 430022, China

glutamine by tryptophan, which is relative rare in collagen, can contribute to a disorder in the collagen properties of intervertebral disc. The increasing proportion of tryptophan in collagen can result in alterations in collagen triple helix, as well as interfering the interaction between collagens IX and II or disturbing the process of lysyl oxidase, which catalyzes cross-link formation, finally leading to disc disease [17–20].

However, recent studies have obtained conflicting results. Some of them, such as Toktas et al. [11] and Paassita et al. [17], found that trp3 gene was a risk fact of IDD or the spinal stenosis with spondylolisthesis which is one type of IDD. Others, such as Eskola et al. [21] and Rathod et al. [22], did not observe a relationship between trp3 and IDD. Besides, Bagheri et al. [18], only got an association of trp3 with IDD in males. A few articles reported the association of trp3 with ethnicity [23]. But no meta-analysis has investigated the association between IDD and *COL9A3* trp3 polymorphism up to now. Therefore, we performed a meta-analysis to evaluate the connection between them. In this study, we aim to identify the association of genetic mutations with IDD, which is likely to be of significant importance and might help identify 'high-risk' individuals of IDD or guide the clinical treatment of some specific individuals.

Methods
Strategy for literature search
In order to identify all articles that studied the association of *COL9A3* Trp3 polymorphism with IDD, we searched electronic databases including PubMed, Web of Science (WOS), Embase and Cochrane library up to January 01, 2018. The search strategy to screen out all possible articles involved the use of the following terms: ("COL9A3" OR "Collagen 9 alpha-3") AND ("Gene polymorphism") AND ("Intervertebral Disk Degeneration" OR "Disk Degeneration, Intervertebral" OR "IDD" OR "Disc Degeneration" OR "disc herniation" OR "low back pain"); ("Trp3" OR "rs61734651" OR "20q13.33" OR "arg103") AND ("Gene polymorphism") AND ("Intervertebral Disk Degeneration" OR "Disk Degeneration, Intervertebral" OR "IDD" OR "Disc Degeneration" OR "disc herniation" OR "low back pain"); ("COL9A3" OR "Collagen 9 alpha-3") AND ("Trp3" OR "rs61734651" OR "20q13.33" OR "arg103") AND ("Intervertebral Disk Degeneration" OR "Disk Degeneration, Intervertebral" OR "IDD" OR "Disc Degeneration" OR "disc herniation" OR "low back pain"). In order to increase the sensitivity of the searching strategy, both MeSH terms and free words were applied.

Inclusion and exclusion criteria
Studies included in this meta-analysis should satisfy the following inclusion criteria: (1) Evaluation of the association between *COL9A3* trp3 polymorphism and the risk of IDD; (2) Human subjects; (3) Case-control study; and (4) Available genotype data were provided to calculate the odds ratios (ORs) and 95% confidence interval (CI).

Correspondingly, the exclusion criteria were defined as: (1) Comments, reviews or animal studies; (2) Duplicate reports with previous publications; (3) the study only described data of case population; (4) Studies without available genotype frequencies.

All retrieved articles were evaluated and discussed to achieve accordance by two junior investigators depending on the inclusion and exclusion strategies independently. If a conflict (among the basic information, data, and the quality of articles separately extracted by two investigators) still existed, a senior author was invited to extract the specific data independently using blind method. Then comparing the results with the two junior investigators to solve the problem and finally come to a consistency.

Data extraction
The following characteristics of each study were collected: (1) name of the first author; (2) year of publication; (3) country of enrollment; (4) ethnicity of the study population; (5) age and gender of individuals included; (6) diagnostic criteria for IDD cases; (7) genotyping methods; (8) source of controls; (9) matching items; (10) number of subjects under IDD cases and controls; (11) Relation with IDD; Data were extracted carefully from all eligible publications independently by two investigators. For conflict resolution, an agreement was reached by discussion.

Methodological quality assessment
The two investigators assessed the qualities of all the included studies separately using the Clark scores system, which contains 10 items [24, 25]. Scores below 5 indicate low quality, while 5–7 scores represent moderate quality and 8–10 scores denote high quality [24, 25].

Statistical analysis
The PRISMA checklists and their guidelines were cautiously followed during the whole process of the study [26]. The association strength between *COL9A3* trp3 polymorphism and IDD risk was assessed by combining ORs with 95%CI. The estimations of pooled ORs were determined by the weighted average OR from each study. Significance was identified by a *P*-value less than 0.05 in Z-test. The pooled ORs and 95%CI were calculated for trp3 positive (the mutation type) versus trp3 negative (the wild type). Because seven studies [11, 14, 18, 23, 27–29] included in this meta-analysis only exhibited data in "Trp3 positive versus Trp3 negative" form. In other words, these studies did not have enough data

to calculate ORs and 95%CI for five comparison models. In addition, although the other four studies [17, 21, 22, 30] included this meta-analysis showed separate data in homozygous type (TGG/TGG), heterozygous type (TGG/CGG) and wild type (the others which not include TGG at this site, such as CGG/CGG) for trp3, the number of subjects for homozygous type (TGG/TGG) was too small with no more than two subjects observed in each study. So we combined homozygous and heterozygous type together as trp3 positive (TGG/TGG, TGG/CGG) and the wild type was defined as trp3 negative (the others which not include TGG at this site). In other words, the trp3 positive was defined as the presence of at least 1 Trp3 allele and the trp3 negative were the types without Trp3 allele. The statistical heterogeneity was verified by I^2 statistics. Fixed-effect model was used to estimate the ORs and 95%CI when heterogeneity was low ($I^2 < 50\%$), while the random effects was adopted when heterogeneity was high ($I^2 > 50\%$) [31]. Sensitivity analyses were also performed to evaluate the function of an individual study on the pooled ORs by removing each study in turn. All analyses were performed using STATA 14 (Stata, College Station, TX). Subgroup analyses were performed to find whether sex or ethnicity of studies was linked to the value of the pooled ORs and 95%CI as well. Because only few studies included separate data of degree of IDD, we do not conduct a subgroup analysis stratified by disease degree. All P-values were two-sided. Publication bias was checked using the Begg funnel plot [32] and the Egger's test [33] ($P < 0.05$ was considered statistically significant).

Results

Characteristics of the studies

A flow chart, presented as Fig. 1, describes the exclusion/inclusion of publications. The comprehensive articles search screened out 381 potentially relevant articles, of which 82 articles were excluded for duplication and 281 articles were removed because of obvious irrelevance after browsing the title and/or abstract. Two articles were excluded because they did not study trp3, COL9A3 or IDD; one article was removed because it is a duplicate report; three articles were excluded because they did not have detailed data; another article was

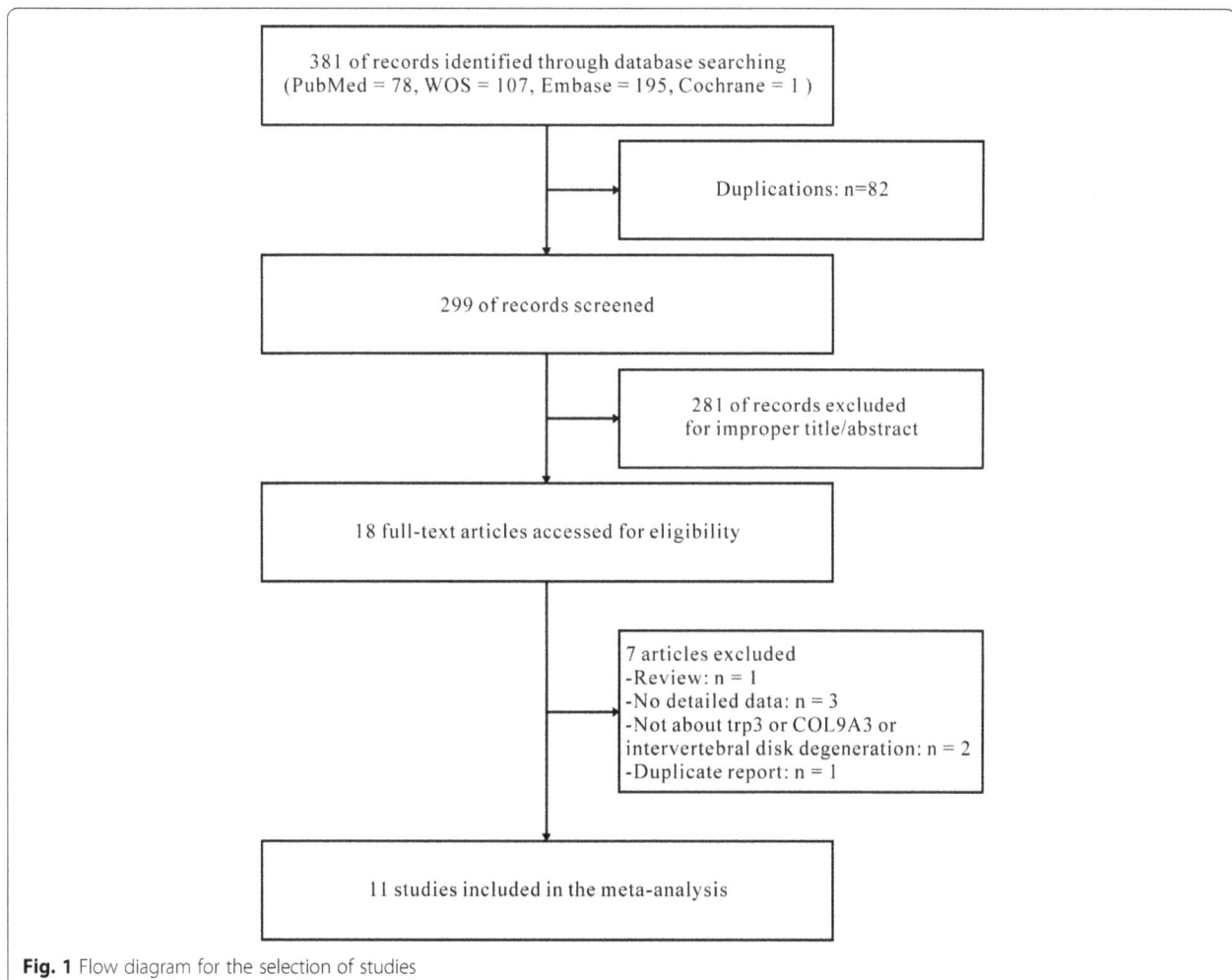

Fig. 1 Flow diagram for the selection of studies

removed because it was a review. Finally, 11 case-control studies [11, 14, 17, 18, 21–23, 27–30] were identified due to the inclusion criteria.

As shown in Tables 1, 11 eligible studies for *COL9A3* trp3 with 1631 cases of IDD and 1366 controls were included in this meta-analysis. The characteristics of all the included studies are also listed in the Tables 1 and 2, including the year, country and continent of studies, the ethnicity, age and gender of subjects, the diagnosis methods, genotyping methods, source of controls, matching items of cases and controls, relation with IDD and the number of subjects in control/case group in each studies. The quality assessment of study was listed in Table 3.

However, Jim et al. [23] measured the 804 subjects with no Trp3 positive subjects neither in case nor in control groups.(Table 2) This proportion is largely deviated from other studies included. We speculate that it might be something wrong in its genotyping method or there might be a selection bias in its subjects. So Jim et al. [23] is excluded in the following analyses.

Association between *COL9A3* trp3 polymorphism and IDD risk in overall

Significant heterogeneity was found among the studies of trp3 in the overall meta-analysis. So the random effects model was applied to evaluate the connection between trp3 polymorphism and IDD risk. The result of the evaluation showed that there was no association of trp3 polymorphism with IDD risk (as shown in Fig. 2a and Table 4, trp3 positive versus trp3 negative: ORs = 1.31, 95%CI = 0.78–2.21, $P = 0.309$; heterogeneity test $\chi^2 = 25.31$, $P < 0.10$, $I^2 = 64.40\%$).

Subgroup analysis between *COL9A3* trp3 polymorphism and IDD risk based on gender

Subgroup meta-analysis of the studies based on gender (male and female) showed no significant heterogeneity. Thus, the fixed effects model was used to assess the relationship between trp3 polymorphism and IDD risk. The result of the evaluation indicated that trp3 polymorphism was not associated with IDD risk in both gender (as shown in Fig. 2b and Table 4, for male subgroup, trp3 positive versus trp3 negative: ORs = 1.30, 95%CI = 0.77–2.17, $P = 0.322$; heterogeneity test $\chi^2 = 11.30$, $P < 0.10$, $I^2 = 46.90\%$; for female subgroup, trp3 positive versus trp3 negative: ORs = 1.11, 95%CI = 0.62–2.01, $P = 0.725$; heterogeneity test $\chi^2 = 1,64$, $P > 0.10$, $I^2 = 0.00\%$).

Subgroup analysis between *COL9A3* trp3 polymorphism and IDD risk based on ethnicity

Subgroup analysis was conducted according to different ethnicity (Asian, Caucasian and unclear) and was observed significant heterogeneity. So the random effects model

was used to test the association between trp3 polymorphism and IDD risk. The result of the calculations indicated that trp3 polymorphism had no associations to IDD risk in any ethnicity (as shown in Fig. 2c and Table 4, for Asian subgroup, trp3 positive versus trp3 negative: ORs = 1.22, 95%CI = 0.52–2.89, $P = 0.645$; heterogeneity test $\chi2 = 1.53$, $P > 0.10$, $I^2 = 34.70\%$. for Caucasian subgroup, trp3 positive versus trp3 negative: ORs = 1.53, 95%CI = 0.55–4.29, $P = 0.417$; heterogeneity test $\chi^2 = 10.17$, $P < 0.10$, $I^2 = 80.30\%$; for unclear subgroup, trp3 positive versus trp3 negative: ORs = 0.96, 95%CI = 0.53–1.75, $P = 0.907$; heterogeneity test $\chi^2 = 4.96$, $P > 0.10$, $I^2 = 19.3\%$).

Sensitivity analysis

Sensitivity analysis was conducted to evaluate the influence set by the individual study on the pooled ORs for *COL9A3* trp3 polymorphism by deleting one study each turn in every genetic model (as shown in Fig. 3). There was no change in the significance of any outcomes, indicating the stability of the results in this meta-analysis.

Publication Bias

The Begg funnel plot (as shown in Fig. 4) and the Egger's test were performed to assess publication bias in the selected literature. No evidence of publication bias was observed in this study (Begg's test: $P = 0.283$, Egger's test: $t = 0.54$, 95%CI = − 2.88–4.64, $P = 0.606$ for *COL9A3* trp3).

Discussion

IDD, a common musculoskeletal disease, is widely considered as multifactorial diseases enforcing economic and medical burdens to society. Genetic factors have been considered as one of the leading causes of IDD [7, 11, 34]. *COL9A3*, an extracellular matrix molecule present in the nucleus pulposus of the intervertebral disc and cartilage, codes for Collagen IX [35]. Collagen IX is vital for the normal cartilage development or maintenance. Mutations in *COL9A3* could cause chondrodysplasias in humans as well as articular cartilage and intervertebral discs degeneration in mice [36]. *COL9A3* gene was observed to be a key genetic influencer in the process of IDD [23]. Previous studies have reported the association between the *COL9A3* trp3 polymorphism and IDD, but with conflicting results. With the studies with larger sample sizes of predisposing gene polymorphism, it would be much more reliable to discover the connection between candidate genes and specific type of diseases. In order to solve the inconsistence, meta-analysis was performed to examine the association of *COL9A3* trp3 polymorphism with IDD risk by critically reviewing 11 studies. Its strength came from the accumulation of various published data, offering more information to explore significant differences.

The pooled ORs (trp3 positive versus trp3 negative) and 95%CI did not show a significant association of

Table 1 Main Characteristics of Studies Included in This Meta-analysis for *COL9A3* trp3 Polymorphisms

Study ID	year	Enrolled Country	Ethnicity	Age	Gender	Diagnosis by	Genotyping Method	Control Source	Matching	Cases	Controls	Relation with IDD
Bagheri et al. [18]	2016	Iran	Iranian	20~66	both	MRI	PCR-seq	individuals with acute trauma and patients without IDD	gender	108	57	only present in male subgroup
Solovieva et al. [14]	2006	Finland	N/D	40~45	men	MRI	PCR-seq	Patients without IDD	HWE, age	77	55	Absent
Kales et al. [27]	2004	Greece	Southern European	<60	both	surgery, MRI or CT	PCR-seq	patients without IDD and visitors to nonsurgical, nonorthopedic units	BMI	105	102	Absent
Paassita et al. [17]	2001	Finland	Finnish	<78	N/D	both clinic and MRI or CT	PCR-seq CSGE	healthy individuals, osteoarthritis, rheumatoid arthritis, chondrodysplasias	N/D	171	321	Present
Kelempisioti et al. [30]	2011	Finland	N/D	young adult, mean age 21	both	MRI	PCR-seq	Patients without IDD	gender, HWE	292	246	Absent
Matsui et al. [28]	2004	USA	most of them are Caucasian	16~87	both	N/D	PCR-seq	Individuals with a vertebral fracture treated by fusion	N/D[a]	97	10	Absent[b]
Eskola et al. [21]	2010	Finland	Caucasian	12~14	both	MRI	PCR-seq	children without IDD	age, weight, BMI, HWE	66	154	Absent
Rathod et al. [22]	2012	India	Indian	15~60	both	both clinic and MRI	PCR-seq and TaqMan assay	Patients without IDD	age	100	100	Absent
Zhu et al. [29]	2011	USA	most of them are Caucasian	16~78	both	N/D	N/D	Individuals with a vertebral fracture treated by fusion	age	26	6	N/D
jim et al. [23]	2005	China	Chinese	18~55	both	MRI	PCR-seq CSGE	Patients without IDD	age, gender	514	290	Absent
Toktas et al. [11]	2015	Turkey	N/D	35~45	male	MRI	PCR-seq	healthy individuals	age, gender	75	25	Absent[c]

Abbreviations: *PCR-seq* restriction analysis polymerase chain reaction sequencing, *N/D* not described, *CSGE* conformation sensitive gel electrophoresis, *MRI* magnetic resonance imaging, *CT* Computed Tomography, *IDD* intervertebral disk degeneration, *HWE* Hardy–Weinberg equilibrium, *BMI* body mass index. [a]This study matched age, gender, race between trp3 positive and trp3 negative groups, but not between control and case groups. [b], although absent relation with IDD, case group was positively associated with the diagnosis of spinal stenosis with spondylolisthesis. [c], although absent relation with IDD, control group has significantly higher scores in Pfirrmann classification than case group

Table 2 Distribution of Genotypes and *COL9A3* trp3 Polymorphisms Among Cases and Controls

Study ID	Year	Continent	Gender	Case		Control	
				Trp3 positive	Trp3 negative	Trp3 positive	Trp3 negative
Bagheri et al. [18]	2016	Asia	male	12	21	2	21
			female	17	58	8	26
			overall	29	79	10	47
Solovieva et al. [14]	2006	Europe	male	15	62	8	47
Kales et al. [27]	2004	Europe	male	6	62	1	46
			female	3	34	4	51
			overall	9	96	5	97
Paassita et al. [17]	2001	Europe	unknown	40	131	30	291
Kelempisioti et al. [30]	2011	Europe	overall	43	249	52	194
Matsui et al. [28]	2004	America	overall	7	90	0	10
Eskola et al. [21]	2010	Europe	male	2	28	14	59
			female	7	29	17	64
			overall	9	57	31	123
Rathod et al. [22]	2012	Asia	male	3	62	7	60
			female	2	33	0	33
			overall	5	95	7	93
Zhu et al. [29]	2011	America	male	3	11	0	2
			female	3	9	0	4
			overall	6	20	0	6
Jim et al. [23]	2005	Asia	overall	0	290	0	514
Toktas et al. [11]	2015	Europe	male	5	70	0	25

COL9A3 trp3 polymorphism with IDD risk in the overall populations. Different *COL9A3* trp3 frequencies have been reported in two genders of subjects (male and female) [18]. So we performed a stratified analysis by gender to determine whether there was an association between trp3 and IDD differed by gender. We also found

Table 3 Quality Assessment of the Included Articles

Author	Year	A	B	C	D	E	F	G	H	I	J	Sum
Bagheri et al. [18]	2016	1	0	1	1	1	0	0	1	1	0	6
Solovieva et al. [14]	2006	1	1	1	1	1	0	0	1	1	0	7
Kales et al. [27]	2004	1	0	1	1	1	0	0	1	1	0	6
Paassita et al. [17]	2001	1	0	1	1	1	0	0	1	0	0	5
Kelempisioti et al. [30]	2011	0	1	1	1	1	0	0	1	1	0	6
Matsui et al. [28]	2004	0	0	1	1	1	1	0	1	0	0	5
Eskola et al. [21]	2010	1	1	1	1	1	0	0	1	1	0	7
Rathod et al. [22]	2012	1	0	1	1	1	0	0	1	1	0	6
Zhu et al. [29]	2011	0	0	1	1	1	0	0	1	1	0	5
Jim et al. [23]	2005	1	0	1	1	1	0	0	1	1	0	6
Toktas et al. [11]	2015	0	0	1	1	1	0	0	1	1	0	5

Abbreviations: *A* Control group, *B* Hardy–Weinberg equilibrium, *C* Case group, *D* Primer, *E* Reproducibility, *F* Blinding, *G* Power calculation, *H* Statistics, *I* Corrected statistics, *J* Independent replication, *Sum* sum of quality assessment score, *1* done, *0* undone or unclear

no association of *COL9A3* trp3 polymorphism with IDD risk both in male or female subgroup. To our limited knowledge, ethnicity may contribute to different genetic characteristics of IDD. Hence, we also performed a subgroup analysis by ethnicity and the outcomes indicated no association of *COL9A3* trp3 polymorphism with IDD risk in any of ethnicity subgroup. Based on the analyses above, we speculated that *COL9A3* trp3 might be a minor factor in genetic etiology of IDD risk due to the small amount of *COL9A3* inside the intervertebral discs [37]. All of the results above do not eliminate the possibility of a clinically vital association that remains to be explored more carefully in convincing studies of larger sample sizes.

No significant heterogeneity was observed in subgroup analysis of gender, whereas there existed heterogeneities in the overall comparisons and subgroup analysis of continent for trp3 and IDD risk. To search the source of heterogeneity, we observed that I^2 values had significantly decreased after excluding Paassita et al. [17] or Kelempisioti et al. [30] in overall analysis. We also found that I^2 values had significantly decreased after excluding a study of Paassita et al. [17] in subgroup analysis of Europe continent. The results indicated that the major source of the heterogeneity might result from these

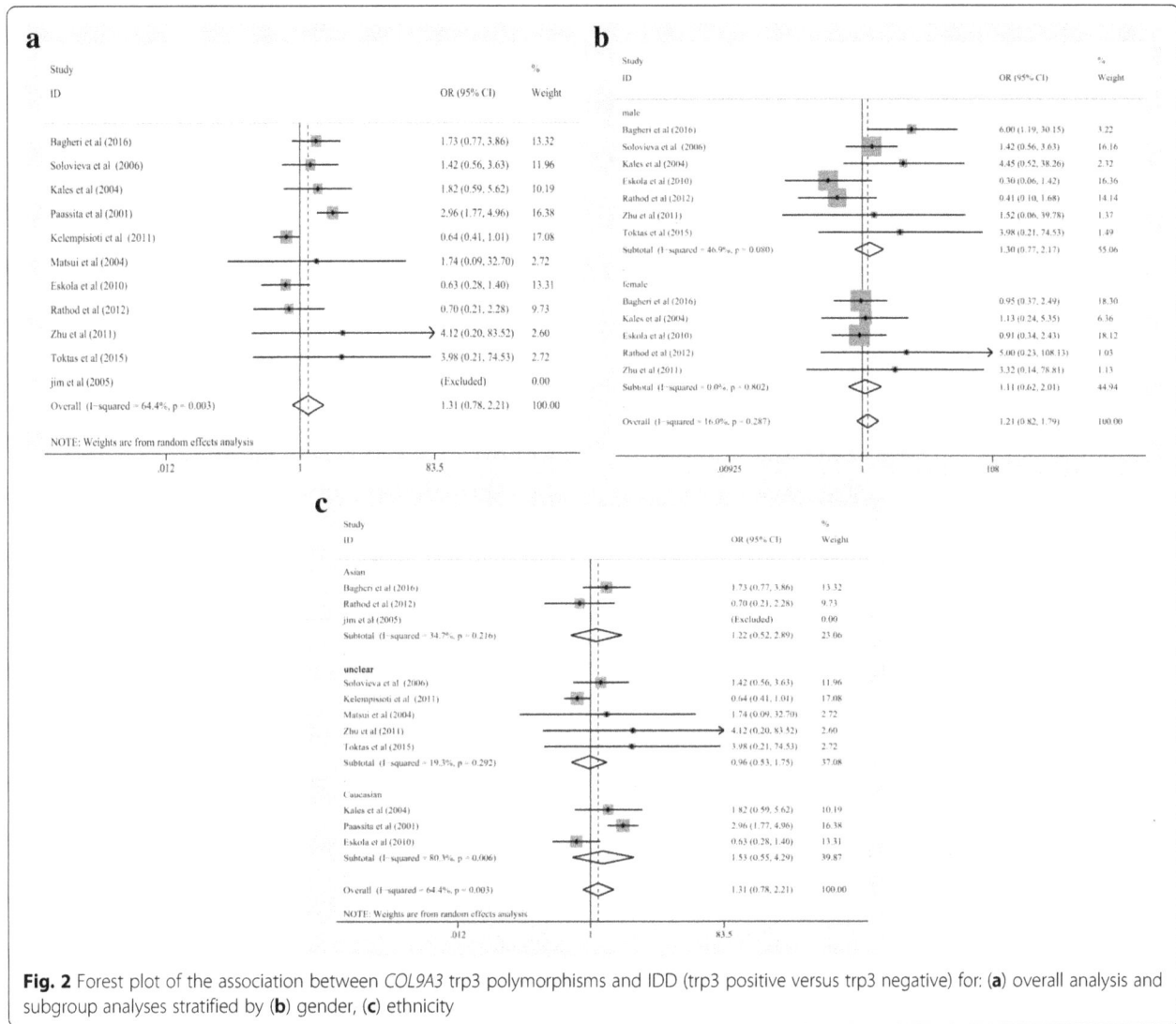

Fig. 2 Forest plot of the association between *COL9A3* trp3 polymorphisms and IDD (trp3 positive versus trp3 negative) for: (**a**) overall analysis and subgroup analyses stratified by (**b**) gender, (**c**) ethnicity

Table 4 Statistics of polled ORs and Heterogeneity for Overall and Sub Group Analyses of *COL9A3* trp3 Polymorphism

COL9A3 trp3		N	ORs analyses		Heterogeneity Analyses			Model Used for Meta-analysis
			polled ORs (95% CI)	P value	χ^2	P_heterogeneity	I^2 (%)	
Overall		11	1.31 (0.78,2.21)	0.309	25.31	0.003	64.40%	Random
sub group analysis by gender	male	7	1.30 (0.77,2.17)	0.322	11.30	0.080	46.90%	Fixed
	female	5	1.11 (0.62,2.01)	0.725	1.64	0.802	0.00%	
sub group analysis by ethnicity	Asian	3	1.22 (0.52,2.89)	0.645	1.53	0.216	34.70%	Random
	Caucasian	3	1.53 (0.55, 4.29)	0.417	10.17	0.006	80.3%	
	unclear	5	0.96 (0.53, 1.75)	0.907	4.96	0.292	19.3%	

Abbreviations: *CI* confidence interval, *ORs* odds ratios, *N* number of studies included in each analysis

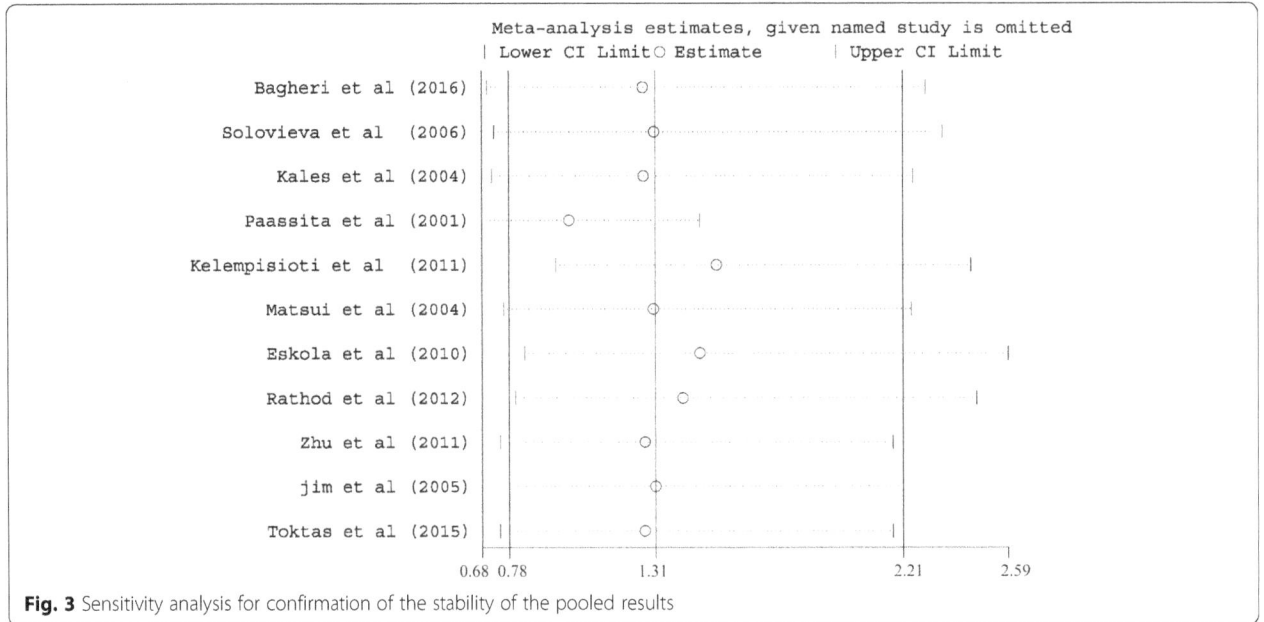

Meta-analysis estimates, given named study is omitted
| Lower CI Limit ○ Estimate | Upper CI Limit

Bagheri et al (2016)
Solovieva et al (2006)
Kales et al (2004)
Paassita et al (2001)
Kelempisioti et al (2011)
Matsui et al (2004)
Eskola et al (2010)
Rathod et al (2012)
Zhu et al (2011)
jim et al (2005)
Toktas et al (2015)

0.68 0.78   1.31   2.21   2.59

Fig. 3 Sensitivity analysis for confirmation of the stability of the pooled results

studies. However, heterogeneity did not seem to influence the results, because the lack of association between trp3 and IDD was not altered after excluding either of study mentioned above.

Moreover, no significant change of results was identified by sensitivity analyses, which indicating the reliability of results. These suggested the reliability of the results. Publication bias was also tested in this study. On the basis that a meta-analysis collects various data from numerous studies, the effect of publication bias among the articles included in the study can influence the meta-analytic results. Neither the Egger's test nor the Begg funnel plot showed significant publication bias for this analysis. Although the results are reliable, more

studies are required to be conducted in order to confirm the outcome of this meta-analysis.

Our meta-analysis has several strengths. Firstly, to our best knowledge, this is the first meta-analysis focusing on the connection between *COL9A3* trp3 polymorphism and the risk of IDD. We suggest that such a method of incorporating the outcomes of related studies may help us to understand the effect of polymorphism on disease development better. Secondly, we also have taken the gender and ethnicity of subjects into account. This study included researches of Asia (Iran, China and India), Europe (Finland, Greece and Turkey) and America (USA), containing different kinds of ethnicities and enrolling both male and female. So the results are much more

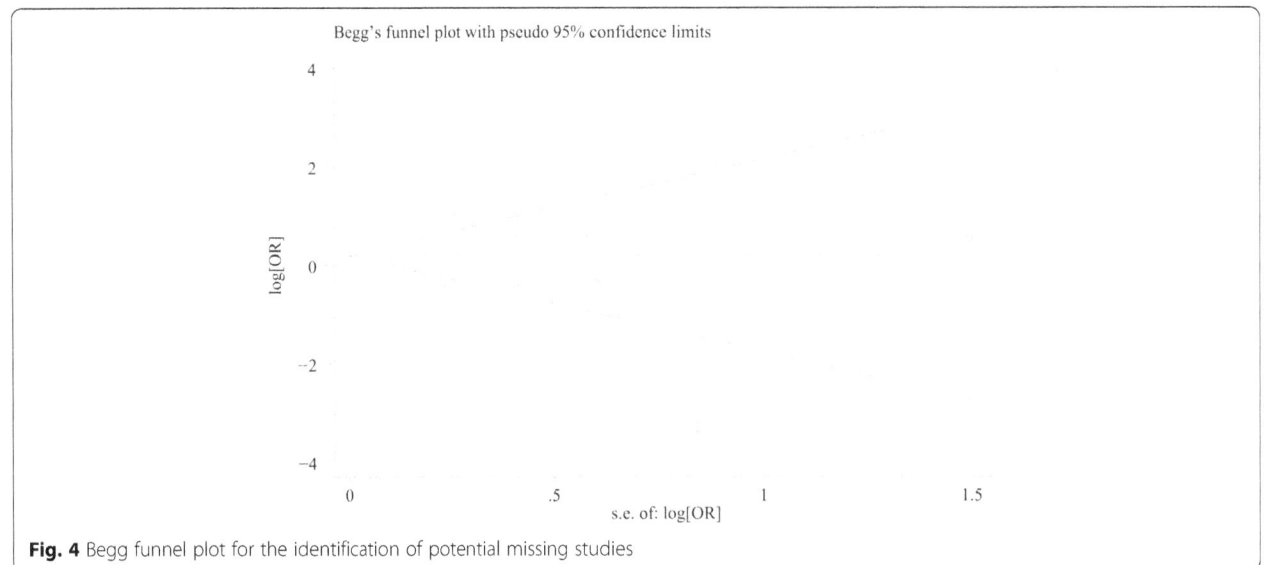

Begg's funnel plot with pseudo 95% confidence limits

Fig. 4 Begg funnel plot for the identification of potential missing studies

comprehensive. Moreover, several strategies and strict principle were applied to evaluate the methodological quality of the studies and most of the studies included in this meta-analysis possessed moderate or high qualities.

The present meta-analysis also has a few limitations that should be taken into account. Firstly, the number of filtered studies for *COL9A3* trp3 polymorphism is a little bit small. Secondly, the heterogeneity was a little bit high when overall and sub group of ethnicity analyses were conducted, contributing to a cautious acceptance of the results. What's more, some studies were removed from our research for lacking detailed data, which may contribute to selection bias. Limited to data, we only analyze trp3 positive versus trp3 negative to estimate the ORs and 95%CI rather than five models (allele, homozygote, recessive, dominant and heterozygote models). This may also influence the reliability of outcomes. Finally, although most of articles in this meta-analysis made a good match of age, gender or other items which might influence the results, some articles did not take certain items into account or even did not mention the match points. These confounding factors might affect the results.

Conclusions

Basing on the epidemiological evidence, our meta-analysis suggested that *COL9A3* trp3 polymorphism did not seem to be connected to risk of IDD in any gender, continent or ethnicity of people. Future researches with larger sample sizes are required to verify this outcome.

Abbreviations
CI: Confidence interval; *COL9A3*: Collagen type IX alpha 3 chain; IDD: Intervertebral disk degeneration; LBP: Low back pain; ORs: Odds ratios; WOS: Web of Science

Acknowledgments
We would like to thank all the people who helped us in the current study.

Funding
This study was supported by the National Key Research and Development Program of China (2016YFC1100100) and the Major Research Plan of National Natural Science Foundation of China (No.91649204).

Authors' contributions
DH contributed to the idea of this study. DH, XD and HL searched literatures and screened them independently. Any disagreement was solved by consulting the senior authors (ZS and KM). XD, DS and HL screened data from the eleven final articles and make Tables. DH, FW and SC played an important role in analyzing the outcomes. XD and DH conducted the data analyses and make graphs. XD and SC wrote the first draft. DS and FW revised the manuscript. ZS and KM polished the draft. ZS approved the final version.

Competing interests
The authors declare that they have no competing interests.

References
1. Mehrdad RMM, Shams-Hosseini NSM, Aghdaei SM, Yousefian MM. Prevalence of low Back pain in health care workers and comparison with other occupational categories in Iran: a systematic review. Iran J Med Sci. 2016;41(6):467–78.
2. Zhang YG, Guo TM, Guo X, Wu SX. Clinical diagnosis for discogenic low back pain. Int J Biol Sci. 2009;5(7):647–58.
3. Zhang YH, Zhao CQ, Jiang LS, Chen XD, Dai LY. Modic changes: a systematic review of the literature. Eur Spine J. 2008;17(10):1289–99.
4. Hoy D, March L, Brooks P, Blyth F, Woolf A, Bain C, Williams G, Smith E, Vos T, Barendregt J, et al. The global burden of low back pain: estimates from the global burden of disease 2010 study. Ann Rheum Dis. 2014;73(6):968–74.
5. Cheung KM, Samartzis D, Karppinen J, Mok FP, Ho DW, Fong DY, Luk KD. Intervertebral disc degeneration: new insights based on "skipped" level disc pathology. Arthritis Rheum. 2010;62(8):2392–400.
6. Rivinoja AE, Paananen MV, Taimela SP, Solovieva S, Okuloff A, Zitting P, Jarvelin MR, Leino-Arjas P, Karppinen JI. Sports, smoking, and overweight during adolescence as predictors of sciatica in adulthood: a 28-year follow-up study of a birth cohort. Am J Epidemiol. 2011;173(8):890–7.
7. Battie MC, Videman T. Lumbar disc degeneration: epidemiology and genetics. J Bone Joint Surg Am. 2006;88(Suppl 2):3–9.
8. Videman T, Sarna S, Battie MC, Koskinen S, Gill K, Paananen H, Gibbons L. The long-term effects of physical loading and exercise lifestyles on back-related symptoms, disability, and spinal pathology among men. Spine. 1995; 20(6):699–709.
9. Heliovaara M. Risk factors for low back pain and sciatica. Ann Med. 1989; 21(4):257–64.
10. Battie MC, Videman T, Gibbons LE, Fisher LD, Manninen H, Gill K. 1995 Volvo award in clinical sciences. Determinants of lumbar disc degeneration. A study relating lifetime exposures and magnetic resonance imaging findings in identical twins. Spine. 1995;20(24):2601–12.
11. Toktas ZO, Eksi MS, Yilmaz B, Demir MK, Ozgen S, Kilic T, Konya D. Association of collagen I, IX and vitamin D receptor gene polymorphisms with radiological severity of intervertebral disc degeneration in southern European ancestor. Eur Spine J. 2015;24(11):2432–41.
12. Valdes AM, Hassett G, Hart DJ, Spector TD. Radiographic progression of lumbar spine disc degeneration is influenced by variation at inflammatory genes: a candidate SNP association study in the Chingford cohort. Spine. 2005;30(21):2445–51.
13. Wrocklage C, Wassmann H, Paulus W. COL9A2 allelotypes in intervertebral disc disease. Biochem Biophys Res Commun. 2000;279(2):398–400.
14. Solovieva S, Lohiniva J, Leino-Arjas P, Raininko R, Luoma K, Ala-Kokko L, Riihimaki H. Intervertebral disc degeneration in relation to the COL9A3 and the IL-1ss gene polymorphisms. Eur Spine J. 2006;15(5):613–9.
15. Urban JP, Roberts S. Degeneration of the intervertebral disc. Arthritis Res Ther. 2003;5(3):120–30.
16. Higashino K, Matsui Y, Yagi S, Takata Y, Goto T, Sakai T, Katoh S, Yasui N. The alpha2 type IX collagen tryptophan polymorphism is associated with the severity of disc degeneration in younger patients with herniated nucleus pulposus of the lumbar spine. Int Orthop. 2007;31(1):107–11.
17. Paassilta P, Lohiniva J, Goring HH, Perala M, Raina SS, Karppinen J, Hakala M, Palm T, Kroger H, Kaitila I, et al. Identification of a novel common genetic risk factor for lumbar disk disease. Jama. 2001;285(14):1843–9.
18. Bagheri MH, Honarpisheh AP, Yavarian M, Alavi Z, Siegelman J, Valtchinov VI. MRI Phenotyping of COL9A2/Trp2 and COL9A3/Trp3 Alleles in Lumbar Disc Disease: A Case-control Study in South-Western Iranian Population Reveals a Significant Trp3-Disease Association in Males. Spine. 2016;41(21):1661–67.
19. Solovieva S, Lohiniva J, Leino-Arjas P, Raininko R, Luoma K, Ala-Kokko L, Riihimaki H. COL9A3 gene polymorphism and obesity in intervertebral disc degeneration of the lumbar spine: evidence of gene-environment interaction. Spine. 2002;27(23):2691–6.
20. Pihlajamaa T, Perala M, Vuoristo MM, Nokelainen M, Bodo M, Schulthess T, Vuorio E, Timpl R, Engel J, Ala-Kokko L. Characterization of recombinant human type IX collagen. Association of alpha chains into homotrimeric and heterotrimeric molecules. J Biol Chem. 1999;274(32):22464–8.

21. Eskola PJ, Kjaer P, Daavittila IM, Solovieva S, Okuloff A, Sorensen JS, Wedderkopp N, Ala-Kokko L, Mannikko M, Karppinen JI. Genetic risk factors of disc degeneration among 12-14-year-old Danish children: a population study. Int J Mol Epidemiol Genet. 2010;1(2):158–65.

22. Rathod TN, Chandanwale AS, Gujrathi S, Patil V, Chavan SA, Shah MN. Association between single nucleotide polymorphism in collagen IX and intervertebral disc disease in the Indian population. Indian J Orthop. 2012; 46(4):420–6.

23. Jim JJ, Noponen-Hietala N, Cheung KM, Ott J, Karppinen J, Sahraravand A, Luk KD, Yip SP, Sham PC, Song YQ, et al. The TRP2 allele of COL9A2 is an age-dependent risk factor for the development and severity of intervertebral disc degeneration. Spine. 2005;30(24):2735–42.

24. Srivastava K, Srivastava A, Sharma KL, Mittal B. Candidate gene studies in gallbladder cancer: a systematic review and meta-analysis. Mutat Res. 2011; 728(1–2):67–79.

25. Clark MF, Baudouin SV. A systematic review of the quality of genetic association studies in human sepsis. Intensive Care Med. 2006;32(11):1706–12.

26. Vrabel M. Preferred reporting items for systematic reviews and meta-analyses. Oncol Nurs Forum. 2015;42(5):552–4.

27. Kales SN, Linos A, Chatzis C, Sai Y, Halla M, Nasioulas G, Christiani DC. The role of collagen IX tryptophan polymorphisms in symptomatic intervertebral disc disease in southern European patients. Spine. 2004;29(11):1266–70.

28. Matsui Y, Mirza SK, Wu JJ, Carter B, Bellabarba C, Shaffrey CI, Chapman JR, Eyre DR. The association of lumbar spondylolisthesis with collagen IX tryptophan alleles. J Bone Joint Surg Br Vol. 2004;86(7):1021–6.

29. Zhu Y, Wu JJ, Weis MA, Mirza SK, Eyre DR. Type IX collagen neo-deposition in degenerative discs of surgical patients whether genotyped plus or minus for COL9 risk alleles. Spine. 2011;36(24):2031–8.

30. Kelempisioti A, Eskola PJ, Okuloff A, Karjalainen U, Takatalo J, Daavittila I, Niinimaki J, Sequeiros RB, Tervonen O, Solovieva S, et al. Genetic susceptibility of intervertebral disc degeneration among young Finnish adults. BMC Med Genet. 2011;12:153.

31. Higgins JP, Thompson SG. Quantifying heterogeneity in a meta-analysis. Stat Med. 2002;21(11):1539–58.

32. Begg CB, Mazumdar M. Operating characteristics of a rank correlation test for publication bias. Biometrics. 1994;50(4):1088–101.

33. Egger M, Davey Smith G, Schneider M, Minder C. Bias in meta-analysis detected by a simple, graphical test. BMJ (Clin Res Ed). 1997;315(7109):629–34.

34. Martirosyan NL, Patel AA, Carotenuto A, Kalani MY, Belykh E, Walker CT, Preul MC, Theodore N. Genetic alterations in intervertebral disc disease. Front Surg. 2016;3:59.

35. Feng H, Danfelter M, Stromqvist B, Heinegard D. Extracellular matrix in disc degeneration. J Bone Joint Surg Am. 2006;88(Suppl 2):25–9.

36. Kimura T, Nakata K, Tsumaki N, Miyamoto S, Matsui Y, Ebara S, Ochi T. Progressive degeneration of articular cartilage and intervertebral discs. An experimental study in transgenic mice bearing a type IX collagen mutation. Int Orthop. 1996;20(3):177–81.

37. Janeczko L, Janeczko M, Chrzanowski R, Zielinski G. The role of polymorphisms of genes encoding collagen IX and XI in lumbar disc disease. Neurol Neurochir Pol. 2014;48(1):60–2.

Permissions

The contributors of this book come from diverse backgrounds, making this book a truly international effort. This book will bring forth new frontiers with its revolutionizing research information and detailed analysis of the nascent developments around the world.

We would like to thank all the contributing authors for lending their expertise to make the book truly unique. They have played a crucial role in the development of this book. Without their invaluable contributions this book wouldn't have been possible. They have made vital efforts to compile up to date information on the varied aspects of this subject to make this book a valuable addition to the collection of many professionals and students.

This book was conceptualized with the vision of imparting up-to-date information and advanced data in this field. To ensure the same, a matchless editorial board was set up. Every individual on the board went through rigorous rounds of assessment to prove their worth. After which they invested a large part of their time researching and compiling the most relevant data for our readers.

The editorial board has been involved in producing this book since its inception. They have spent rigorous hours researching and exploring the diverse topics which have resulted in the successful publishing of this book. They have passed on their knowledge of decades through this book. To expedite this challenging task, the publisher supported the team at every step. A small team of assistant editors was also appointed to further simplify the editing procedure and attain best results for the readers.

Apart from the editorial board, the designing team has also invested a significant amount of their time in understanding the subject and creating the most relevant covers. They scrutinized every image to scout for the most suitable representation of the subject and create an appropriate cover for the book.

The publishing team has been an ardent support to the editorial, designing and production team. Their endless efforts to recruit the best for this project, has resulted in the accomplishment of this book. They are a veteran in the field of academics and their pool of knowledge is as vast as their experience in printing. Their expertise and guidance has proved useful at every step. Their uncompromising quality standards have made this book an exceptional effort. Their encouragement from time to time has been an inspiration for everyone.

The publisher and the editorial board hope that this book will prove to be a valuable piece of knowledge for researchers, students, practitioners and scholars across the globe.

List of Contributors

Danielle D. P. Berghmans and Antoine F. Lenssen
Department of Physical therapy, Maastricht University Medical Center +, PO 5800, 6202, AZ, Maastricht, The Netherlands
Maastricht University/CAPHRI School for Public Health and Primary Care, 6200, MD, Maastricht, The Netherlands

Pieter J. Emans
Department of Orthopedics, Maastricht University Medical Center +, PO 5800, 6202, AZ, Maastricht, The Netherlands
Maastricht University/CAPHRI School for Public Health and Primary Care, 6200, MD, Maastricht, The Netherlands

Rob A. de Bie
Department of Epidemiology, Maastricht University, MD, Maastricht, The Netherlands
Maastricht University/CAPHRI School for Public Health and Primary Care, 6200, MD, Maastricht, The Netherlands

Lei Wang, Deqing Luo and Kejian Lian
Orthopaedic Center of People's Liberation Army, The Affiliated Southeast Hospital of Xiamen University, Zhangzhou 363000, China

Dasheng Lin
Orthopaedic Center of People's Liberation Army, The Affiliated Southeast Hospital of Xiamen University, Zhangzhou 363000, China
Department of Surgery, Experimental Surgery and Regenerative Medicine, Ludwig-Maximilians-University (LMU), 80336 Munich, Germany

Zhaoliang Yu
Weigao Orthopaedic Device Co., Ltd, Weihai 264200, China

Xigui Zhang
Double Engine Medical Material Co., Ltd, Xiamen 361000, China

E. Smith and F. Blyth
University of Sydney, Sydney, Australia

L. March
University of Sydney, Sydney, Australia
Global Alliance for Musculoskeletal Health, Truro, UK

D. G. Hoy
University of Sydney, Sydney, Australia

Global Alliance for Musculoskeletal Health, Truro, UK
Pacific Community (SPC), Noumea, New Caledonia

A. Woolf
Global Alliance for Musculoskeletal Health, Truro, UK
Royal Cornwall Hospital, Truro, UK

T. Raikoti, K. Matikarai, A. Jorari and C. Lepers
Pacific Community (SPC), Noumea, New Caledonia

A. Tuzakana, J. Tako, A. Pitaboe and I. Kalauma
Solomon Islands National Statistics Office, Honiara, Solomon Islands

T. Gill
University of Adelaide, Adelaide, Australia

R. Buchbinder
Monash University, Melbourne, Australia

P. Brooks
University of Melbourne, Melbourne, Australia

A. Briggs
Curtin University, Perth, Australia

Belinda Beck and Rod Barrett
Menzies Health Institute Queensland, School of Allied Health Sciences, Griffith University, Gold Coast, QLD 4222, Australia

Maria Constantinou
Menzies Health Institute Queensland, School of Allied Health Sciences, Griffith University, Gold Coast, QLD 4222, Australia
Australian Catholic University, Brisbane, QLD 4014, Australia

Laura E. Diamond
Menzies Health Institute Queensland, School of Allied Health Sciences, Griffith University, Gold Coast, QLD 4222, Australia
Centre of Clinical Research Excellence in Spinal Pain, Injury and Health, School of Health and Rehabilitation Sciences, The University of Queensland, Brisbane, QLD, Australia

Aderson Loureiro
Menzies Health Institute Queensland, School of Allied Health Sciences, Griffith University, Gold Coast, QLD 4222, Australia
Pontifical Catholic University (PUCRS), Porto Alegre, Brazil

University of Rio dos Sinos (UNISINOS), São Leopoldo, Brazil

Benjamin J. F. Dean and Jennifer C. E. Lane
Nuffield Department of Orthopaedics, Rheumatology and Musculoskeletal Sciences (NDORMS), University of Oxford, Botnar Research Centre, Windmill road, Oxford OX3 7LD, UK
Nuffield Orthopaedic Centre, Windmill road, Oxford OX3 7LD, UK

Nicholas D. Riley and Earl Robert McCulloch
Nuffield Orthopaedic Centre, Windmill road, Oxford OX3 7LD, UK

Amy Beth Touzell
Frankston Hospital, Frankston, VIC, Australia

Alastair J. Graham
Buckinghamshire Hospitals NHS Trust, High Wycombe Hospital, High Wycombe, Amersham HP11 2TT, UK

Ceylan H. H.
Lutfiye Nuri Burat Devlet Hastanesi, 50.Yil Mah., 2107 Sok, 34256 Sultangazi, Istanbul, Turkey

Caypinar B.
Gelisim University, Istanbul, Turkey

Xinnan Bao
Department of Orthopedics, The First People's Hospital of Changzhou, No.185 Juqian Street, Changzhou, Jiangsu Province 213003, China

Xinyu Hu
Orthopedic Trauma Department, The First People's Hospital of Changzhou, No.185 Juqian Street, Changzhou, Jiangsu Province 213003, China

Wei Li, Liang Yuan, Guojun Tong, Youhua He, Yue Meng, Song Hao, Jianting Chen and Dehong Yang
Department of Spinal Surgery, Nanfang Hospital, Southern Medical University, Guangzhou 510515, China

Jun Guo and Richard Bringhurst
Endocrine Unit, Massachusetts General Hospital, Boston, MA 02114, USA

Hjörtur F. Hjartarson
Dept of Orthopedics, Landspitali University Hospital, E-4 Fossvogur, 101, Reykjavik, Iceland
Lund University, Lund, Sweden

Sören Toksvig-Larsen
Dept of Orthopedics, Hässleholm hospital, Esplanadgatan 19, 281 38 Hässleholm, Sweden Lund University, Lund, Sweden

Jun Qiao, Leilei Xu, Zhen Liu, Xu Sun, Bangping Qian, Zezhang Zhu and Yong Qiu
Department of Spine Surgery, the Affiliated Drum Tower Hospital of Nanjing University Medical School, 321 Zhongshan Road, Nanjing, China

Lingyan Xiao
Intensive care unit, the Second Hospital of Nanjing, Southeast University, Nanjing, China

Aurore Hermet, Adrien Gautier and Jonathan Linieres
Service de rééducation et réadaptation de l'appareil locomoteur et des pathologies du rachis, Hôpital Cochin AP-HP, Université Paris Descartes, PRES Sorbonne Paris Cité, Paris, France

Alexandra Roren, Marie-Martine Lefevre-Colau, Serge Poiraudeau and Clémence Palazzo
Service de rééducation et réadaptation de l'appareil locomoteur et des pathologies du rachis, Hôpital Cochin AP-HP, Université Paris Descartes, PRES Sorbonne Paris Cité, Paris, France
CRESS, UMR 1153, INSERM, Paris, Institut fédératif de recherche handicap, INSERM/CNRS, Paris, France
Institut Fédératif de Recherche Handicap, INSERM/CNRS, Paris, France

Asaduzzaman Khan
School of Health and Rehabilitation Sciences, University of Queensland, Brisbane, Australia

Shaun O'Leary
School of Health and Rehabilitation Sciences, University of Queensland, Brisbane, Australia
Physiotherapy Department, Royal Brisbane and Women's Hospital, Brisbane, Australia

Michelle Cottrell
School of Health and Rehabilitation Sciences, University of Queensland, Brisbane, Australia
Physiotherapy Department, Ipswich Hospital, Ipswich, Australia

Maree Raymer
Physiotherapy Department, Royal Brisbane and Women's Hospital, Brisbane, Australia

David Smith
Physiotherapy Department, Ipswich Hospital, Ipswich, Australia

Jessica A. Walsh, Gopi K. Penmetsa and Daniel O. Clegg
Division of Rheumatology School of Medicine, 30 North 1900 East, Salt Lake City, UT 84132, USA

Shaobo Pei, Jianwei Leng, Grant W. Cannon and Brian C. Sauer
George E. Wahlen Veteran Affairs Medical Center, 500 Foothill Boulevard, Salt Lake City, UT 84148, USA

Ali Jabran, Zhenmin Zou and Lei Ren
School of Mechanical, Aerospace and Civil Engineering, University of Manchester, Sackville Street, Manchester M13 9PL, UK

Chris Peach
School of Mechanical, Aerospace and Civil Engineering, University of Manchester, Sackville Street, Manchester M13 9PL, UK
Department of Shoulder and Elbow Surgery, University Hospital of South Manchester, Southmoor Road, Wythenshawe, Manchester M23 9LT, UK

Julia Jurkutat, Dirk Zajonz, Gerald Sommer and Stefan Schleifenbaum
Department of Orthopaedics, Trauma and Plastic Surgery, University Hospital Leipzig, Liebigstrasse 20, D-04103 Leipzig, Germany
ZESBO – Zentrum zur Erforschung der Stütz- und BewegungsOrgane, Semmelweisstrasse 14, D-04103, Leipzig, Germany

Ronny Grunert
Department of Orthopaedics, Trauma and Plastic Surgery, University Hospital Leipzig, Liebigstrasse 20, D-04103 Leipzig, Germany
ZESBO – Zentrum zur Erforschung der Stütz- und BewegungsOrgane, Semmelweisstrasse 14, D-04103, Leipzig, Germany
Fraunhofer Institute for Machine Tools and Forming Technology, 44, Nöthnitzer Straße, D-01187 Dresden, Germany

Torsten Prietzel
Department of Orthopaedics and Trauma Surgery, HELIOS Clinic Blankenhain, Wirthstrasse 5, D-99444 Blankenhain, Germany
ZESBO – Zentrum zur Erforschung der Stütz- und BewegungsOrgane, Semmelweisstrasse 14, D-04103, Leipzig, Germany

Robert Möbius
ZESBO – Zentrum zur Erforschung der Stütz- und BewegungsOrgane, Semmelweisstrasse 14, D-04103, Leipzig, Germany
Department of Anatomy, University of Leipzig, Semmelweisstraße 14, D-04103 Leipzig, Germany

Niels Hammer
Department of Anatomy, University of Otago, Lindo Ferguson Building, 270 Great King St, Dunedin 9016, New Zealand

Kejie Wang
Department of Sports Medicine and Adult Reconstructive Surgery, Drum Tower Hospital Clinical College of Nanjing Medical University, Zhongshan Road 321, Nanjing 210008, Jiangsu, People's Republic of China
Department of Orthopaedics, Changzhou No.1 People's Hospital, Changzhou 213003, Jiangsu, People's Republic of China

Qing Jiang
Department of Sports Medicine and Adult Reconstructive Surgery, Drum Tower Hospital Clinical College of Nanjing Medical University, Zhongshan Road 321, Nanjing 210008, Jiangsu, People's Republic of China
The Center of Diagnosis and Treatment for Joint Disease, Drum Tower Hospital Affiliated to Medical School of Nanjing University, Nanjing 210008, Jiangsu, People's Republic of China

Wenge Ding
Department of Orthopaedics, Changzhou No.1 People's Hospital, Changzhou 213003, Jiangsu, People's Republic of China

Minjie Chu
Department of Epidemiology, School of Public Health, Nantong University, Nantong 226019, Jiangsu, People's Republic of China

Carole Fortin
École de réadaptation, Faculté de médecine, Université de Montréal, C.P. 6128, succursale Centre-ville, Montréal, Québec H3C 3J7, Canada
Research center, CHU Sainte-Justine, Montreal, Quebec, Canada

Debbie Ehrmann Feldman
École de réadaptation, Faculté de médecine, Université de Montréal, C.P. 6128, succursale Centre-ville, Montréal, Québec H3C 3J7, Canada
Institut de Recherche en santé publique de l'Université de Montréal and Centre for interdisciplinary research in rehabilitation, Montreal, Quebec, Canada

Jean-François Aubin-Fournier
Research center, CHU Sainte-Justine, Montreal, Quebec, Canada

Paul van Schaik
Department of Psychology, Teesside University, Middlesbrough, UK

Josette Bettany-Saltikov
Institute of Health and Social Care, Teesside University, Middlesbrough, UK

Jean-Claude Bernard
Centre Médico-Chirurgical de Réadaptation des Massues, Croix Rouge française, Lyon, France

S. P. Boelch, A. Jakuscheit, S. Doerries, L. Fraissler, M. Hoberg, J. Arnholdt and M. Rudert
Department of Orthopaedic Surgery, Julius-Maximilians University Wuerzburg, Koenig-Ludwig-Haus, 11 Brettreichstrasse, 97074 Wuerzburg, Germany

Yuya Kodama, Takayuki Furumatsu, Tomohito Hino, Yusuke Kamatsuki, Yoshiki Okazaki, Shin Masuda, Yuki Okazaki and Toshifumi Ozaki
Department of Orthopaedic Surgery, Okayama University Graduate School of Medicine, Dentistry, and Pharmaceutical Sciences, 2-5-1 Shikatacho, Kitaku, Okayama 700-8558, Japan

Irazú Contreras-Yáñez, G. Guaracha-Basáñez and V. Pascual-Ramos
Department of Immunology and Rheumatology, Instituto Nacional de Ciencias Médicas y Nutrición Salvador Zubirán, Vasco de Quiroga 15, Colonia Sección XVI, Belisario Domínguez, 14500 Ciudad de México, CP, Mexico

E. Díaz-Borjón
Department of Surgery, Orthopedic Unit, Instituto Nacional de Ciencias Médicas y Nutrición Salvador Zubirán, Mexico City, Mexico

M. Iglesias
Department of Surgery, Plastic Surgery Unit, Instituto Nacional de Ciencias Médicas y Nutrición Salvador Zubirán, Mexico City, Mexico

Tatiana de Oliveira Sato
Physical Therapy Department, Federal University of São Carlos (UFSCar), Rodovia Washington Luís, km 235, São Carlos, SP 13565-905, Brazil

David M. Hallman
Centre for Musculoskeletal Research, Department of Occupational and Public Health Sciences, University of Gävle, 801-76 Gävle, SE, Sweden

Jesper Kristiansen
National Research Centre for the Working Environment (NRCWE), Lersø Parkallé 105, 2100 Copenhagen Ø, DK, Denmark

Andreas Holtermann
National Research Centre for the Working Environment (NRCWE), Lersø Parkallé 105, 2100 Copenhagen Ø, DK, Denmark
Department of Sports Science and Clinical Biomechanics, University of Southern Denmark, Odense, Denmark

L. Tarallo, M. Lombardi, F. Zambianchi, A. Giorgini and F. Catani
Orthopaedics and Traumatology Department, University of Modena and Reggio Emilia, Via del Pozzo 71, 41124 Modena, Italy

Fan Yang, Sheng Yao, Kai-fang Chen, Feng-zhao Zhu, Ze-kang Xiong, Yan-hui Ji, Ting-fang Sun and Xiao-dong Guo
Department of Orthopaedics, Union Hospital, Tongji Medical College, Huazhong University of Science and Technology, Wuhan 430022, China

Catherine D. Hughes, David L. Scott and Fowzia Ibrahim
Department of Rheumatology, King's College London School of Medicine, Weston Education Centre, King's College London, Cutcombe Road, London SE5 9RJ, UK

Annelise A. Slater, Todd J. Hullfish and Josh R. Baxter
Human Motion Laboratory, Department of Orthopaedic Surgery, University of Pennsylvania, 3737 Market Street, Suite 702, Philadelphia, PA 19104, USA

Donghua Huang, Xiangyu Deng, Kaige Ma, Fashuai Wu, Deyao Shi, Hang Liang, Sheng Chen and Zengwu Shao
Department of Orthopaedics, Union Hospital, Tongji Medical College, Huazhong University of Science and Technology, Wuhan 430022, China

Index

www.ingramcontent.com/pod-product-compliance
Lightning Source LLC
Chambersburg PA
CBHW080253230326

41458CB00097B/4437